Precision Nutrition and Metabolic Syndrome Management

Special Issue Editors

J. Alfredo Martínez
M. Angeles Zulet

MDPI • Basel • Beijing • Wuhan • Barcelona • Belgrade

MDPI

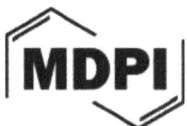

Special Issue Editors
J. Alfredo Martínez
University of Navarra; IMDEAfood
Spain

M. Angeles Zulet
University of Navarra; IMDEAfood
Spain

Editorial Office
MDPI
St. Alban-Anlage 66
Basel, Switzerland

This edition is a reprint of the Special Issue published online in the open access journal *Nutrients* (ISSN 2072-6643) from 2017–2018 (available at: http://www.mdpi.com/journal/nutrients/special_issues/precision_nutrition_metabolic).

For citation purposes, cite each article independently as indicated on the article page online and as indicated below:

Lastname, F.M.; Lastname, F.M. Article title. *Journal Name* **Year**, *Article number*, page range.

First Editon 2018

ISBN 978-3-03842-859-6 (Pbk)
ISBN 978-3-03842-860-2 (PDF)

Table of Contents

About the Special Issue Editors

J. Alfredo Martínez, MD, holds a PhD in Nutrition. He is co-author or has been involved in several landmark intervention trials, such as SEAFOODplus, DIOGENES, NUGENOB, FOOD4ME, PREDIMED, and PREVIEW, whose results have been published in the most relevant medical and scientific journals, including NEJM, Lancet, Nature, BMJ, AJCN, Circulation, etc., producing more than 25.000 citations. Prof Martínez has supervised more than 70 PhD students and published more than 800 peer-reviewed papers in the area of Obesity and Nutrition, including precision nutritional omics (H-index > 60). He is currently president of the International Union of Nutritional Sciences and has been the recipient of several important awards including the Hippocrates and Dupont prizes. He is also a member of CIBERobn (Pathophysiology of Obesity and Nutrition-ISCIII, Madrid, Spain), IMDEA (Madrid Institute of Advanced Studies), CIN (Center for Nutrition Research, University of Navarra). During his scientific career, Prof. J. Alfredo Martínez has enjoyed training or invited stays at Nottingham, Berkeley, MIT, Harvard, Oxford, and King's College, London.

M. Angeles Zulet is BPharm and PharmD, Lecturer of Nutrition, and senior researcher at the Department of Nutrition, Food Science, and Physiology of the University of Navarra. Her research activity has focused on the mechanisms of obesity and associated complications. She is co-author of more than 100 articles indexed in the JCR and of 25 book chapters. She has led and collaborated on different Autonomous Community, National, International, and European research projects and has contributed to studies in partnership with different Laboratories and Companies. She is also a member of CIBERobn (Pathophysiology of Obesity and Nutrition-ISCIII, Madrid, Spain), IdiSNA (Institute of Sanitary Research of Navarra), CIN (Center for Nutrition Research, University of Navarra) and has been European Master's Degree (E-MENU, University of Navarra) coordinator for more than 10 years. She received a National Award (General Council of Official Associations of Pharmacists, 1998) and an International Award (Nestlé Nutrition Institute / NSERF / Nutrition (2015), conjointly with Prof. J. Alfredo Martínez.

Preface to "Precision Nutrition and Metabolic Syndrome Management"

Precision Nutrition is a recent endeavor seeking to individualize dietary advice and nutritional prescription taking into account not only the genetic makeup, but also a number of features such as age, sex, phenotype, lifestyles, likes and dislikes, clinical backgrounds, social issues, allergies, intolerances, and other personal factors. This approach is supported by omics technologies, such as genomics, nutrigenetics, epigenomics, metabolomic, metagenomics etc., which are able to characterize the individual in a personalized manner. Of course, advances in understanding the metabolic pathways at the cellular level as well as investigations in animal models and humans and epidemiological studies are enormously contributing to develop precision nutrition.

In this context, metabolic syndrome management requires particular attention and the consideration of a number of features, which are different between individuals with obesity, such as hypertension, hypercholesterolemia, hyperglycemia, and other associated manifestations related to excessive adiposity and fat accumulation. This Special Issue book involves a number of chapters including the integration of traditional and metabolomics biomarkers for predicting the responsiveness to nutritional interventions against oxidative stress and inflammation. In addition, it also presents a review concerning personalized nutritional approaches for the prevention and management of metabolic syndrome and addressing precision nutrition in regard to lipid metabolism in colorectal cancer patients. A review of personalized bariatric surgery prescription is also included in this issue. Furthermore, the role of the Japanese traditional diet as a sustainable dietary pattern orientated to precision nutrition is considered. Other important chapters are focused on fatty acid consumption affecting obesity and associated disorders together with the design of a protein diet score including animal and vegetal proteins for individualized nutrition. The involvement of fruit fiber consumption in liver health status and the properties of the bioactive compound genistein are addressed as important issues concerning liver steatosis and cardiac function in postmenopausal women with metabolic syndrome, respectively. The role of hydroxytyrosol in the prevention of the metabolic syndrome and related disorders is also reported. Alterations in circulating amino acid metabolite ratio are described as potential biomarkers of metabolic syndrome manifestations related to arginase activity. Finally, novel miRNAs involved in the prevention of liver steatosis induced by resveratrol and the developmental programming of obesity and liver metabolism by maternal perinatal precision nutrition are discussed.

Summing up, this recompilation offers the reader a selection of important chapters considering diverse aspects of precision nutrition at the cellular level and in in vivo models and hopefully contributes a better understanding of the value of precision nutrition.

The editors wish to thank all the authors for contributing their time to the production of this volume and address specific thanks to the University of Navarra, IMDEA, CIBERobn, and IUNS.

J. Alfredo Martínez, M. Angeles Zulet
Special Issue Editors

![nutrients logo] *nutrients*

Article

Integration of Traditional and Metabolomics Biomarkers Identifies Prognostic Metabolites for Predicting Responsiveness to Nutritional Intervention against Oxidative Stress and Inflammation

You Jin Kim [1], Iksoo Huh [2], Ji Yeon Kim [3], Saejong Park [4], Sung Ha Ryu [5], Kyu-Bong Kim [5], Suhkmann Kim [6], Taesung Park [2,*] and Oran Kwon [1,*]

[1] Department of Nutritional Science and Food Management, Ewha Womans University, Seoul 03760, Korea; eugene841226@gmail.com
[2] Department of Statistics, Seoul National University, Seoul 08826, Korea; huhixoo@gmail.com
[3] Department of Food Science and Technology, Seoul National University of Science and Technology, Seoul 01811, Korea; jiyeonk@seoultech.ac.kr
[4] Department of Sport Science, Korea Institute of Sport Science, Seoul 01794, Korea; saejpark@sports.re.kr
[5] College of Pharmacy, Dankook University, Chungnam 31116, Korea; shryu@glpt.co.kr (S.H.R.); kyubong@dankook.ac.kr (K.-B.K.)
[6] Department of Chemistry and Chemistry Institute for Functional Materials, Pusan National University, Busan 46241, Korea; suhkmann@pusan.ac.kr
* Correspondence: tspark@stats.snu.ac.kr (T.P.); orank@ewha.ac.kr (O.K.);
 Tel.: +82-2-888-6693 (T.P.); +82-2-3277-6860 (O.K.)

Received: 16 January 2017; Accepted: 28 February 2017; Published: 4 March 2017

Abstract: Various statistical approaches can be applied to integrate traditional and omics biomarkers, allowing the discovery of prognostic markers to classify subjects into poor and good prognosis groups in terms of responses to nutritional interventions. Here, we performed a prototype study to identify metabolites that predict responses to an intervention against oxidative stress and inflammation, using a data set from a randomized controlled trial evaluating Korean black raspberry (KBR) in sedentary overweight/obese subjects. First, a linear mixed-effects model analysis with multiple testing correction showed that four-week consumption of KBR significantly changed oxidized glutathione (GSSG, $q = 0.027$) level, the ratio of reduced glutathione (GSH) to GSSG ($q = 0.039$) in erythrocytes, malondialdehyde (MDA, $q = 0.006$) and interleukin-6 ($q = 0.006$) levels in plasma, and seventeen NMR metabolites in urine compared with those in the placebo group. A subsequent generalized linear mixed model analysis showed linear correlations between baseline urinary glycine and N-phenylacetylglycine (PAG) and changes in the GSH:GSSG ratio ($p = 0.008$ and 0.004) as well as between baseline urinary adenine and changes in MDA ($p = 0.018$). Then, receiver operating characteristic analysis revealed that a two-metabolite set (glycine and PAG) had the strongest prognostic relevance for future interventions against oxidative stress (the area under the curve (AUC) = 0.778). Leave-one-out cross-validation confirmed the accuracy of prediction (AUC = 0.683). The current findings suggest that a higher level of this two-metabolite set at baseline is useful for predicting responders to dietary interventions in subjects with oxidative stress and inflammation, contributing to the emergence of personalized nutrition.

Keywords: oxidative stress; inflammation; prognostic marker; metabolomics; sedentary overweight/obese adults

1. Introduction

ROS overproduction and subsequent low-grade inflammation are believed to be reasons for the acceleration of age-related chronic diseases [1]. Epidemiological evidence has indicated that foods and their constituents have been associated with reducing oxidative stress and inflammation, thus implicating them in preventing the onset of chronic disease [2,3]. However, many randomized human intervention studies to assess the benefits of foods or food constituents have often led to negative results. It is partly because differences between study subjects may be much larger than differences directly related to nutritional intervention [4]. To address this issue, the concept of precision nutrition or personalized nutrition has been introduced, where the understanding of individual's response to an intervention is required to be achieved [5]. Fortunately, advances in omics technologies and statistical analysis have now begun to make it possible to obtain holistic and systemic information from even a single nutritional intervention study, thus making precision nutrition a realistic goal [6,7].

Particularly, metabolomics are known as powerful and sensitive tools that can reveal crucial information that is closely related to an individual's current health status and responses to nutritional interventions [8]. The promising field of metabolomics involves the estimation of exposure to specific foods, such as methylglutarylcarnitine for cocoa [9], proline betaine for citrus [10], resveratrol for wine [11], 2-furoylglycine for coffee [12], alkylresorcinols for whole grains [13], and furan fatty acids (3-carboxy-4-methyl-5-propyl-2-furanpropionic acid) for fish [14], to name a few examples. Alternatively, metabolomics approach may be useful for the development of precision nutrition. To accomplish precision nutrition, the identification of desired health outcomes and valid biomarkers to measure how response changes are critically important. Moreover, biomarker should be sufficiently accurate and have a relationship in the predicted direction [15]. It has been portrayed that an appropriate prognostic markers will be useful to predict future response and enable target interventions to those who need or respond to them [5]. At present, however, only a few studies have focused on the use of metabolomics in the search for prognostic markers [16,17].

Black raspberry is one of the most economically important crops and has become a popular food because it is a rich source of vitamins and polyphenolic compounds with high antioxidant capacities [18]. Black raspberry is a common name for three *Rubus* species: *Rubus coreanus*, native to Eastern Asia; *Rubus occidentalis*, native to Midwestern and Eastern North America; and *Rubus leucodermis*, native to the Pacific Northwest [19]. In Korea, *Rubus coreanus* (Korean black raspberry (KBR)) and *Rubus occidentalis* (Northern American black raspberry (NAB)) have been widely used with confusion. Two recent studies compared bioactive component in KBR and NAB using fingerprinting techniques and revealed that each varied in proportions and total concentration of bioactive components [20,21]. However, thus far a comparison of biological effect between KBR and NAB remains poorly understood in a clinical setting, providing a rationale to initiate a human intervention study.

In this work, we first conducted a preliminary study to compare the antioxidative and anti-inflammatory properties of KBR with those of NAB in a randomized controlled trial with sedentary overweight/obese adults challenged with treadmill exercise at 60% VO_2 maximum for 30 min. This approach is based on the previous findings, which indicated that acute moderate exercise is known to induce transient inflammation and oxidative stress [22]. Then, we performed a prototype study to explore the practical use of metabolites as a method for classifying subjects into poor and good prognosis groups in response to a nutritional intervention. To this end, we obtained ^{1}H-NMR metabolomics data derived from the KBR group and applied various statistical analyses to integrate traditional and metabolomics biomarkers.

2. Materials and Methods

2.1. Test Materials

Freeze-dried powder of KBR and NAB and a color/flavor-matched placebo containing lactose were provided by the Korean Rural Development Administration (Suwon, Gyunggi-do, Korea). The full chemical signatures and in vitro antioxidant capacities of KBR and NAB have been reported in previous publications [23,24]. The daily dose (30 g/day; equivalent to 100 g/day of fresh fruits) was determined based on previous studies from other researchers [25,26]. The daily dose of KBR represented 0.9 g of total phenol, including 17.5 mg of myricetin, 9.6 mg of genistin, 7.2 mg of quercetin, 1.2 mg of daidzein, and 1.2 mg of eriodictyol, as well as 126 kcal (65.5% as carbohydrate, 10.1% as protein, and 5.4% as fat). The daily dose of NAB represented 1.3 g of total phenol, including 25.2 mg of myricetin, 16.6 mg of genistin, 7.4 mg of kaempferol, 3.9 mg of quercetin, 1.8 mg of eriodictyol, and 0.6 mg of daidzein, as well as 111 kcal (67.8% as carbohydrate, 7.5% as protein, and 7.6% as fat) [21].

2.2. Participants

One hundred and two subjects (30–60 years) with a body mass index (BMI) between 23 and 30 kg/m^2 and a sedentary lifestyle were recruited from the general public by poster advertisements. According to the recommendation of World Health Organization for Asian populations, 82% of subjects were classified as overweight (23–27.5 kg/m^2) and 18% as obese (>27.5 kg/m^2) [27]; and according to the recommendation of the Institute of Medicine, all subjects were classified as sedentary (2.5 h of exercise/week) [28]. The exclusion criteria included the current use of dietary supplements; inflammatory disease, liver disease, renal disease, cardiovascular disease, hypertension, stroke, diabetes mellitus, or any other disease affecting the results of the study; difficulty engaging in treadmill exercises; cigarette smoking; known hypersensitivity to the study product; and pregnancy or lactation. After providing written informed consent, participants underwent anthropometric measurements, a complete blood count analysis, and an exercise treadmill test to evaluate their eligibility status. The maximal oxygen consumption (VO$_{2max}$) and maximum heart rate were determined during an incremental exercise program (2% grade increase every 2 min at a constant pace, 5–8 km/h) using a treadmill (T150; COSMED, Albano Laziale, Rome, Italy) and a respiratory gas analyzer (Quark CPET; COSMED, Albano Laziale, Rome, Italy).

2.3. Experimental Design

Seventy-two eligible subjects were enrolled at Ewha Womans University, which had three arms (placebo, KBR, and NAB). During a two-week lead-in period, participants were recommended to maintain their usual dietary and exercise habits and to avoid high-flavonoid foods and beverages including berries, fruits, vegetables, juices, microalgae, and teas for minimizing between-subject variability of bioactive components at baseline. Upon completion of a two-week lead-in period, subjects were randomly assigned to each group for 14 days using computer-generated random numbers at a ratio of 1:1:1 via stratified block randomization. Investigators and participants were blind to group allocation. During the treatment period, subjects were required to consume one sachet of corresponding test materials before each meal. Subject compliance was assessed by counting returned sachets and questioning the subjects. Changes in dietary habits and physical activity were monitored using a three-day (two weekdays and one weekend day) dietary record and were analyzed using a computerized nutritional analysis program (Can-Pro 3.0, The Korean Nutrition Society, Seoul, Korea).

At baseline and at the end of the trial, a treadmill exercise challenge was administered for 30 min at 60% VO$_{2max}$ to perturb the subject's homeostasis and then to quantify the responsiveness to test materials. Venous blood samples were collected in K2-EDTA-coated tubes (Becton Dickinson, Franklin Lakes, NJ, USA) before and immediately after the completion of exercise, followed by the separation of erythrocytes from plasma by centrifugation at 1500× *g* for 10 min. Spot urine samples were collected in polypropylene containers before and immediately after the completion of exercise. The samples were stored at −70 °C until analysis.

The study protocol was approved by the Institutional Review Boards of Ewha Womans University (Seoul, Korea) and was registered with the WHO International Clinical Trials Registry Platform under the following identification number: KCT0000644.

2.4. Measurements of Traditional Biomarkers

Plasma malondialdehyde (MDA; intra-Coefficients of Variance (CV): 13.1%; inter-CV: 5.2%) levels were determined by HPLC fluorescence (emission = 515 nm, excitation = 553 nm; SHISEIDO, Tokyo, Japan) with a Capcell Pak C18 column (UG120 type, 5 μm × 4.6 mm × 150 mm, Shiseido). Plasma oxidized LDL (ox-LDL; intra-CV: 7.9%; inter-CV: 9.6%), interleukin-6 (IL-6; intra-CV: 7.4%; inter-CV: 7.8%), and tumor necrosis factor-α (TNF-α; intra-CV: 4.9%; inter-CV: 7.6%) were measured with ELISA kits (Mercodia, Uppsala, Sweden for ox-LDL; R&D Systems, Minneapolis, MN, USA for IL-6 and TNF-α). Reduced (GSH; intra-CV: 4.0%; inter-CV: 5.9%) and oxidized glutathione (GSSG; intra-CV: 9.9%; inter-CV: 4.9%) levels in erythrocytes were measured as described by Rahman et al. [29]. Erythrocyte antioxidant enzyme activities (glutathione peroxidase, GPx (intra-CV: 5.7%; inter-CV: 7.2%); superoxide dismutase, SOD (intra-CV: 3.2%; inter-CV: 3.7%); and catalase, CAT (intra-CV: 3.8%; inter-CV: 9.9%)) and total hemoglobin (Hb) were measured spectrophotometrically using commercially available kits (Cayman, Ann Arbor, MI, USA). All measurements were performed in duplicate.

2.5. ^1H NMR Spectroscopy and Pre-Processing of NMR Spectra

After the plasma and urine samples were thawed and centrifuged, aliquot of each sample was transferred to a microcentrifuge tube containing phosphate buffer and deuterium oxide with 0.05% 3-(trimethylsilyl)-propionic-(2,2,3,3-d4) acid sodium salt as an internal standard for plasma and 2,2-dimethyl-2-silapentane-5-sulfonate for urine. Each sample was vortexed for 60 s and centrifuged for 10 min at 7000 rpm, and then an aliquot was used for analysis.

^{1}H-NMR spectroscopy was conducted on a Varian 600 MHz spectrometer (Varian, Palo Alto, CA, USA) at Pusan National University (Pusan, Korea). One-dimensional NMR spectra were acquired with the following parameters: spectral width 24,038.5 Hz, 3 s acquisition time, and 128 nt. Additional conditions of a relaxation delay time of 1 s and a saturation power of 4 were set to suppress massive water peaks. NMR spectra of each sample were acquired once since NMR is a highly reproducible technique [30]. NMR spectra were reduced to data using the Chenomx NMR Suite program 7.6 (Chenomx, Edmonton, AB, Canada). The spectral ^{1}H NMR region of δ 0.0–10.0 was segmented into regions with a width of 0.04 ppm, providing 250 integrated chemical shift regions in each NMR spectrum. The spectral regions corresponding to water (δ 4.5–5.0) were removed before normalization and spectra alignment. Metabolite concentrations were annotated and quantified manually in the NMR spectra using the Chenomx NMR Suite Professional software package 7.6 (Chenomx). For urine samples, metabolite concentrations were adjusted to the creatinine concentration because spot urine measurements, rather than 24 h urine samples, were used in this study [31].

2.6. Statistical Analysis

The sample size was estimated at 24 subjects per group to provide a power of 80% to detect a difference in GPx activity based on a previous KBR study [26] with a two-sided α-level of 0.05, allowing for an attrition rate of 20%.

Skewed data were logarithmically or square root transformed, but the results are expressed as the arithmetic means ± standard errors of the mean (SEMs) for ease of understanding. SAS 9.3 (SAS Institute, Cary, NC, USA), and the glmer function of the lme4 package [32], the heatmap.2 function of the gplots package [33], and the auc function of the pROC package [34] in R were used for the analysis.

Differences in means for the traditional and metabolomics biomarkers were analyzed using a linear mixed-effects (LME) model, taking into account a random effect (participant), a random error (within-participant), fixed effects (group, week, and the interaction between group and week), and a covariate (exercise). Corrected *p*-values (*q*-values) were calculated using Storey's false discovery rate (FDR) approach (95% confidence intervals) [35,36] to correct for multiple testing. An expected pathway of differential metabolites was drawn according to the Kyoto Encyclopedia of Genes and Genomes website (http://www.genome.jp/kegg/) and the MetaCyc Encyclopedia of Metabolic Pathways (http://www.metacyc.org/) and referring to Zgoda-Pols JR et al. [37]. Then, to explore prognostic metabolites for classifying the subjects into poor and good prognosis groups in terms of oxidative and inflammatory stress, a generalized linear mixed (GLM) model was applied to the data set with a logit link function and backward elimination optimization. In this model, ^{1}H NMR baseline metabolites were dichotomized (coded as 1 or 0) using median value and changes in traditional biomarkers were dichotomized to reflect positive or negative responses. Correlations between the variables were visualized using a heat map scaled by the t-value of GLM. The accuracy of predictions was tested by an area under the receiver operating characteristics (ROC) analysis. ROC curves were obtained by plotting the true-positive rates (sensitivity) against the false-positive rates (1-specificity). Areas under the curve (AUCs) with 95% CIs were calculated for sensitivity and specificity values. *P*-values were calculated for the comparison of the area under the ROC curve of each model with the reference line of 0.5. Finally, the validation of the most likely prognostic marker was performed with a leave-one-out cross-validation (LOOCV) technique.

3. Results

3.1. Preliminary Study to Compare Oxidative Stress and Inflammation in the KBR and NAB Groups Using Traditional Biomarkers

A total of 72 subjects were enrolled and 67 subjects were evaluable for response in a preliminary study (Supplemental Figure S1). All the participants were documented to fit the protocol and the groups were well matched for age and sex (Supplemental Table S1). From the three-day dietary records completed during the intervention, no significant group effect was detected across the baseline and four-week intervention among the dietary intake variables in terms of calories or micronutrients (Supplemental Table S2). The overall compliance was estimated at 96%. No serious or severe adverse events were observed.

The MDA, oxidized LDL, TNF-α, and IL-6 were measured in plasma. However, endogenous antioxidants and enzymes including GSH, GSSG, GPx, SOD, and CAT were measured in erythrocytes, because they are abundant in erythrocytes, which are constantly subjected to oxidative stress. The data demonstrated that the overall effect was similar for both KBR and NAB, but KBR showed a more significant effect than NAB in terms of GSSG (*q* = 0.036), GSH:GSSG (*q* = 0.050), and MDA (*q* = 0.008) levels (Supplemental Table S3).

3.2. Selection of Traditional Biomarkers and Metabolites for Integration

The ^{1}H-NMR metabolomics data were obtained from the KBR group: 63 metabolites were identified in the urine samples (Supplemental Table S4) and the 31 metabolites were identified in the plasma samples (Supplemental Table S5). A LME model was used to assess differences in the KBR and the control group. As a result, four traditional biomarkers and sixteen urinary metabolites with FDR *q*-values less than 0.05 were selected to be included in further analysis (Table 1). Four traditional biomarkers were GSSG (*q* = 0.027) and GSH:GSSG ratio (*q* = 0.039) in erythrocytes and MDA (*q* = 0.006) and IL-6 (*q* = 0.006) in plasma; and sixteen metabolites were amino acids (alanine, asparagine, glutamine, glycine, histidine, lysine, serine, and carnitine), organic acids (citrate and formate), purine nucleotide (adenine), and other metabolites (N6-acetyllysine, betaine, 3-indoxylsulfate, *N*-phenylacetylglycine (PAG), and phenylacetate).

Pathway analysis using KEGG database identified the tricarboxylic acid (TCA) cycle/oxidative phosphorylation (citrate, formate, and glutamine), glycerophospholipid metabolism (serine, betaine, glycine, and choline), purine metabolism (adenine, glutamine, and glycine), and amino acid metabolism (alanine, asparagine, aspartate, glutamine, glycine, histidine, isoleucine, leucine, lysine, and serine) (Figure 1).

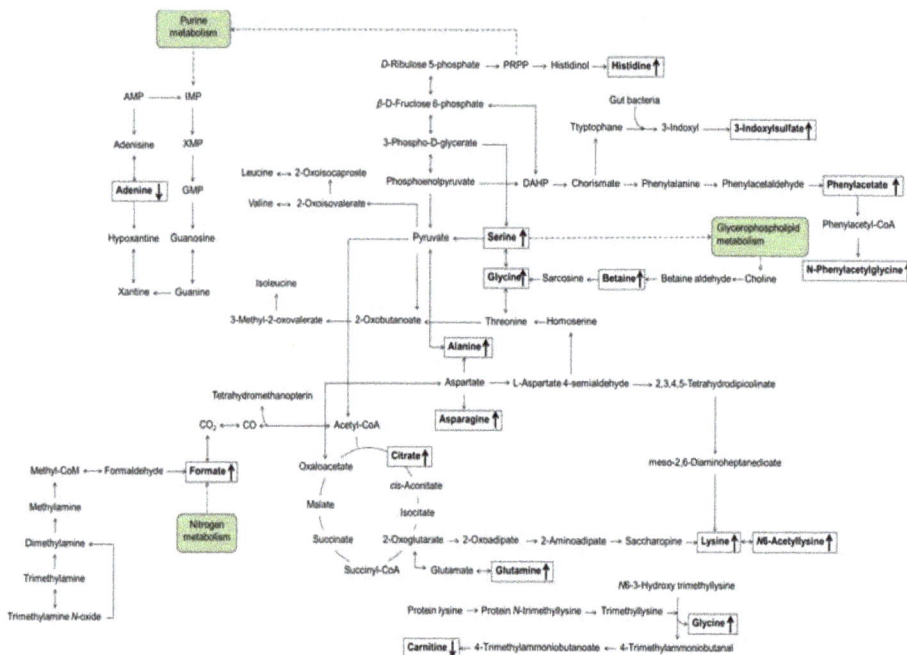

Figure 1. Proposed metabolic pathways related to endogenous urinary metabolites that were significantly changed in response to KBR administration over four weeks compared with those in the placebo group. Arrows indicate the directions of alterations. KBR, Korean black raspberry.

Table 1. Significantly altered traditional metabolomics biomarkers in response to KBR consumption in sedentary overweight/obese adults [1].

Variables	Placebo		KBR		β [2]	*q*-Value [3]
	Baseline	Delta Change	Baseline	Delta Change		
Traditional biomarkers						
GSSG (μM/g Hb)	12.9 ± 0.6 [4]	1.8 ± 0.3	12.9 ± 0.7	0.3 ± 0.4	−1.117	0.027
GSH:GSSG ratio	3.0 ± 0.2	−0.3 ± 0.1	2.8 ± 0.2	0.2 ± 0.2	0.045	0.039
MDA (nM)	14.5 ± 1.5	0.0 ± 0.4	16.4 ± 1.6	−2.5 ± 0.6	−0.058	0.006
IL-6 (pg/mL)	196.1 ± 22.8	51.4 ± 31.8	182.7 ± 24.4	−52.1 ± 17.9	−0.199	0.006
Urinary metabolites (μM)						
3-Indoxylsulfate	2.31 ± 0.16	0.11 ± 0.21	2.16 ± 0.18	0.81 ± 0.2	0.399	0.009
Adenine	1.26 ± 0.11	0.09 ± 0.18	1.64 ± 0.21	−0.6 ± 0.2	−0.286	0.041
Alanine	2.79 ± 0.18	−0.14 ± 0.17	2.49 ± 0.16	0.35 ± 0.13	0.194	0.021
Asparagine	1.62 ± 0.09	0.16 ± 0.13	1.55 ± 0.09	0.47 ± 0.12	0.199	0.041
Betaine	1.63 ± 0.12	−0.07 ± 0.13	1.55 ± 0.14	0.31 ± 0.15	0.295	0.024
Carnitine	0.95 ± 0.11	0.22 ± 0.14	0.91 ± 0.09	−0.13 ± 0.11	−0.555	0.009
Citrate	11.49 ± 0.78	−1.15 ± 0.5	11.19 ± 1.16	0.53 ± 0.68	0.029	0.037
Formate	3.22 ± 0.28	0.01 ± 0.32	2.58 ± 0.19	1.31 ± 0.48	0.314	0.034

Table 1. *Cont.*

Variables	Placebo		KBR		β [2]	*q*-Value [3]
	Baseline	Delta Change	Baseline	Delta Change		
Urinary metabolites (µM)						
Glutamine	5.29 ± 0.29	−0.26 ± 0.24	4.61 ± 0.22	0.95 ± 0.22	0.220	0.0001
Glycine	10.51 ± 1.29	−0.83 ± 0.81	8.63 ± 0.75	1.18 ± 0.56	0.200	0.021
Histidine	4.33 ± 0.4	−0.55 ± 0.4	3.76 ± 0.34	1.25 ± 0.38	0.018	0.013
Lysine	1.83 ± 0.25	−0.27 ± 0.2	1.11 ± 0.1	0.3 ± 0.12	0.329	0.021
N-Phenylacetylglycine	3.05 ± 0.15	−0.16 ± 0.2	2.62 ± 0.13	0.53 ± 0.14	0.007	0.016
N6-Acetyllysine	1.04 ± 0.03	0.02 ± 0.04	0.99 ± 0.03	0.14 ± 0.04	0.001	0.028
Phenylacetate	1.04 ± 0.04	0.01 ± 0.05	1.07 ± 0.06	0.21 ± 0.06	0.002	0.021
Serine	5.19 ± 0.31	0.42 ± 0.35	4.05 ± 0.18	1.51 ± 0.31	0.248	0.021

GSH, reduced glutathione; GSSG, oxidized glutathione: GPx, glutathione peroxidase; Hb, hemoglobin; SOD, superoxide dismutase; MDA, malondialdehyde; IL-6, interleukin-6, TNF-α: tumor necrosis factor-alpha; KBR, Korean black raspberry. [1] Data are expressed as the means ± SEM; [2] The beta estimates (β; estimated slope) of each variable were determined using a linear mixed-effects model. The beta estimate describes the effect of the KBR group versus the placebo group on the linear change over the supplementation period; [3] Storey's positive false discovery rate (pFDR) was calculated as *q*-values to account for multiple testing; [4] The absolute delta change was calculated by subtracting the measurement at baseline from that at the end of four weeks.

3.3. Identification of Candidate Prognostic Metabolites

The selected biomarkers were integrated to identify associations between alterations in four traditional biomarkers and those in seventeen urinary metabolites at baseline using a GLM analysis. The key statistical measures (Supplemental Table S6) and the resulting heat map (Figure 2) revealed that urinary glycine and PAG levels were positively associated with an increase in the erythrocyte GSH:GSSG ratio ($p = 0.008$ and 0.004, respectively). In contrast, the urinary adenine level was negatively associated with a decrease in the plasma MDA level ($p = 0.018$).

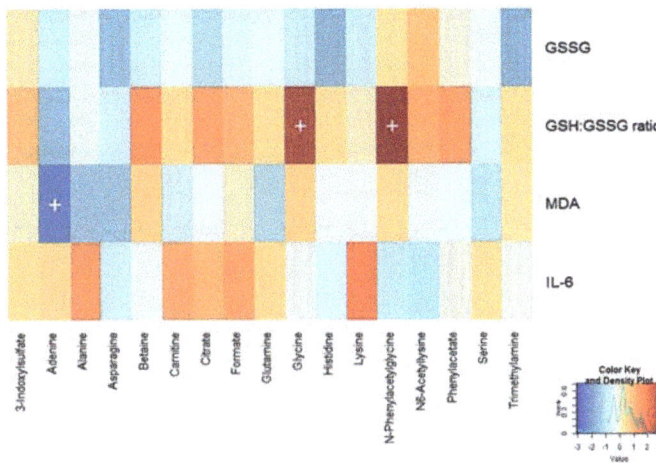

Figure 2. Correlation heat map generated by a generalized linear mixed model analysis of four traditional biomarkers with seventeen urinary metabolomic signatures. Red and blue colors indicate negative and positive t-values, respectively. A cross indicates a *p*-value < 0.05.

3.4. Validation of Prognostic Metabolites

An ROC analysis was performed on the three single candidate metabolites (glycine, PAG, and adenine) and a two-metabolite set (glycine + PAG) to test the prognostic performance (Figure 3). A two-metabolite set demonstrated the highest prognostic value, with a sensitivity of 86.4% and a specificity of 58.1% (AUC = 0.778, *p* < 0.0001). Therefore, the predictive ability of this two-metabolite set was further validated using an LOOCV analysis, demonstrating an AUC of 0.683 with a sensitivity of 86.4% and a specificity of 58.1% (Figure 4).

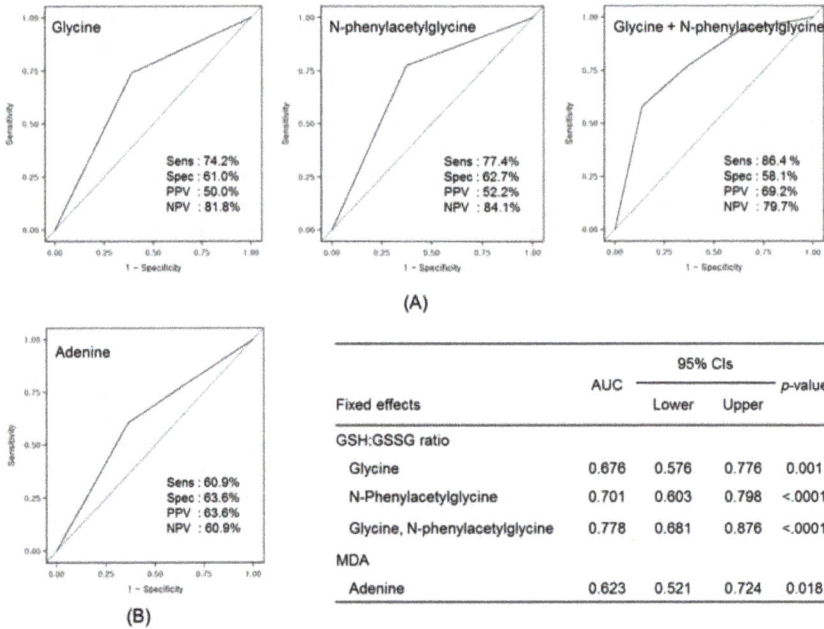

(A)

Fixed effects	AUC	95% CIs		*p*-value
		Lower	Upper	
GSH:GSSG ratio				
Glycine	0.676	0.576	0.776	0.001
N-Phenylacetylglycine	0.701	0.603	0.798	<.0001
Glycine, N-phenylacetylglycine	0.778	0.681	0.876	<.0001
MDA				
Adenine	0.623	0.521	0.724	0.018

(B)

Figure 3. ROC curves of three single metabolite and a two-metabolite set for predicting changes in traditional biomarkers: (**A**) erythrocyte GSH:GSSG ratio; and (**B**) plasma MDA level. The gray diagonal line represents the reference line of 0.5. Sensitivity, specificity, PPV, and NPV are shown in each box, and AUC, CI, and *p*-value are presented in the inset. ROC, receiver operating characteristic; GSH, glutathione; GSSG, oxidized glutathione; MDA, malondialdehyde; PPV, positive predictive value; NPV, negative predictive value; AUC, area under the curve; CI, confidence intervals.

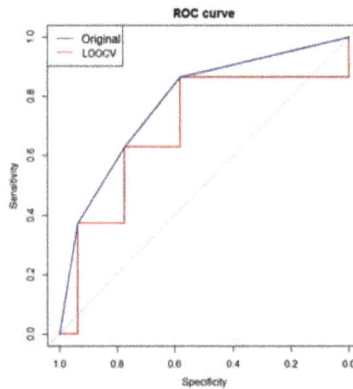

Figure 4. ROC curve of a two-metabolite set (glycine + N-phenylacetylglycine) by LOOCV. The blue and red ROC curves were generated using the original data set and the LOOCV data set. The gray diagonal line represents the reference line of 0.5. LOOCV, leave-one-out cross-validation.

4. Discussion

This study was composed of two parts. We first performed a preliminary study to compare anti-oxidative/anti-inflammatory properties of KBR with those of NAB in a clinical setting. Participants in the study were sedentary overweight/obese subjects presented with an exercise challenge because existing data indicate that such individuals are vulnerable to oxidative stress and have low-level chronic inflammation [38]. Using metabolic profiling, Park et al. [21] showed that myricetin, genistin, quercetin, daidzein, eridictyol are the major components both in KBR and NAB, but the proportions and contents of individual components were different each other. Based on fingerprinting of anthocyanins, Lee et al. [20] demonstrated that cyanidin-3-glucoside, cyanidin-3-rutinoside, and pelargonidin-3-glucoside were three major components in KBR, while cyanidin-3-sambubioside and cyanidin-3-xylosylrutinoside were major components in NAB. However, a bioassay for comparing the anti-oxidant capacities of KBR and NAB in vitro revealed that the level of general antioxidant activities of KBR was indistinguishable from that of NAB [24]. In this clinical trial, we demonstrated a consistent result that KBR and NAB had an almost equivalent efficacy on oxidative stress and inflammation, although KBR exhibited more or less superior activities to NAB in terms of GSH:GSSG ratio, MDA, and IL-6 levels. Taken together, we could conclude that the distinct profiles of bioactive components can be used as marker compounds to confirm the identity between KBR and NAB, but may not be good enough to be used as exclusive active components for protecting oxidative stress and inflammation.

Second part was the main study, in which we performed a pioneering study to explore whether baseline levels of metabolites in biofluids would predict a change in traditional biomarkers related to oxidative stress and inflammation in response to a nutritional intervention on an individual level. Two biofluids, plasma and urine, were used to collect relevant information on endogenous metabolites. Urine samples are known to be advantageous to study due to the ease of sample collection, large sample volumes, high concentrations, and few interfering proteins [39,40], implicating that the urinary metabolites could be more useful for identifying individuals who are at risk for progression of disease [41]. In the present study, we demonstrated that urinary metabolites were more responsive to KBR administration than plasma metabolites.

Endogenous metabolites are quite different from food metabolites in terms of characteristics and applications [42]. Endogenous metabolites are defined as low-molecular-weight chemicals derived from the host, and provide a rich source of information regarding physiological responses to foods or their constituents. Thus, endogenous metabolites are useful for either discriminating responders from non-responders who are likely to benefit from a nutritional intervention [16,17] or predicting effectiveness for maintaining or improving health at the individual level [43]. In contrast, food metabolites are defined as chemicals derived from the digestion, absorption, and biotransformation of foods, and thus can be used for the accurate monitoring of food exposure [44]. Among the analytical techniques that can be employed for the quantitative detection of multiple metabolites in biofluids, NMR spectroscopy and mass spectrometry are the most common. ^{1}H NMR spectroscopic techniques have inherently low sensitivity; thus, they cannot detect components at low concentrations below the range of micromoles per liter [42]. The major bioactive components found KBR are rapidly eliminated or transformed, thus it is not possible to detect them in biofluids collected after overnight fasting, thus metabolites cannot be used to define compliance [45]. However, NMR spectroscopy allows the detection of a wide range of endogenous metabolites. In this study, a total of 63 metabolites in urine samples and 31 metabolites in plasma samples were detected. Of these, 26 metabolites (3-hydroxybutyrate, acetate, acetone, alanine, arginine, betaine, choline, citrate, creatine, formate, glucose, glutamine, glycerol, glycine, histidine, isoleucine, lactate, leucine, lysine, methanol, phenylalanine, pyruvate, serine, succinate, tyrosine, and valine) were detected in both biofluids.

To identify candidate prognostic metabolites and enhance the prognostic power, various statistical approaches were used. First, signature biomarkers were identified, which were then integrated to obtain associations between baseline metabolites and changes of traditional biomarkers. Similar approaches were employed to identify plasma metabolite signatures for predicting glucose tolerance changes in sedentary women after high-intensity interval training [17] and to develop predictive models for prostate carcinoma recurrence [46]. However, to our knowledge, no previous study has investigated the use of prognostic markers for screening potential responders to maximize the benefits of nutritional intervention against oxidative stress. In addition, we tested whether changing the baseline metabolites could increase the diagnostic validity by ROC analysis. The ROC curve for a two-metabolite set (glycine and PAG) outperformed single markers (glycine, PAG, or adenine), highlighting that this set is a promising biomarker that possesses the greatest discriminatory power to predict individual responses to KBR consumption in sedentary overweight/obese adults. Several other studies have supported an association between urinary glycine or PAG levels and status of oxidative stress [47–52] or inflammatory stress [52]. Finally, the predictive accuracy of this two-metabolite set was further validated with the LOOCV procedure, because the ROC curve may lead to an overestimation of the AUC if it is constructed using all samples [53]. The LOOCV procedure has an advantage of reducing the likelihood of developing an overly optimistic predictive model given the relatively small sample in our study [54]. As a result, we concluded that the predictive accuracy was fair, indicating that a higher level of glycine and PAG set may serve as a prognostic marker for planning strategic personalized interventions on oxidative stress and inflammation.

Metabolic pathway analysis revealed that urinary levels of glycine, PAG, and adenine are involved in purine [55,56] and phenylalanine metabolism [57], conceivably resulting in changes in the GSH redox state and suppression of oxidative stress. Glycine is a precursor to GSH, thus indirectly contributing to the role of a cytoprotective agent by ROS scavenging mechanisms [48,58]. In the case where glycine availability is reduced, for example by protein malnutrition, sepsis, and diabetes, reduced glycine availability may become a limiting factor for GSH synthesis [59]. A couple of studies supported the notion that a high level of urinary glycine is associated with accelerating GSH restoration against the oxidative stress [48,58,60]. PAG is a glycine conjugate, which is expected to respond in the same direction with glycine [50]. In contrast, however, when adenine is present in excess, xanthine oxidase is activated, inducing oxidative stress by hydroxyl free radicals and hydrogen peroxide [61]. It was also reported that excessive adenine found in a chronic renal failure animal model was related to oxidative damages and inflammation [55,62]. Collectively, these data may explain our finding that background levels of three urinary metabolites were associated with internal capacity to overcome oxidative stress and thus useful to differentiate responders from non-responders to a nutritional intervention as prognostic markers.

It is important to note the limitations of this study. Firstly, for validation of the predictive ability of a proposed metabolite, we used the LOOCV procedure. However, it could not be a substitute for external validation on an independent sample set. Therefore, the next step will be to validate this result in a large cohort or other clinical studies. Secondly, in the present study, we only suggested that the subjects who have a statistically higher mean value of background urinary glycine and PAG levels may have a good prognosis following a nutritional intervention against oxidative stress. Further evidence seems to be necessary for establishing the cut-off point for the examination, rather than the performance of the test as a whole. Lastly, translational works are needed to gain future insights into the use of a two-metabolite set as a simple laboratory diagnostic kit for identifying responders to create personalized nutritional interventions that maximize the salutary benefits on an individual level. However, even with these limitations, the model we have proposed may provide fundamental understanding of the process and insight in developing prognostic metabolites for identification of potential responders who can magnify the salutary benefits of nutritional intervention against oxidative stress on an individual level. Afterwards, when aiming at an antioxidant intervention, subjects would be selected using the proposed prognostic markers to implement the individually tailored nutritional intervention.

5. Conclusions

The metabolites may not only be limited to assessing overall dietary exposure, but also may be useful when selecting individuals who are most likely to benefit from nutritional interventions. The results obtained in this study provided insight into the opportunities involved in identifying prognostic metabolic markers, which may be useful for classifying responders and non-responders to nutritional interventions in subjects with oxidative stress and inflammation. Together with further studies, these results may be contributing to the emergence of personalized nutrition.

Supplementary Materials: The following are available online at http://www.mdpi.com/2072-6643/9/3/233/s1, Figure S1: The Consolidated Standards of Reporting Trials flow diagram representing the phases of the randomized study for comparing the two species of raspberries, Table S1: Baseline characteristics of subjects participated in a preliminary study, Table S2: Daily dietary energy and nutrient intake at baseline and Week 4, Table S3: Comparison of anti-oxidant and anti-inflammatory effects of KBR and NAB in sedentary overweight/obese adults challenged with exercise, Table S4: Summary of urinary ^{1}H NMR metabolites before and after placebo or KBR administration in sedentary overweight/obese adults challenged with exercise, Table S5: Summary of plasma ^{1}H NMR metabolites before and after placebo or KBR administration in sedentary overweight/obese adults challenged with exercise, Table S6: Associations between the changes in traditional biomarkers and urinary metabolomic signatures at baseline.

Acknowledgments: This study was supported by the Ministry of Education, Science and Technology of Korea (NRF Project No. 2012M3A9C4048761 and 2013M3A9C4078158).

Author Contributions: Y.J.K., J.Y.K., S.P., T.P. and O.K. designed and conducted the research; Y.J.K., I.H., S.H.R., K.B.K. and S.K. analyzed samples and performed statistical analyses; Y.J.K. and O.K. wrote the manuscript; and O.K. and T.P. assume primary responsibility for the final content of the manuscript. All authors read and approved the final version of the manuscript.

Conflicts of Interest: The authors declare no conflict of interest. The founding sponsors had no role in the design of the study; in the collection, analyses, or interpretation of data; in the writing of the manuscript, and in the decision to publish the results.

References

1. Sarkar, D.; Fisher, P.B. Molecular mechanisms of aging-associated inflammation. *Cancer Lett.* **2006**, *236*, 13–23. [CrossRef] [PubMed]
2. Holt, E.M.; Steffen, L.M.; Moran, A.; Basu, S.; Steinberger, J.; Ross, J.A.; Hong, C.P.; Sinaiko, A.R. Fruit and vegetable consumption and its relation to markers of inflammation and oxidative stress in adolescents. *J. Am. Diet. Assoc.* **2009**, *109*, 414–421. [CrossRef] [PubMed]
3. Pan, M.H.; Lai, C.S.; Dushenkov, S.; Ho, C.T. Modulation of inflammatory genes by natural dietary bioactive compounds. *J. Agric. Food Chem.* **2009**, *57*, 4467–4477. [CrossRef] [PubMed]
4. van Dorsten, F.A.; Grun, C.H.; van Velzen, E.J.; Jacobs, D.M.; Draijer, R.; van Duynhoven, J.P. The metabolic fate of red wine and grape juice polyphenols in humans assessed by metabolomics. *Mol. Nutr. Food Res.* **2010**, *54*, 897–908. [CrossRef] [PubMed]
5. Srinivasan, B.; Lee, S.; Erickson, D.; Mehta, S. Precision nutrition - review of methods for point-of-care assessment of nutritional status. *Curr. Opin. Biotechnol.* **2016**, *44*, 103–108. [CrossRef] [PubMed]
6. van Ommen, B.; Keijer, J.; Kleemann, R.; Elliott, R.; Drevon, C.A.; McArdle, H.; Gibney, M.; Müller, M. The challenges for molecular nutrition research 2: Quantification of the nutritional phenotype. *Genes Nutr.* **2008**, *3*, 51–59. [CrossRef] [PubMed]
7. van Ommen, B.; Keijer, J.; Heil, S.G.; Kaput, J. Challenging homeostasis to define biomarkers for nutrition related health. *Mol. Nutr. Food Res.* **2009**, *53*, 795–804. [CrossRef] [PubMed]
8. Gibney, M.J.; Walsh, M.; Brennan, L.; Roche, H.M.; German, B.; van Ommen, B. Metabolomics in human nutrition: Opportunities and challenges. *Am. J. Clin. Nutr.* **2005**, *82*, 497–503. [PubMed]
9. Garcia-Aloy, M.; Llorach, R.; Urpi-Sarda, M.; Jauregui, O.; Corella, D.; Ruiz-Canela, M.; Salas-Salvado, J.; Fito, M.; Ros, E.; Estruch, R.; et al. A metabolomics-driven approach to predict cocoa product consumption by designing a multimetabolite biomarker model in free-living subjects from the predimed study. *Mol. Nutr. Food Res.* **2015**, *59*, 212–220. [CrossRef] [PubMed]

10. Heinzmann, S.S.; Brown, I.J.; Chan, Q.; Bictash, M.; Dumas, M.E.; Kochhar, S.; Stamler, J.; Holmes, E.; Elliott, P.; Nicholson, J.K. Metabolic profiling strategy for discovery of nutritional biomarkers: Proline betaine as a marker of citrus consumption. *Am. J. Clin. Nutr.* **2010**, *92*, 436–443. [CrossRef] [PubMed]

11. Zamora-Ros, R.; Urpi-Sarda, M.; Lamuela-Raventos, R.M.; Estruch, R.; Martinez-Gonzalez, M.A.; Bullo, M.; Aros, F.; Cherubini, A.; Andres-Lacueva, C. Resveratrol metabolites in urine as a biomarker of wine intake in free-living subjects: The predimed study. *Free Radic. Biol. Med.* **2009**, *46*, 1562–1566. [CrossRef] [PubMed]

12. Heinzmann, S.S.; Holmes, E.; Kochhar, S.; Nicholson, J.K.; Schmitt-Kopplin, P. 2-furoylglycine as a candidate biomarker of coffee consumption. *J. Agric. Food chem.* **2015**, *63*, 8615–8621. [CrossRef] [PubMed]

13. McKeown, N.M.; Marklund, M.; Ma, J.; Ross, A.B.; Lichtenstein, A.H.; Livingston, K.A.; Jacques, P.F.; Rasmussen, H.M.; Blumberg, J.B.; Chen, C.Y. Comparison of plasma alkylresorcinols (ar) and urinary ar metabolites as biomarkers of compliance in a short-term, whole-grain intervention study. *Eur. J. Nutr.* **2015**, *55*, 1235–1244. [CrossRef] [PubMed]

14. Hanhineva, K.; Lankinen, M.A.; Pedret, A.; Schwab, U.; Kolehmainen, M.; Paananen, J.; de Mello, V.; Sola, R.; Lehtonen, M.; Poutanen, K.; et al. Nontargeted metabolite profiling discriminates diet-specific biomarkers for consumption of whole grains, fatty fish, and bilberries in a randomized controlled trial. *J. Nutr.* **2015**, *145*, 7–17. [CrossRef] [PubMed]

15. Betts, J.; Gonzalez, J. Personalised nutrition: What makes you so special? *Nutr. Bull.* **2016**, *41*, 353–359. [CrossRef]

16. Elnenaei, M.O.; Chandra, R.; Mangion, T.; Moniz, C. Genomic and metabolomic patterns segregate with responses to calcium and vitamin D supplementation. *Br. J. Nutr.* **2011**, *105*, 71–79. [CrossRef] [PubMed]

17. Kuehnbaum, N.L.; Gillen, J.B.; Gibala, M.J.; Britz-McKibbin, P. Personalized metabolomics for predicting glucose tolerance changes in sedentary women after high-intensity interval training. *Scientific reports* **2014**, *4*, 6166. [CrossRef] [PubMed]

18. Hyun, T.K.; Lee, S.; Rim, Y.; Kumar, R.; Han, X.; Lee, S.Y.; Lee, C.H.; Kim, J.Y. De-novo rna sequencing and metabolite profiling to identify genes involved in anthocyanin biosynthesis in korean black raspberry (rubus coreanus miquel). *PLoS ONE* **2014**, *9*, e88292. [CrossRef] [PubMed]

19. Finn, C.; Wennstrom, K.; Link, J.; Ridout, J. Evaluation of rubus leucodermis populations from the pacific northwest. *HortScience* **2003**, *38*, 1169–1172.

20. Lee, J.; Dossett, M.; Finn, C.E. Anthocyanin fingerprinting of true bokbunja (rubus coreanus miq.) fruit. *J. Funct. Foods* **2013**, *5*, 1985–1990. [CrossRef]

21. Park, S.J.; Hyun, S.-H.; Suh, H.W.; Lee, S.-Y.; Min, T.-S.; Auh, J.-H.; Lee, H.-J.; Kim, J.-H.; Cho, S.-M.; Choi, H.-K. Differentiation of black raspberry fruits according to species and geographic origins by genomic analysis and 1h-nmr-based metabolic profiling. *J. Korean Soc. Appl. Biol. Chem.* **2012**, *55*, 633–642. [CrossRef]

22. Fisher-Wellman, K.; Bloomer, R.J. Acute exercise and oxidative stress: A 30 year history. *Dyn. Med. DM* **2009**, *8*, 1. [CrossRef] [PubMed]

23. Kim, H.-S.; Park, S.J.; Hyun, S.-H.; Yang, S.-O.; Lee, J.; Auh, J.-H.; Kim, J.-H.; Cho, S.-M.; Marriott, P.J.; Choi, H.-K. Biochemical monitoring of black raspberry (rubus coreanus miquel) fruits according to maturation stage by 1h nmr using multiple solvent systems. *Food Res. Int.* **2011**, *44*, 1977–1987. [CrossRef]

24. Kim, L.S.; Youn, S.H.; Kim, J.Y. Comparative study on antioxidant effects of extracts from rubus coreanus and rubus occidentalis. *J. Korean Soc. Food Sci. Nutr.* **2014**, *43*, 1357–1362. [CrossRef]

25. Suh, H.W.; Kim, S.-H.; Park, S.J.; Hyun, S.-H.; Lee, S.-Y.; Auh, J.-H.; Lee, H.J.; Cho, S.-M.; Kim, J.-H.; Choi, H.-K. Effect of korean black raspberry (rubus coreanus miquel) fruit administration on DNA damage levels in smokers and screening biomarker investigation using 1h-nmr-based metabolic profiling. *Food Res. Int.* **2013**, *54*, 1255–1262. [CrossRef]

26. Lee, J.E.; Park, E.; Lee, J.E.; Auh, J.H.; Choi, H.K.; Lee, J.; Cho, S.; Kim, J.H. Effects of a rubus coreanus miquel supplement on plasma antioxidant capacity in healthy Korean men. *Nutr. Res. Pract.* **2011**, *5*, 429–434. [CrossRef] [PubMed]

27. WHO Expert Consultation. Appropriate body-mass index for Asian populations and its implications for policy and intervention strategies. *Lancet* **2004**, *363*, 157–163.

28. Food & Nutrition Information Center. Food & Nutrition Information Center. Physical Activity. In *Dietary Reference Intakes*; The National Academies Press: Washington, DC, USA, 2005; Chapter 12; pp. 880–935.

29. Rahman, I.; Kode, A.; Biswas, S.K. Assay for quantitative determination of glutathione and glutathione disulfide levels using enzymatic recycling method. *Nat. Protoc.* **2006**, *1*, 3159–3165. [CrossRef] [PubMed]

30. Loureiro, C.C.; Duarte, I.F.; Gomes, J.; Carrola, J.; Barros, A.S.; Gil, A.M.; Bousquet, J.; Bom, A.T.; Rocha, S.M. Urinary metabolomic changes as a predictive biomarker of asthma exacerbation. *J. Allergy Clin. Immunol.* **2014**, *133*, 261–263 e261–265. [CrossRef] [PubMed]

31. Carrieri, M.; Trevisan, A.; Bartolucci, G.B. Adjustment to concentration-dilution of spot urine samples: Correlation between specific gravity and creatinine. *Int. Arch. Occup. Environ. Health* **2001**, *74*, 63–67. [CrossRef] [PubMed]

32. Pinheiro, J.; Bates, D.; DebRoy, S.; Sarkar, D. R Development Core Team. Nlme: Linear and Nonlinear Mixed Effects Models. 2015, 3.1-122. Available online: https://CRAN.R-project.org/package=nlme (accessed on 10 January 2016).

33. Warnes, G.R.; Bolker, B.; Bonebakker, L.; Gentleman, R.; Huber, W.; Liaw, A.; Lumley, T.; Maechler, M.; Magnusson, A.; Moeller, S. Gplots: Various R Programming Tools for Plotting Data. R Package Version 2.12. 1. 2013. Available online: https://CRAN.R-project.org/package=gplots (accessed on 10 January 2016).

34. Robin, X.; Turck, N.; Hainard, A.; Tiberti, N.; Lisacek, F.; Sanchez, J.C.; Muller, M. Proc: An open-source package for r and s+ to analyze and compare roc curves. *BMC Bioinform.* **2011**, *12*, 77. [CrossRef] [PubMed]

35. Franceschi, P.; Giordan, M.; Wehrens, R. Multiple comparisons in mass-spectrometry-based-omics technologies. *TrAC Trends Anal. Chem.* **2013**, *50*, 11–21. [CrossRef]

36. Storey, J.D.; Tibshirani, R. Statistical significance for genomewide studies. *Proc. Natl. Acad. Sci. USA* **2003**, *100*, 9440–9445. [CrossRef] [PubMed]

37. Zgoda-Pols, J.R.; Chowdhury, S.; Wirth, M.; Milburn, M.V.; Alexander, D.C.; Alton, K.B. Metabolomics analysis reveals elevation of 3-indoxyl sulfate in plasma and brain during chemically-induced acute kidney injury in mice: Investigation of nicotinic acid receptor agonists. *Toxicol. Appl. Pharmacol.* **2011**, *255*, 48–56. [CrossRef] [PubMed]

38. Vincent, H.K.; Innes, K.E.; Vincent, K.R. Oxidative stress and potential interventions to reduce oxidative stress in overweight and obesity. *Diabetes Obes. Metab.* **2007**, *9*, 813–839. [CrossRef] [PubMed]

39. Lenz, E.M.; Bright, J.; Wilson, I.D.; Morgan, S.R.; Nash, A.F. A 1h nmr-based metabonomic study of urine and plasma samples obtained from healthy human subjects. *J. Pharm. Biomed. Anal.* **2003**, *33*, 1103–1115. [CrossRef]

40. Stella, C.; Beckwith-Hall, B.; Cloarec, O.; Holmes, E.; Lindon, J.C.; Powell, J.; van der Ouderaa, F.; Bingham, S.; Cross, A.J.; Nicholson, J.K. Susceptibility of human metabolic phenotypes to dietary modulation. *J. Proteome Res.* **2006**, *5*, 2780–2788. [CrossRef] [PubMed]

41. Pena, M.J.; Lambers Heerspink, H.J.; Hellemons, M.E.; Friedrich, T.; Dallmann, G.; Lajer, M.; Bakker, S.J.; Gansevoort, R.T.; Rossing, P.; de Zeeuw, D.; et al. Urine and plasma metabolites predict the development of diabetic nephropathy in individuals with type 2 diabetes mellitus. *Diabet. Med.* **2014**, *31*, 1138–1147. [CrossRef] [PubMed]

42. Scalbert, A.; Brennan, L.; Manach, C.; Andres-Lacueva, C.; Dragsted, L.O.; Draper, J.; Rappaport, S.M.; van der Hooft, J.J.; Wishart, D.S. The food metabolome: A window over dietary exposure. *Am. J. Clin. Nutr.* **2014**, *99*, 1286–1308. [CrossRef] [PubMed]

43. Rezzi, S.; Ramadan, Z.; Fay, L.B.; Kochhar, S. Nutritional metabonomics: Applications and perspectives. *J. Proteome Res.* **2007**, *6*, 513–525. [CrossRef] [PubMed]

44. Manach, C.; Hubert, J.; Llorach, R.; Scalbert, A. The complex links between dietary phytochemicals and human health deciphered by metabolomics. *Mol. Nutr. Food Res.* **2009**, *53*, 1303–1315. [CrossRef] [PubMed]

45. Rechner, A.R.; Kuhnle, G.; Bremner, P.; Hubbard, G.P.; Moore, K.P.; Rice-Evans, C.A. The metabolic fate of dietary polyphenols in humans. *Free Radic. Biol. Med.* **2002**, *33*, 220–235. [CrossRef]

46. Stephenson, A.J.; Smith, A.; Kattan, M.W.; Satagopan, J.; Reuter, V.E.; Scardino, P.T.; Gerald, W.L. Integration of gene expression profiling and clinical variables to predict prostate carcinoma recurrence after radical prostatectomy. *Cancer* **2005**, *104*, 290–298. [CrossRef] [PubMed]

47. Wang, X.Y.; Lin, J.C.; Chen, T.L.; Zhou, M.M.; Su, M.M.; Jia, W. Metabolic profiling reveals the protective effect of diammonium glycyrrhizinate on acute hepatic injury induced by carbon tetrachloride. *Metabolomics* **2011**, *7*, 226–236. [CrossRef]

48. Bonvallot, N.; Tremblay-Franco, M.; Chevrier, C.; Canlet, C.; Warembourg, C.; Cravedi, J.P.; Cordier, S. Metabolomics tools for describing complex pesticide exposure in pregnant women in brittany (France). *PLoS ONE* **2013**, *8*, e64433. [CrossRef] [PubMed]

49. Liu, G.; Xiao, L.; Cao, W.; Fang, T.; Jia, G.; Chen, X.; Zhao, H.; Wu, C.; Wang, J. Changes in the metabolome of rats after exposure to arginine and *N*-carbamylglutamate in combination with diquat, a compound that causes oxidative stress, assessed by h nmr spectroscopy. *Food Funct.* **2016**, *7*, 964–974. [CrossRef] [PubMed]

50. Jiang, L.; Zhao, X.; Huang, C.; Lei, H.; Tang, H.; Wang, Y. Dynamic changes in metabolic profiles of rats subchronically exposed to mequindox. *Mol. Biol. Syst.* **2014**, *10*, 2914–2922. [CrossRef] [PubMed]

51. Gonzalez-Guardia, L.; Yubero-Serrano, E.M.; Delgado-Lista, J.; Perez-Martinez, P.; Garcia-Rios, A.; Marin, C.; Camargo, A.; Delgado-Casado, N.; Roche, H.M.; Perez-Jimenez, F.; et al. Effects of the mediterranean diet supplemented with coenzyme q10 on metabolomic profiles in elderly men and women. *J. Gerontol. A Biol. Sci. Med. Sci.* **2015**, *70*, 78–84. [CrossRef] [PubMed]

52. Wang, K.C.; Kuo, C.H.; Tian, T.F.; Tsai, M.H.; Chiung, Y.M.; Hsiech, C.M.; Tsai, S.J.; Wang, S.Y.; Tsai, D.M.; Huang, C.C.; et al. Metabolomic characterization of laborers exposed to welding fumes. *Chem. Res. Toxicol.* **2012**, *25*, 676–686. [CrossRef] [PubMed]

53. Ducena, K.; Abols, A.; Vilmanis, J.; Narbuts, Z.; Tars, J.; Andrejeva, D.; Line, A.; Pirags, V. Validity of multiplex biomarker model of 6 genes for the differential diagnosis of thyroid nodules. *Thyroid Res.* **2011**, *4*, 11. [CrossRef] [PubMed]

54. Molinaro, A.M.; Simon, R.; Pfeiffer, R.M. Prediction error estimation: A comparison of resampling methods. *Bioinformatics* **2005**, *21*, 3301–3307. [CrossRef] [PubMed]

55. Ali, B.H.; Al-Husseni, I.; Beegam, S.; Al-Shukaili, A.; Nemmar, A.; Schierling, S.; Queisser, N.; Schupp, N. Effect of gum arabic on oxidative stress and inflammation in adenine-induced chronic renal failure in rats. *PLoS ONE* **2013**, *8*, e55242. [CrossRef] [PubMed]

56. Belmonte, M.; Stasolla, C.; Loukanina, N.; Yeung, E.C.; Thorpe, T.A. Glutathione modulation of purine metabolism in cultured white spruce embryogenic tissue. *Plant Sci.* **2003**, *165*, 1377–1385. [CrossRef]

57. Luan, H.; Liu, L.F.; Tang, Z.; Zhang, M.; Chua, K.K.; Song, J.X.; Mok, V.C.; Li, M.; Cai, Z. Comprehensive urinary metabolomic profiling and identification of potential noninvasive marker for idiopathic parkinson's disease. *Sci. Rep.* **2015**, *5*, 13888. [CrossRef] [PubMed]

58. Lee, Y.K.; Park, E.Y.; Kim, S.; Son, J.Y.; Kim, T.H.; Kang, W.G.; Jeong, T.C.; Kim, K.B.; Kwack, S.J.; Lee, J.; et al. Evaluation of cadmium-induced nephrotoxicity using urinary metabolomic profiles in sprague-dawley male rats. *J. Toxicol. Environ. Health Part A* **2014**, *77*, 1384–1398. [CrossRef] [PubMed]

59. Wu, G.; Fang, Y.Z.; Yang, S.; Lupton, J.R.; Turner, N.D. Glutathione metabolism and its implications for health. *J. Nutr.* **2004**, *134*, 489–492. [PubMed]

60. Noctor, G.; Arisi, A.C.M.; Jouanin, L.; Valadier, M.H.; Roux, Y.; Foyer, C.H. The role of glycine in determining the rate of glutathione synthesis in poplar. Possible implications for glutathione production during stress. *Physiol. Plant.* **1997**, *100*, 255–263. [CrossRef]

61. Higgins, P.; Dawson, J.; Walters, M. The potential for xanthine oxidase inhibition in the prevention and treatment of cardiovascular and cerebrovascular disease. *Cardiovasc. Psychiatry Neurol.* **2009**, *2009*, 282059. [CrossRef] [PubMed]

62. Goyal, R.N.; Chatterjee, S.; Rana, A.R.S. Electrochemical sensor based on oxidation of 2,8-dihydroxyadenine to monitor DNA damage in calf thymus DNA. *Electroanalysis* **2011**, *23*, 1383–1390. [CrossRef]

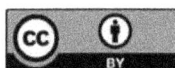

nutrients

Review

Hydroxytyrosol in the Prevention of the Metabolic Syndrome and Related Disorders

Julien Peyrol [1], Catherine Riva [1,*] and Marie Josèphe Amiot [2,3,4,5,6,7,8,*]

[1] Laboratory of Cardiovascular Pharm-Ecology EA4278, Department of Sport Sciences, Faculty of Sciences, Avignon University, F-84000 Avignon, France; julien.peyrol@univ-avignon.fr
[2] Unité Mixte de Recherche (UMR), Nutrition, Obesity and Risk of Thrombosis, Aix-Marseille University, F-13005 Marseille, France
[3] Unité Mixte de Recherche (UMR), Markets, Organisations, Institutions, Stakeholder Strategies, F-34060 Montpellier, France
[4] Centre de Coopération Internationale en Recherche Agronomique pour le Développement, F-34060 Montpellier, France
[5] Centre International de Hautes Études Agronomiques Méditerranéennes, F-34060 Montpellier, France
[6] Montpellier SupAgro, F-34060 Montpellier, France
[7] Institut National de la Recherche Agronomique; Division of Nutrtition, Chemical Food Safety and Consumer Behaviour, F-75015 Paris, France
[8] Institut National de la Santé et de la Recherche Médicale, F-75015 Paris, France
* Correspondence: catherine.riva@univ-avignon.fr (C.R.); marie-josephe.amiot.carlin@inra.fr (M.J.A.); Tel.: +33-4-9016-2933 (C.R.); +33-4-9961-2246 (M.J.A.)

Received: 15 February 2017; Accepted: 16 March 2017; Published: 20 March 2017

Abstract: Virgin olive oil (VOO) constitutes the main source of fat in the Mediterranean diet. VOO is rich in oleic acid, displaying health-promoting properties, but also contains minor bioactive components, especially phenolic compounds. Hydroxytyrosol (HT), the main polyphenol of olive oil, has been reported to be the most bioactive component. This review aims to compile the results of clinical, animal and cell culture studies evaluating the effects of HT on the features of Metabolic Syndrome (MetS) (body weight/adiposity, dyslipidemia, hypertension, and hyperglycemia/insulin resistance) and associated complications (oxidative stress and inflammation). HT was able to improve the lipid profile, glycaemia, and insulin sensitivity, and counteract oxidative and inflammatory processes. Experimental studies identified multiple molecular targets for HT conferring its beneficial effect on health in spite of its low bioavailability. However, rodent experiments and clinical trials with pure HT at biologically relevant concentrations are still lacking. Moreover, the roles of intestine and its gut microbiota have not been elucidated.

Keywords: olive oil; oleuropein; hydroxytyrosol; tyrosol; body weight; dyslipidemia; hyperglycemia; hypertension; oxidative stress; inflammation

1. Introduction

Metabolic syndrome (MetS), a cluster of several interrelated cardiovascular risk factors (hyperglycemia, hypertension, dyslipidemia, insulin resistance and central adiposity) [1] lead to an increased prevalence of cardiovascular diseases (CVD) and type 2 diabetes mellitus (T2DM). A report published in 2015 claimed that the mortality for T2DM is around five millions persons per year, and it is expected that 23.6 million will die of CVD in the world by 2030 [2]. Olive oil, a natural juice from olive, is the primary source of fat in the Mediterranean diet, which is associated with a lower incidence of CVD mortality [3] and contains minor components, especially phenolic compounds, which are recognized as health beneficial components [4]. Hydroxytyrosol (HT), a non-flavonoid polyphenolic compound derived from oleuropein (OLE) and, notably present in olive and olive oil, could be involved in lower incidence of CVD and T2DM in the Mediterranean region, despite a high intake of fat as olive oil. HT could be an efficient bioactive phenolic candidate, owing to its protective action of health towards inflammation and oxidative stress. Despite its well-described actions, the low plasmatic concentrations of HT after 25 mL extra-virgin olive oil (EVOO) consumption, ranging from 50 to 160 nM [5,6] questioned the assessment of its bioactivity. In addition, among the exponential increase of published studies on HT, few are related to its effects on MetS key components and the associated complications. Herein, this review discusses the effects of HT on MetS key components and the molecular mechanisms exerting its health protective effects.

2. Mediterranean Diet and Olive Oil as Primary and Secondary Preventive Nutritional Strategies

The Mediterranean diet pattern is characterized by a high consumptions of fruits, vegetables, beans, nuts, unrefined grains, and fish; a lower intake of meats and full-fat dairy products; and a daily consumption of olive oil as the mostly used fat in culinary practices. Fatty acid consumption, characterized by a higher rate of monounsaturated (MUFAs) and polyunsaturated (PUFAs) fatty acids consumption than saturated fatty acid (SFAs), is central in the consumption of VOO in the Mediterranean population countries. Indeed, Greece, Italy and Spain are characterized by a higher consumption of MUFAs compared to SFAs, whereas, in the US, the ratio MUFA/SFA is ~1 [7,8].

Lifestyle interventions using a Mediterranean-type diet reported inverse associations between a good adherence to this pattern and the risk of CVD [9] or T2DM [10] and showed a reduction in the incidence of key components of MetS including obesity [11–13], hypertension [14–16], glucose tolerance [17], dyslipidemia [18] and insulin resistance [19]. Olive oil, the main MUFAs in the Mediterranean diet, has been widely identified as the initiator of these health benefits with increasing consumption of virgin olive oil (VOO) enhancing lipid profile, reducing blood pressure and endothelial dysfunction, improving inflammatory and prothrombotic environment through reduced Low Density Lipoprotein (LDL) oxidizability [20]. Recently, the Prevencion con Dieta mediterránea study (PREDIMED) [21] showed that patients with a Mediterranean diet supplemented with extra-virgin olive oil (EVOO) or nuts had a lower incidence of T2DM and a reduced associated-mortality. EVOO provided in the Mediterranean diet was beneficial for blood pressure, glycemia, dyslipidemia, oxidative stress and inflammation [22,23]. Interestingly, the EUROLIVE (Effect of Olive Oils on Oxidative Damage in European Populations) study highlighted inverse relationships between the total cholesterol/High Density Lipoprotein (HDL)-cholesterol ratio or oxidative stress markers and the phenolic content of the olive oil [24]. The cardio-protective actions of olive oil components have been reported [25–27] and the non-saponifiable minor bioactive compounds [28–30] such as phenolic compounds including HT and its precursor OLE, rather than oleic acid, were reported responsible for the protective properties [31].

3. Olive Oil Composition and Polyphenolic Fraction

The olive oil composition can be divided into two fractions, saponifiable and unsaponifiable fractions. The saponifiable fraction of olive oil corresponds to the total amount of SFAs, MUFAs and PUFAs. Olive oil is characterized by a high content of MUFAs, whereas the concentrations of SFAs and PUFAs range from 8% to 26% and from 3% to 22%, respectively. Oleic acid is present up to 83% in virgin olive oil [32].

The unsaponifiable fraction contains more than 200 compounds; among them, phenolic compounds account for 3% of the total oil composition [33]. This fraction contributes to the specific characteristics of olive oil, such as aroma, taste, color and oxidative stability [34]. The most abundant fraction of the unsaponifiable fraction is hydrocarbons (squalene, β-carotene and lutein). Other compounds are phytosterols, triterpenic compounds in the form of dialcohols or acids and fat-soluble phenols including tocopherol and tocotrienols. The most polar fraction consists in phenolic compounds, which can be classified into several groups: phenolic acids (caffeic, ferulic, gallic, gentisic, *o*-coumaric, *p*-coumaric, *p*-hydroxybenzoic and protocatehuic acids), phenolic alcohols 3,4-dihydroxyphenylethanol named HT and tyrosol (Tyr), phenolic secoiridoids, hydroxyl-isocromans (formed by the reaction between HT and benzaldehyde or vanillin), flavonoids and lignans [35]. In olive fruit, phenolic compounds are present as glycosylated forms. Oleuropein aglycone is a phenolic secoiridoid liberated from the glucoside form, OLE, upon the action of a β-glucosidase during olive ripening. In olive oil, oleuropein aglycone is degraded into elenolic acid, the secoiridoid moiety, and HT, the phenolic moiety.

4. Virgin Olive Oil Phenols Concentration

Not less than 30 polyphenols have been identified in olive oil and considerable variations have been noted in the concentrations of these phenolic compounds. Phenolic concentration in EVOO ranges from 50 to 800 mg/kg [36] with a mean of 230 mg/kg, whereas in refined olive oil it is much lower [37].

HT and their corresponding secoiridoid derivatives constitute around 90% of the total phenolic content of VOO [38]. Olive oil phenol concentration depends of olive variety [39], agricultural environment and practices [39], the maturity stages of the fruit [39], storage conditions and processing [40,41].

5. Bioavailability of Hydroxytyrosol and Metabolism

A consensus indicated that HT does not exert any cytotoxic effect on cells [42], or animals [43,44]. In 2000, Visioli et al. [45] showed that olive oil phenols, especially HT and Tyr, are dose-dependently absorbed in humans after ingestion and excreted in urine. However, the levels of free HT and Tyr in urine were lower compared with their glucuronide metabolites. In addition to glucuronides, other metabolites of HT were found in plasma and urine such as the methylated or sulfated forms [46]. It has been reported that there is a significant absorption (40%–95%) of HT [45–48] indicating that human intestine absorbs a major part of ingested VOO phenolic compounds. Moreover, HT is more assimilated when given as an olive oil compared to an aqueous solution [49], and its absorption was greater when ingested in its natural form present in extra-virgin olive oil rather than added in refined olive oil or incorporated into a yoghurt, as shown by its urinary recoveries being 44%, 23% and 5.8%, respectively [50]. Such results suggested that the olive oil matrix could act as a protective factor preventing the degradation of phenolic compounds in the gastrointestinal tract. The range levels of circulating metabolites of OLE was 10–60 μg post-ingestion of a 50 mL high-phenol-containing VOO [51,52].

Consumption of VOO in the Mediterranean countries is expected to be around 30–50 g/day [53] leading to an intake of 200 μg of phenolic compounds. Taking into account that the absorption rate of phenols is in the range of 40%–95%, it results an amount of 4–9 mg/day of olive oil phenols. Note that, in the gastrointestinal tract, HT and Tyr result from the degradation of aglycones of OLE and its monophenolic form ligstrosides. Its degradation is incomplete and OLE can be readily absorbed across the intestine [54] by possible implication of glucose transporter [55]. Besides, glucuronidation of HT was previously reported in intestinal Caco-2 and in HepG2 cells [56–58].

Note that D'Angelo et al. [43] have found that intravenous administration of HT led to a fast and extensive uptake of this molecule within 5 min after injection in several tissues such as skeletal muscle, heart, liver, lungs and kidney.

6. Hydroxytyrosol, Body Weight and Development of Adipose Tissue

Body weight is the main outcome to define obesity and body mass index increase is positively correlated with MetS. Only one clinical study assessed the effect of HT supplementation on body weight showing that 12-week supplementation of HT (9.67 mg/day) associated with OLE (51.1 mg/day) did not exert any effect on body weight in overweight men [59]. The absence of effect was confirmed in numerous rodent experiments [60–64], except for one study that showed a beneficial effect of HT (50 mg/kg/day × 17 weeks) supplementation against diet-induced obesity [65].

Whereas no in vivo studies experienced the impact of VOO phenolic compounds on adipose tissue development, in vitro, VOO phenolic compounds have been shown to influence adipocyte hyperplasia and hypertrophy through the expression of genes related to obesity. It was reported that HT (25 and 150 μM) reduced hyperplasia and hypertrophy by reducing triglycerides content by downregulating adipogenesis-related genes, peroxisome proliferator-activated receptors α and γ, peroxisome proliferator-activated receptor γ coactivator 1-α (PGC-1α), lipoprotein lipase, hormone sensitive lipase, acetyl CoA carboxylase-1, carnitine palmitoyltransferase-1, CCAAT/enhancer binding protein α, and sterol regulatory element-binding transcription factor-1 transcription factors and downstream genes (glucose transporter-4, CD36 and fatty acid synthase) [66,67]. Taken together, these data suggested that HT might reduce the size of adipocytes and be beneficial for reducing the risk of obesity.

The processes of adipose hypertrophy and hyperplasia are associated with mitochondrial stress and dysfunction observed by a reduction of adenosine triphosphate (ATP) formation and a reduction of mitochondrial complex expression subunits. In a murine model of high fat diet (HFD)-induced obesity, it has been shown that HT (50 mg/kg/day × 17 weeks) could normalize mitochondrial complex subunit expression and mitochondrial fission marker dynamin-related protein-1 [65]. The high amount of subunit expression could be attributed to an enhancement of mitochondria quantity. Indeed, Hao et al. [68] have found that HT allows to enhance Mitochondrial transcription factor A (1 μM), Nuclear respiratory factors 1 and 2 (Nrf1 and Nrf2) (1 μM) mRNA, key activators of mitochondrial transcription and genome replication, thus increasing protein levels of complexes 1, 2, and 3 in adipocytes (0.1, 1 and 10 μM). The authors also found an increase of peroxisome proliferator-activated receptors α and γ (1 and 10 μM) and carnitine palmitoyltransferase I (1 and 10 μM) expressions, which are implicated in mitochondria biogenesis, suggesting a possible better oxidative status in adipocytes.

Furthermore, it seems that HT (1 μM) acts as a starving agent, since an increase in adenosine monophosphate kinase (AMPK), acetyl CoA carboxylase, hormone-sensitive lipase and lipase phosphorylation were reported in adipocytes [68].

7. Hydroxytyrosol and Lipid Metabolism

The prospective EUROLIVE study demonstrated that olive oils with different levels of polyphenols led to a reduction in LDL-c and TG [24] in a dose-dependent manner. The absence of body weight gain suggested that HT could possess a lipolytic function, especially in adipose tissue. Whereas clinical trials were not undertaken, some experimental studies, performed in rodent and murine models (0.03% × 8 weeks and 50 mg/kg/day × 17 weeks) [63,65] or adipocytes (150 μM and 1 μM) [66,68] reported that HT attenuates TGs accumulation in adipocytes, blood, liver and skeletal muscles (50 mg/kg/day × 17 weeks and 25 μM) [65,69]; glycerol release (75 μM) [69]; and lowers serum cholesterol in HFD-rats (10 mg/kg/day × 5 weeks) [70], and LDL and HDL-c levels (50 mg/kg/day × 17 weeks) [65] and plasma cholesterol in control rats (0.03% × 8 weeks) [63]. Moreover, HT treatment inhibited epididymal and perirenal fat formation and limited liver weight gain (50 mg/kg/day × 17 weeks) [65]. On the other hand, it has been demonstrated in a *db/db* model of mice, that HT (10 mg/kg/day × 8 weeks) increased the activity of mitochondrial complex, and lipolysis fatty acid oxidation-related genes [65]. In contrast, Acin et al. [71] reported that HT (10 mg/kg/day × 10 weeks) had deleterious effects with increasing plasma cholesterol, very low density lipoprotein-cholesterol, and LDL-c and reducing ApoA-1 resulting in an increased atheroma plaque formation.

In vitro, HT was reported to increase oxygen consumption, suggesting a higher oxidative rate to produce ATP [65], proteins implicated in mitochondria biogenesis, mitochondria mass and size [68]. AMPK was decreased during chronic stress situation, thus reducing glycolysis and fatty acid oxidation. Moreover, Cao et al. [65] have reported, in obese mice, that HT supplementation (50 mg/kg/day × 17 weeks) leads to a reduction in SREBP-1c level, a well-known regulator of fatty acid and cholesterol synthesis in liver.

8. Hydroxytyrosol, Glucose Homeostasis and Insulin-Resistance

The strength of olive oil to reduce the incidence of all the glucose-associated disorders is no longer to be demonstrated. Moreover, the enhancement of glucose tolerance was shown to be dependent of the concentration of polyphenols and olive oil [72]. Clinical trials regarding the impact of HT on carbohydrate metabolism are still lacking but experiments in rodent models of MetS are available and suggested that HT is able to reduce plasmatic glucose concentration (50 mg/kg/day × 17 weeks, 20 mg/kg × 2 months and 0.04% × 8 weeks) [65,73,74] and insulin secretion (50 μg/mL) [73] leading to a decrease of insulin-resistance [65,74]. Moreover, Pirozzi et al. [70] found that HT (10 mg/kg/ day × 5 weeks) enhances glucose tolerance and increases insulin sensitivity leading to a decrease of homeostatic model assessment-insulin resistance. Interestingly, in a *db/db* model of mice, Cao et al. [65] have reported that HT given at 10 mg/kg/day for 8 weeks decreases fasting glucose level.

9. Hydroxytyrosol and Hypertension

Clinical trials have demonstrated that olive oil is more efficient than any other oil at reducing blood pressure [75–78]. It has been hypothesized that the effect of olive oil on blood pressure was not only mediated through its MUFAs content but also through its polyphenol content. Indeed, some studies mentioned that the polyphenols of olive oil were responsible of the anti-hypertensive effect of olive oils, as demonstrated in hypercholesterolemic [79] or pre-hypertensive subjects [80] after consuming polyphenols enriched olive oil. Ruiz-Gutierrez et al. [81] reported a reduction of both systolic (SBP) and diastolic (DBP) blood pressures after an olive oil-rich diet but not after a high-oleic-acid sunflower diet. In this sense, clinical trials proved that consumption of OLE was able to reduce SBP and DBP after consumption of OLE in both pre-hypertensive subjects (136 mg/day + 6 mg/day HT × 6 weeks) [82] and hypertensive rats (30 mg/day × 5 weeks) [83]. Given the fact that OLE is degraded into HT, the question arose if the blood pressure lowering effect was due to OLE or HT. Lopez-Villodres et al. [84] found that HT supplementation (10 mg/kg/day × 2 months) increased in diabetic rats the levels of nitrites and nitrates, potent donors of NO acting as vasorelaxing agent. In addition, Storniolo et al. [85] demonstrated that HT (10 μM) counteracted hyperglycemia-induced endothelin-1 expression, a well-known hypertensive agent, in a more extend than oleic acid.

10. Associated Complications: Oxidative Stress, Inflammation and Cardiovascular Dysfunction

10.1. Antioxidative Properties

Oxidative stress is a central physiologic process playing an important role in the maintenance of intracellular homeostasis. However, despite intracellular protective mechanisms, including superoxide dismustase (SOD), Catalase (Cat) and reduced glutathione, excess reactive oxygen species (ROS) is detrimental to cellular physiology. Obesity and T2DM are characterized by an excessive amount of ROS overwhelming intracellular defenses and leading to reinforce MetS associated complications. Polyphenols have been used as nutraceutical antioxidant for several years since an increased amount of fruits and vegetables were linked to the reduction of oxidative pathologies.

10.1.1. Hydroxytyrosol and LDL Oxidizability

Oxidation of the lipid part of LDL leads to a change in the lipoprotein conformation by which LDL is better able to enter into monocytes/macrophage of the arterial wall and develop the atherosclerotic process. Human studies suggested that olive oil protects LDL against oxidation as indicated by decreased LDL oxidizability [86,87] and this strong effect prevails on linoleate-rich particles [88]. It has been well demonstrated that phenolic compounds, especially HT, are protective against LDL oxidation. Based on this protective effect, the European Food Safety Authority claimed that 5 mg of HT (as free and derived forms) should be consumed daily. To prove that HT is efficient, its supplementation (45–50 mg/day × 3 weeks) in sunflower oil was shown to reduce oxLDL [89], suggesting that HT could prevent CVD. These results in clinical trials were corroborated by animal experiments [74,90].

Increase of lag-time [91,92] is the main outcome of reduction in LDL oxidizability and this change could be attributed to an increase in oleic acid [88] or HT [38,60,93] rate in LDL. Such mechanism occurs rapidly and increases with phenolic compounds in olive oil [94].

Mateos et al. [95] reported that consumption of polyphenol-rich VOO leads to a reduction of the expression of pro-atherogenic genes such as CD40 antigen ligand and oxLDL receptor-1 when compared with the refined olive oil, which was depleted in polyphenols [87]. Another mechanism that can be implicated in the protection of LDL by olive oil could be the enhancement of arylesterase plasma activity, an enzyme presents on HDL surface, suggested to contribute to the antioxidant protection conferred by HDL on LDL oxidation [96,97]. However, the scavenging properties of HT cannot be excluded in the protection of LDL oxidizability (10 μM) [98,99]. In fact, Briante et al. [100] reported that HT protects, in vitro, LDL from oxidation at a concentration >18 μg/mg of LDL.

10.1.2. Hydroxytyrosol and Mitochondria

There is evidence that mitochondrial dysfunction in MetS is associated with T2DM [101,102]. Genetic factors, oxidative stress, mitochondrial biogenesis and aging may affect mitochondrial function, leading to insulin resistance. Fewer and smaller-sized mitochondria have been found in skeletal muscles of insulin-resistance, obese, or T2DM subjects and are linked with a lower mitochondrial oxidative capacity [103]. The decreased mitochondrial oxidative capacity is associated with the reduction in expression of mitochondrial genome [104]. To counteract such effect and enhance oxidative metabolism, HT was supposed to be a good candidate. Although no clinical trial investigated the effect of HT supplementation, studies in obese- and diabetic-rendered rats and in doxorubicin-induced cardiotoxicity rats revealed that HT (0.5, 10 and 50 mg/kg/day) is able to increase mitochondrial function through an enhancement of mitochondrial complex subunit expression [65,105] and activity [105,106]. Enhanced mitochondrial activity was associated with an increase of uncoupling protein-2 protein expression (100 μM) [107]. All the animal experiments supported the impact of HT in the protection of mitochondria from oxidative damages, which operates a shift towards a more efficient oxidative metabolism. Furthermore, it has been demonstrated that HT increases the mitochondrial deoxyribonucleic acid content (1 μM and 10 and 50 mg/kg/day) [68,108], the mitochondria function and membrane potential (0.1 and 10 μg/mL) [109] and density (1 μM) [68]. Mitochondrial biogenesis and respiration were stimulated by PGC-1α by strongly inducing its gene expression. Rodent and culture cell experiments reported also that HT was able to increase PGC-1α and Nrf2 expression (0.1, 1 and 10 μM and 100 μM) [68,107] and AMPK, an upstream regulator of PGC-1α [68,107]. Note that an increase in maximal oxygen consumption was found (1 and 10 μM) [68].

10.1.3. Hydroxytyrosol and Antioxidant Protein Expression

There is a recognized link between oxidative stress and key components of MetS. Besides LDL oxidation, other oxidative markers also showed improvements. HT was reported to prevent the increase of protein carbonyl levels and lipid peroxidation markers, and to normalize liver glutathione level, liver glutathione *S*-transferase, and total SOD activity in obese mice (10 and 50 mg/kg/day) [65]. In cell culture, it was also demonstrated that HT increases Cu/SOD expression (100 μM) [107]; normalizes glutathione concentrations; increases glutathione peroxidase, glutathione reductase and glutathione-*S*-transferase protein expression (0.5 to 10 μM) [110]; increases CAT activity (50 μM) [111]; and reduces the reduced glutathione/oxidized glutathione (known as GSH:GSSG ratio) (1 and 5 μM) in presence of hydrogen peroxide, suggesting a reduction in the oxidative status [63]. The antioxidative capacities are not limited to the expression of type 2 detoxifying proteins as SOD, Cat, and glutathione peroxidase. Indeed, it exists adaptive systems as those implying heme oxygenase-1, the expression of which is regulated by Nrf2. The positive impact of HT on Nrf2 nuclear translocation was shown and associated to phosphoinositide/protein kinase B and extracellular signal-regulated kinase pathway (0.5 to 10 μM) [110] and also AMPK/forkhead box 3a (50 μM) [111].

Moreover, it has been found that HT (20 µg/day) for four weeks was able to reduce plasma hydroperoxide concentrations, normalize plasma malondialdehyde and conjugated dienes, and increase plasma antioxidant capacity in a rat model of HFD-induced obesity [64].

10.1.4. Hydroxytyrosol and Superoxide ($O_2^{\bullet-}$) Scavenging Properties

In an acute model of oxidative stress driven in rat aortas, Rietjens et al. [98] showed that HT acts as a scavenging agent. Since, numerous studies were published and confirmed that HT protect against ROS production in human vascular endothelial cells, erythrocytes and renal epithelial tubular cells (5 to 80 µM) [111–113], displays scavenger activity for peroxynitrous acid (5 µM to 1 mM) [114,115] and has a protective role on deoxyribonucleic acid damages associated to peroxinitrous acid (0.05 to 1 mM) [114]. Moreover, it can inhibit superoxide anion burst from macrophages but not from neutrophils where it can only scavenge hydrogen peroxide (1 to 50 µM) [116]. It also protects erythrocytes from hemolysis (50 to 200 µM) [117], endothelial cells from monocytes adhesion (0.5 to 2.5 µM) [118] and hepatocytes (10 to 40 µM) [119], and protects from lipid peroxidation in rat livers (5 to 60 µM) [120] as well as from lipid oxidation (10 µM) [91].

10.2. Hydroxytyrosol and Inflammation

It is well known that the pathophysiology of MetS causes chronic inflammation. HT has been reported to possess significant anti-inflammatory capacity. In fact, in clinical trial, HT (25 mg/day × one week) led to a reduction of plasma CRP and isoprostane levels, but did not exert any effect on other inflammatory markers as interleukin-6, monocytes chemoattractant protein-1 and tumor necrosis factor-α (TNF-α) [121]. In rodent experiments, it was demonstrated that HT reduces TNF-α, IL-6 and cyclooxygenase-2 expression in liver (50 mg/kg/day × 17 weeks) [65], increases the anti-inflammatory IL-10 expression (12.5 µg/mL and 10 mg/kg/day × 10 days) [122,123], reduces inducible nitric oxide synthase (iNOS) expression (12.5 µg/mL and 5 mg/kg/day × 30 days) [122,124,125] and cyclooxygenase-2 expression [125]. Considering that leptin, a well-known protein acting on satiety and having inflammatory property, HT was shown to lower leptin level in mice thus suggesting that could act as a starving and anti-inflammatory agent (0.03% × 8 weeks and 50 mg/kg/day × 17 weeks) [63,65] and attenuate TNF-α and IL-1β expression in animal model [125,126]. In vitro, HT has been reported to increase adiponectin expression and secretion in the presence of TNF-α (1 to 20 µM) [127], reduce iNOS, cyclooxygenase-2 and TNF-α expressions (25 to 100 µM) [128], reduce nuclear factor-κB (NF-κB) binding activity (50 and 100 µM) [129] and, interestingly, increase iκBα expression, an inhibitor of NF-κB binding activity [129]. Moreover, a reduction of metalloproteinase-9 activity and secretion (1 and 10 µM) [130] and a reduction of prostaglandin E_2 secretion and expression were found (1 and 10 µM) [130].

10.3. Hydroxytyrosol and Atherosclerosis

Phenolic compounds in VOO were shown to improve endothelial dysfunction and reduce oxidative stress plasma parameters, both playing a key role in the development of atherosclerosis [131,132]. Moreover, VOO phenolic compounds could counteract inflammation, which is an important trigger in the development of atherosclerosis though the expression of adhesion molecules. In a clinical trial enrolling healthy volunteers, it has been demonstrated that sunflower oil supplemented with HT decreased vascular cell adhesion protein (VCAM-1) plasmatic concentration (45–50 mg/kg/ day × 3 weeks) [89] and monocyte chemoattractant protein-1 and interleukin-8 receptor expression (366 mg/kg/day × 3 weeks) [87]. Such results were confirmed in rodent models, where HT reduced platelet aggregation, VCAM-1 and IL-1β expressions (0.5 to 10 mg/kg/day × 2 months) [84] and TNF-α expression (0.04%) [74]. Interestingly, Gonzalez et al. [60] reported that HT (4 mg/kg/ day × 2 months) reduced the size of atherosclerotic lesions in rabbits fed with a high fat and high cholesterol diet.

Several in vitro studies confirmed the anti-inflammatory capacity of HT by reducing VCAM-1, intercellular adhesion protein expressions (0.5 to 75 µM) [22,118,133]. Molecular mechanisms leading to this reduction probably involved the reduction of NF-κB activation (0.5 to 75 µM) [22,23]. Despite the great interest surrounding HT as a nutraceutical, Acin et al. [71] reported that HT supplementation (10 mg/kg/day) for 10 weeks led to an increase in atherosclerotic plaque, in monocyte activation and a reduction in ApoA-I from HDL in ApoE-deficient mice. However, these mice did not develop obesity, low-grade inflammation and oxidative stress, thus explaining this deleterious effect because HT could act as an oxidant.

10.4. Hydroxytyrosol and Vascular Dysfunction

Nitric oxide (NO•) plays a pivotal role in endothelial function and its decreased bioavailability is correlated with altered vascular tone. Lopez-Villodres et al. [84] found that in streptozotocin-induced model of diabetes, HT supplementation (10 mg/kg/day × 2 months) increased the level of nitrates and nitrites. HT was reported to be ineffective on eNOS expression and activity (i.e., phosphorylation on its Ser1177) in absence of oxidative stress in HUVECs (0.1 to 100 µM) [134]. In an endothelial cell culture model of hyperglycemia, Storniolo et al. [85] showed that HT (10 µM) increases NO• production, which is correlated to an increase of endothelial nitric oxide synthase phosphorylation (P-eNOS)/endothelial nitric oxide synthase (eNOS) ratio. When stimulated by acetylcholine, an activator of eNOS/NO• signaling pathway, HT increased NO• production, more than oleic acid; this increase was linked to higher intracellular calcium concentration. Rietjens et al. [98] evidenced that HT (10 µM) enhances endothelium-dependent relaxation in addition to increase P-eNOS/eNOS ratio. This enhancement was associated with a cGMP increase, a downstream molecule of eNOS acting on smooth muscle cells relaxation. In a vascular endothelial cell culture model, Zrelli et al. [135] found that HT (50 µM) increases P-eNOS resulting in increasing NO• production, associated to the decreased of NF-κB and iκBα phosphorylation in the presence of TNF-α. These results suggest that eNOS could decrease inflammatory response, and thereafter, decrease thrombus formation. Furthermore, it was demonstrated that HT reduced iNOS expression (25 to 100 µM) [128], known for its inflammatory, and oxidative properties in monocytes.

10.5. Hydroxytyrosol and Cardiac Dysfunction

All of the cardiovascular risk factors of MetS are associated with increased risk of heart failure. HT was revealed as cardiac protective after olive oil consumption. Bayram et al. [136] have found that female SAMP8 mice fed with a Western diet enriched with a high-polyphenol content (mainly tyrosol (20.8 mg/kg oil) and hydroxytyrosol (18.9 mg/kg oil)) had lower TBARS levels in cardiac muscle. Alterations of cardiac function were correlated with cardiac remodeling leading to blood pressure increase thus raising CVD. Mnafgui et al. [137] showed that a HT supplementation (2 and 5 mg/kg/day × 1 week) in a rodent CVD model leads to a reduction of heart weight and heart weight/body weight ratio. These morphological changes were followed by the reductions of SBP, DBP and mean arterial blood pressure, heart rate and ST segment elevation. Moreover, these authors [137] found an increase of lactate dehydrogenase and creatine kinase protein expressions showing an enhancement of glucose consumption, probably producing higher ATP. Granados-Principal et al. [106] found in cardiac tissue that HT (0.5 mg/kg, 5 days/week × 6 weeks) increases expression of mitochondria complexes 1, 2 and 3 and reduces specific markers of oxidative damages to proteins. These HT beneficial effects on cardiac function are probably due to its antioxidative properties (0.1 and 10 µg/mL) [109], since HT was not found in rat heart (1, 10 and 100 mg/kg) [138].

11. Functional Applications in Food Processing

Nowadays, several antioxidants are used to reduce food oxidation and thus extend shelf life. Adding 100 mg/kg HT in frankfurters was effective against lipid oxidation during storage, to a greater extent than a mix of butylated hydroxyanisole/butylated hydroxytoluene [139]. Nieto et al. [140] also showed a reduced lipid oxidation in sausages with HT (50 ppm). Thus HT added in fat used could help to maintain the nutritional and sensorial qualities of processed food products.

12. Limitations of Experimental Studies

Ex vivo and in vitro studies with HT are well documented, but question the extrapolation to human relevancy. In fact, high concentrations were usually used in cell models [22,111,135], certainly due to the oxidation of HT [141]. HT has been tested as a sole molecule, and not with other antioxidant compounds (phenolic compounds, tocopherols, carotenoids and vitamin C) that occur in human context. Moreover, the influence of food matrix on the bioactivity of HT is avoided in most of experimental studies.

13. Conclusions

To conclude, the beneficial effects of HT were extensively studied in rodent experiments and clinical trials evidencing the role of HT in the reduction of MetS and its associated complications, which are briefly presented in Figure 1. Both experimental and clinical studies demonstrated that HT reduced oxidative stress and inflammation, thus altering positively MetS key components. However, contradictory results for obesity were reported, probably resulting from differences in the study design, administered doses and type of animals. Moreover, actually, no experiment assesses the impact of pure HT on blood pressure in normotensive or hypertensive subjects. In this sense, larger and more experimental studies and clinical trials are needed.

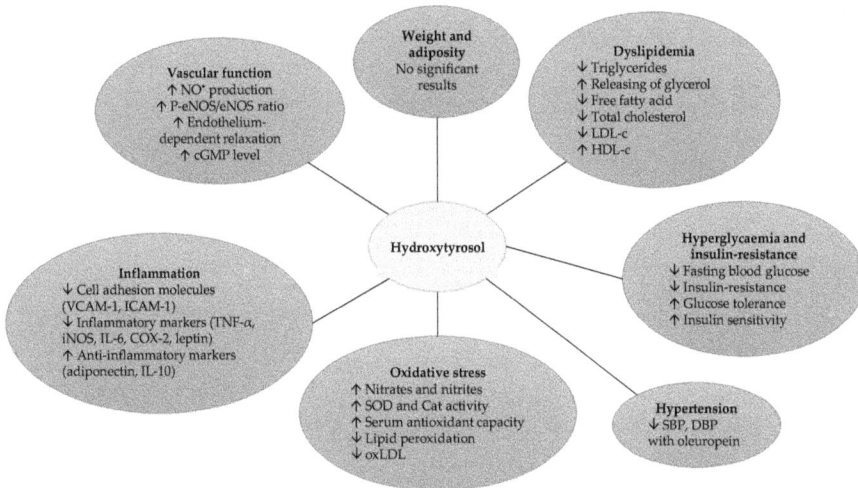

Figure 1. Effect of hydroxytyrosol on metabolic syndrome-associated complications and metabolic syndrome. ↑: Increase in; ↓: Decrease in. LDL-c: Low-Density Lipoprotein-cholesterol; HDL-c: High Density Lipoprotein-cholesterol; SBP: Systolic Blood Pressure; DBP: Diastolic Blood Pressure; SOD: Super Oxide Dismutase; Cat: Catalase; oxLDL: oxidized Low-Density Lipoprotein; VCAM-1: Vascular Cell Adhesion Molecule-1; ICAM-1: Intercellular Adhesion Molecule-1; TNF-α: Tumor Necrosis Factor alpha; iNOS: inducible Nitric Oxide Synthase; IL-6: Interleukin-6; COX-2: Cyclooxygenase-2; IL-10: Interleukin-10; NO•: Nitric Oxide; P-eNOS/eNOS: Phosphorylated Endothelial Nitric Oxide Synthase/endothelial Nitric Oxide Synthase ratio; cGMP: cyclic Guanosine Monophosphate.

The role of dietary polyphenols in human health depends largely on their bioavailability and, because HT bioavailability is reduced, with systemic concentration ranging in the nanomolar levels, it could be expected that HT exerts its effects directly in the gastrointestinal tract before being absorbed.

Nutrients **2017**, *9*, 306

Indeed, the concentration of phenolic compounds may reach the millimolar range. In this sense, modulation of gut microbiota could be the most remarkable local effect exerted by HT. Recently, another component of the Mediterranean diet, resveratrol, has been shown to modulate positively gut microbiota enhancing glucose tolerance in a mice model of obesity [142] and also through a duodenal Sirt-1 pathway into the hypothalamus [143] enhancing hypothalamic insulin-resistance. Sirt-1 is an energy sensitizer upregulating antioxidative and anti-inflammatory gene expression and improving mitochondrial biogenesis through PGC-1α. Direct effects of HT on duodenal Sirt-1 pathway cannot be excluded.

Acknowledgments: The authors declare that they have received no grants in support of their research work and no funds for covering the costs to publish in open access.

Author Contributions: All authors analyzed the data and wrote the paper.

Conflicts of Interest: The authors declare no conflict of interest.

Abbreviations

The following abbreviations are used in this manuscript:

AMPK	Adenosine monophosphate kinase
ATP	Adenosine triphosphate
Cat	Catalase
CVD	Cardiovascular diseases
eNOS	Endothelial nitric oxide synthase
EVOO	Extra-virgin olive oil
HDL	High-density lipoprotein
HFD	High Fat Diet
IL	interleukin
iNOS	Inducible nitric oxide synthase
LDL	Low density lipoprotein
MUFA	Monounsaturated fatty acid
NO	Nitric oxide
Nrf2	Nuclear factor 2
OLE	Oleuropein
P-eNOS	Phosphorylated endothelial nitric oxide synthase
PGC1α	Peroxisome proliferator-activated receptor gamma coactivator 1-alpha
PUFA	Polyunsaturated fatty acid
ROS	Reactive oxygen species
SFA	Saturated fatty acid
SOD	Superoxide dismustase
TBARS	Thiobarbituric acid reactive substances
TNF-α	Tumor necrosis factor-alpha
VCAM-1	Vascular adhesion molecule-1
VOO	Virgin olive oil

References

1. Alberti, K.G.M.M.; Eckel, R.H.; Grundy, S.M.; Zimmet, P.Z.; Cleeman, J.I.; Donato, K.A.; Fruchart, J.-C.; James, W.P.T.; Loria, C.M.; Smith, S.C., Jr.; et al. Harmonizing the metabolic syndrome: A joint interim statement of the International Diabetes Federation Task Force on Epidemiology and Prevention; National Heart, Lung, and Blood Institute; American Heart Association; World Heart Federation; International Atherosclerosis Society; and International Association for the Study of Obesity. *Circulation* **2009**, *120*, 1640–1645. [PubMed]
2. Laslett, L.J.; Alagona, P.; Clark, B.A.; Drozda, J.P.; Saldivar, F.; Wilson, S.R.; Poe, C.; Hart, M. The worldwide environment of cardiovascular disease: Prevalence, diagnosis, therapy, and policy issues: A report from the American College of Cardiology. *J. Am. Coll. Cardiol.* **2012**, *60*, S1–S49. [CrossRef] [PubMed]

Nutrients **2017**, *9*, 306

3. Estruch, R.; Ros, E.; Salas-Salvadó, J.; Covas, M.-I.; Corella, D.; Arós, F.; Gómez-Gracia, E.; Ruiz-Gutiérrez, V.; Fiol, M.; Lapetra, J.; et al. Study Investigators Primary prevention of cardiovascular disease with a Mediterranean diet. *N. Engl. J. Med.* **2013**, *368*, 1279–1290. [CrossRef] [PubMed]
4. Covas, M.-I.; Ruiz-Gutiérrez, V.; de la Torre, R.; Kafatos, A.; Lamuela-Raventós, R.M.; Osada, J.; Owen, R.W.; Visioli, F. Minor Components of Olive Oil: Evidence to Date of Health Benefits in Humans. *Nutr. Rev.* **2006**, *64*, S20–S30. [CrossRef]
5. Miro-Casas, E.; Covas, M.-I.; Farre, M.; Fito, M.; Ortuño, J.; Weinbrenner, T.; Roset, P.; de la Torre, R. Hydroxytyrosol disposition in humans. *Clin. Chem.* **2003**, *49*, 945–952. [CrossRef] [PubMed]
6. Weinbrenner, T.; Fitó, M.; de la Torre, R.; Saez, G.T.; Rijken, P.; Tormos, C.; Coolen, S.; Albaladejo, M.F.; Abanades, S.; Schroder, H.; et al. Olive oils high in phenolic compounds modulate oxidative/antioxidative status in men. *J. Nutr.* **2004**, *134*, 2314–2321. [PubMed]
7. Freisling, H.; Fahey, M.T.; Moskal, A.; Ocké, M.C.; Ferrari, P.; Jenab, M.; Norat, T.; Naska, A.; Welch, A.A.; Navarro, C.; et al. Region-specific nutrient intake patterns exhibit a geographical gradient within and between European countries. *J. Nutr.* **2010**, *140*, 1280–1286. [CrossRef] [PubMed]
8. Harika, R.K.; Eilander, A.; Alssema, M.; Osendarp, S.J.M.; Zock, P.L. Intake of fatty acids in general populations worldwide does not meet dietary recommendations to prevent coronary heart disease: A systematic review of data from 40 countries. *Ann. Nutr. Metab.* **2013**, *63*, 229–238. [CrossRef] [PubMed]
9. Sofi, F.; Macchi, C.; Abbate, R.; Gensini, G.F.; Casini, A. Mediterranean diet and health status: An updated meta-analysis and a proposal for a literature-based adherence score. *Public Health Nutr.* **2014**, *17*, 2769–2782. [CrossRef] [PubMed]
10. Panagiotakos, D.B.; Pitsavos, C.H.; Chrysohoou, C.; Skoumas, J.; Papadimitriou, L.; Stefanadis, C.; Toutouzas, P.K. Status and management of hypertension in Greece: Role of the adoption of a Mediterranean diet: The Attica study. *J. Hypertens.* **2003**, *21*, 1483–1489. [CrossRef] [PubMed]
11. Barbaro, B.; Toietta, G.; Maggio, R.; Arciello, M.; Tarocchi, M.; Galli, A.; Balsano, C. Effects of the olive-derived polyphenol oleuropein on human health. *Int. J. Mol. Sci.* **2014**, *15*, 18508–18524. [CrossRef] [PubMed]
12. Brown, L.; Poudyal, H.; Panchal, S.K. Functional foods as potential therapeutic options for metabolic syndrome. *Obes. Rev.* **2015**, *16*, 914–941. [CrossRef] [PubMed]
13. Covas, M.-I.; de la Torre, R.; Fitó, M. Virgin olive oil: A key food for cardiovascular risk protection. *Br. J. Nutr.* **2015**, *113* (Suppl. S2), S19–S28. [CrossRef] [PubMed]
14. Buckland, G.; Bach, A.; Serra-Majem, L. Obesity and the Mediterranean diet: A systematic review of observational and intervention studies. *Obes. Rev.* **2008**, *9*, 582–593. [CrossRef] [PubMed]
15. Núñez-Córdoba, J.M.; Valencia-Serrano, F.; Toledo, E.; Alonso, A.; Martínez-González, M.A. The Mediterranean diet and incidence of hypertension: The Seguimiento Universidad de Navarra (SUN) Study. *Am. J. Epidemiol.* **2009**, *169*, 339–346. [CrossRef] [PubMed]
16. Toledo, E.; Hu, F.B.; Estruch, R.; Buil-Cosiales, P.; Corella, D.; Salas-Salvadó, J.; Covas, M.I.; Arós, F.; Gómez-Gracia, E.; Fiol, M.; et al. Effect of the Mediterranean diet on blood pressure in the PREDIMED trial: Results from a randomized controlled trial. *BMC Med.* **2013**, *11*, 207. [CrossRef] [PubMed]
17. Esposito, K.; Marfella, R.; Ciotola, M.; Di Palo, C.; Giugliano, F.; Giugliano, G.; D'Armiento, M.; D'Andrea, F.; Giugliano, D. Effect of a mediterranean-style diet on endothelial dysfunction and markers of vascular inflammation in the metabolic syndrome: A randomized trial. *JAMA* **2004**, *292*, 1440–1446. [CrossRef] [PubMed]
18. Mekki, K.; Bouzidi-bekada, N.; Kaddous, A.; Bouchenak, M. Mediterranean diet improves dyslipidemia and biomarkers in chronic renal failure patients. *Food Funct.* **2010**, *1*, 110–115. [CrossRef] [PubMed]
19. Georgoulis, M.; Kontogianni, M.D.; Yiannakouris, N. Mediterranean diet and diabetes: Prevention and treatment. *Nutrients* **2014**, *6*, 1406–1423. [CrossRef] [PubMed]
20. López-Miranda, J.; Pérez-Jiménez, F.; Ros, E.; De Caterina, R.; Badimón, L.; Covas, M.I.; Escrich, E.; Ordovás, J.M.; Soriguer, F.; Abiá, R.; et al. Olive oil and health: Summary of the II international conference on olive oil and health consensus report, Jaén and Córdoba (Spain) 2008. *Nutr. Metab. Cardiovasc. Dis.* **2010**, *20*, 284–294. [CrossRef] [PubMed]
21. Salas-Salvadó, J.; Martinez-González, M.Á.; Bulló, M.; Ros, E. The role of diet in the prevention of type 2 diabetes. *Nutr. Metab. Cardiovasc. Dis.* **2011**, *21* (Suppl. S2), B32–B48. [CrossRef] [PubMed]

22. Carluccio, M.A.; Siculella, L.; Ancora, M.A.; Massaro, M.; Scoditti, E.; Storelli, C.; Visioli, F.; Distante, A.; de Caterina, R. Olive oil and red wine antioxidant polyphenols inhibit endothelial activation: Antiatherogenic properties of Mediterranean diet phytochemicals. *Arterioscler. Thromb. Vasc. Biol.* **2003**, *23*, 622–629. [CrossRef] [PubMed]

23. Salas-Salvadó, J.; Garcia-Arellano, A.; Estruch, R.; Marquez-Sandoval, F.; Corella, D.; Fiol, M.; Gómez-Gracia, E.; Viñoles, E.; Arós, F.; Herrera, C.; et al. Investigators Components of the Mediterranean-type food pattern and serum inflammatory markers among patients at high risk for cardiovascular disease. *Eur. J. Clin. Nutr.* **2008**, *62*, 651–659. [CrossRef] [PubMed]

24. Covas, M.-I.; Nyyssönen, K.; Poulsen, H.E.; Kaikkonen, J.; Zunft, H.-J.F.; Kiesewetter, H.; Gaddi, A.; de la Torre, R.; Mursu, J.; Bäumler, H.; et al. The effect of polyphenols in olive oil on heart disease risk factors: A randomized trial. *Ann. Intern. Med.* **2006**, *145*, 333–341. [CrossRef] [PubMed]

25. Panagiotakos, D.B.; Pitsavos, C.; Polychronopoulos, E.; Chrysohoou, C.; Zampelas, A.; Trichopoulou, A. Can a Mediterranean diet moderate the development and clinical progression of coronary heart disease? A systematic review. *Med. Sci. Monit.* **2004**, *10*, RA193–RA198. [PubMed]

26. Poudyal, H.; Campbell, F.; Brown, L. Olive leaf extract attenuates cardiac, hepatic, and metabolic changes in high carbohydrate-, high fat-fed rats. *J. Nutr.* **2010**, *140*, 946–953. [CrossRef] [PubMed]

27. Babio, N.; Toledo, E.; Estruch, R.; Ros, E.; Martínez-González, M.A.; Castañer, O.; Bulló, M.; Corella, D.; Arós, F.; Gómez-Gracia, E.; et al. Mediterranean diets and metabolic syndrome status in the PREDIMED randomized trial. *Can. Med. Assoc. J.* **2014**, *186*, E649–E657. [CrossRef] [PubMed]

28. Pérez-Jiménez, F.; Ruano, J.; Perez-Martinez, P.; Lopez-Segura, F.; Lopez-Miranda, J. The influence of olive oil on human health: Not a question of fat alone. *Mol. Nutr. Food Res.* **2007**, *51*, 1199–1208. [CrossRef] [PubMed]

29. Cicerale, S.; Conlan, X.A.; Sinclair, A.J.; Keast, R.S.J. Chemistry and health of olive oil phenolics. *Crit. Rev. Food Sci. Nutr.* **2009**, *49*, 218–236. [CrossRef] [PubMed]

30. Visioli, F.; Bernardini, E. Extra virgin olive oil's polyphenols: Biological activities. *Curr. Pharm. Des.* **2011**, *17*, 786–804. [CrossRef] [PubMed]

31. Rafehi, H.; Ververis, K.; Karagiannis, T.C. Mechanisms of action of phenolic compounds in olive. *J. Diet. Suppl.* **2012**, *9*, 96–109. [CrossRef] [PubMed]

32. Hodson, L.; Fielding, B.A. Stearoyl-CoA desaturase: Rogue or innocent bystander? *Prog. Lipid Res.* **2013**, *52*, 15–42. [CrossRef] [PubMed]

33. De la Lastra Romero, C.A. An up-date of olive oil and bioactive constituents in health: Molecular mechanisms and clinical implications. *Curr. Pharm. Des.* **2011**, *17*, 752–753. [CrossRef] [PubMed]

34. Frankel, E.; Bakhouche, A.; Lozano-Sánchez, J.; Segura-Carretero, A.; Fernández-Gutiérrez, A. Literature review on production process to obtain extra virgin olive oil enriched in bioactive compounds. Potential use of byproducts as alternative sources of polyphenols. *J. Agric. Food Chem.* **2013**, *61*, 5179–5188. [CrossRef] [PubMed]

35. Montserrat-de la Paz, S.; Bermudez, B.; Cardelo, M.P.; Lopez, S.; Abia, R.; Muriana, F.J.G. Olive oil and postprandial hyperlipidemia: Implications for atherosclerosis and metabolic syndrome. *Food Funct.* **2016**, *7*, 4734–4744. [CrossRef]

36. Vissers, M.N.; Zock, P.L.; Katan, M.B. Bioavailability and antioxidant effects of olive oil phenols in humans: A review. *Eur. J. Clin. Nutr.* **2004**, *58*, 955–965. [CrossRef] [PubMed]

37. Owen, R.W.; Mier, W.; Giacosa, A.; Hull, W.E.; Spiegelhalder, B.; Bartsch, H. Phenolic compounds and squalene in olive oils: The concentration and antioxidant potential of total phenols, simple phenols, secoiridoids, Lignansand squalene. *Food Chem. Toxicol.* **2000**, *38*, 647–659. [CrossRef]

38. De la Torre-Carbot, K.; Chávez-Servín, J.L.; Jaúregui, O.; Castellote, A.I.; Lamuela-Raventós, R.M.; Fitó, M.; Covas, M.-I.; Muñoz-Aguayo, D.; López-Sabater, M.C. Presence of virgin olive oil phenolic metabolites in human low density lipoprotein fraction: Determination by high-performance liquid chromatography-electrospray ionization tandem mass spectrometry. *Anal. Chim. Acta* **2007**, *583*, 402–410. [CrossRef] [PubMed]

39. Esti, M.; Cinquanta, L.; La Notte, E. Phenolic Compounds in Different Olive Varieties. *J. Agric. Food Chem.* **1998**, *46*, 32–35. [CrossRef] [PubMed]

40. Okogeri, O.; Tasioula-Margari, M. Changes occurring in phenolic compounds and alpha-tocopherol of virgin olive oil during storage. *J. Agric. Food Chem.* **2002**, *50*, 1077–1080. [CrossRef] [PubMed]

41. Kalua, C.M.; Bedgood, D.R.; Bishop, A.G.; Prenzler, P.D. Changes in volatile and phenolic compounds with malaxation time and temperature during virgin olive oil production. *J. Agric. Food Chem.* **2006**, *54*, 7641–7651. [CrossRef] [PubMed]

42. Auñon-Calles, D.; Giordano, E.; Bohnenberger, S.; Visioli, F. Hydroxytyrosol is not genotoxic in vitro. *Pharmacol. Res.* **2013**, *74*, 87–93. [CrossRef] [PubMed]

43. D'Angelo, S.; Manna, C.; Migliardi, V.; Mazzoni, O.; Morrica, P.; Capasso, G.; Pontoni, G.; Galletti, P.; Zappia, V. Pharmacokinetics and metabolism of hydroxytyrosol, a natural antioxidant from olive oil. *Drug Metab. Dispos.* **2001**, *29*, 1492–1498. [PubMed]

44. Auñon-Calles, D.; Canut, L.; Visioli, F. Toxicological evaluation of pure hydroxytyrosol. *Food Chem. Toxicol.* **2013**, *55*, 498–504. [CrossRef]

45. Visioli, F.; Galli, C.; Bornet, F.; Mattei, A.; Patelli, R.; Galli, G.; Caruso, D. Olive oil phenolics are dose-dependently absorbed in humans. *FEBS Lett.* **2000**, *468*, 159–160. [CrossRef]

46. Tuck, K.L.; Hayball, P.J. Major phenolic compounds in olive oil: Metabolism and health effects. *J. Nutr. Biochem.* **2002**, *13*, 636–644. [CrossRef]

47. Visioli, F.; Caruso, D.; Plasmati, E.; Patelli, R.; Mulinacci, N.; Romani, A.; Galli, G.; Galli, C. Hydroxytyrosol, as a component of olive mill waste water, is dose dependently absorbed and increases the antioxidant capacity of rat plasma. *Free Radic. Res.* **2001**, *34*, 301–305. [CrossRef] [PubMed]

48. Vissers, M.N.; Zock, P.L.; Roodenburg, A.J.C.; Leenen, R.; Katan, M.B. Olive oil phenols are absorbed in humans. *J. Nutr.* **2002**, *132*, 409–417. [PubMed]

49. Tuck, K.L.; Freeman, M.P.; Hayball, P.J.; Stretch, G.L.; Stupans, I. The in vivo fate of hydroxytyrosol and tyrosol, antioxidant phenolic constituents of olive oil, after intravenous and oral dosing of labeled compounds to rats. *J. Nutr.* **2001**, *131*, 1993–1996. [PubMed]

50. Visioli, F.; Galli, C.; Grande, S.; Colonnelli, K.; Patelli, C.; Galli, G.; Caruso, D. Hydroxytyrosol excretion differs between rats and humans and depends on the vehicle of administration. *J. Nutr.* **2003**, *133*, 2612–2615. [PubMed]

51. García-Villalba, R.; Carrasco-Pancorbo, A.; Nevedomskaya, E.; Mayboroda, O.A.; Deelder, A.M.; Segura-Carretero, A.; Fernández-Gutiérrez, A. Exploratory analysis of human urine by LC-ESI-TOF MS after high intake of olive oil: Understanding the metabolism of polyphenols. *Anal. Bioanal. Chem.* **2010**, *398*, 463–475. [CrossRef] [PubMed]

52. García-Villalba, R.; Larrosa, M.; Possemiers, S.; Tomás-Barberán, F.A.; Espín, J.C. Bioavailability of phenolics from an oleuropein-rich olive (*Olea europaea*) leaf extract and its acute effect on plasma antioxidant status: Comparison between pre- and postmenopausal women. *Eur. J. Nutr.* **2014**, *53*, 1015–1027. [CrossRef] [PubMed]

53. Corona, G.; Spencer, J.P.E.; Dessì, M.A. Extra virgin olive oil phenolics: Absorption, metabolism, and biological activities in the GI tract. *Toxicol. Ind. Health* **2009**, *25*, 285–293. [CrossRef] [PubMed]

54. Edgecombe, S.C.; Stretch, G.L.; Hayball, P.J. Oleuropein, an antioxidant polyphenol from olive oil, is poorly absorbed from isolated perfused rat intestine. *J. Nutr.* **2000**, *130*, 2996–3002. [PubMed]

55. Gee, J.M.; DuPont, M.S.; Rhodes, M.J.; Johnson, I.T. Quercetin glucosides interact with the intestinal glucose transport pathway. *Free Radic. Biol. Med.* **1998**, *25*, 19–25. [CrossRef]

56. Spencer, J.P.; Chowrimootoo, G.; Choudhury, R.; Debnam, E.S.; Srai, S.K.; Rice-Evans, C. The small intestine can both absorb and glucuronidate luminal flavonoids. *FEBS Lett.* **1999**, *458*, 224–230. [CrossRef]

57. Manna, C.; Galletti, P.; Maisto, G.; Cucciolla, V.; D'Angelo, S.; Zappia, V. Transport mechanism and metabolism of olive oil hydroxytyrosol in Caco-2 cells. *FEBS Lett.* **2000**, *470*, 341–344. [CrossRef]

58. Mateos, R.; Goya, L.; Bravo, L. Metabolism of the Olive Oil Phenols Hydroxytyrosol, Tyrosol, and Hydroxytyrosyl Acetate by Human Hepatoma HepG2 Cells. *J. Agric. Food Chem.* **2005**, *53*, 9897–9905. [CrossRef] [PubMed]

59. De Bock, M.; Derraik, J.G.B.; Brennan, C.M.; Biggs, J.B.; Morgan, P.E.; Hodgkinson, S.C.; Hofman, P.L.; Cutfield, W.S. Olive (*Olea europaea* L.) leaf polyphenols improve insulin sensitivity in middle-aged overweight men: A randomized, placebo-controlled, crossover trial. *PLoS ONE* **2013**, *8*, e57622. [CrossRef] [PubMed]

60. González-Santiago, M.; Martín-Bautista, E.; Carrero, J.J.; Fonollá, J.; Baró, L.; Bartolomé, M.V.; Gil-Loyzaga, P.; López-Huertas, E. One-month administration of hydroxytyrosol, a phenolic antioxidant present in olive oil, to hyperlipemic rabbits improves blood lipid profile, antioxidant status and reduces atherosclerosis development. *Atherosclerosis* **2006**, *188*, 35–42. [CrossRef] [PubMed]

61. Jemai, H.; Fki, I.; Bouaziz, M.; Bouallagui, Z.; El Feki, A.; Isoda, H.; Sayadi, S. Lipid-lowering and antioxidant effects of hydroxytyrosol and its triacetylated derivative recovered from olive tree leaves in cholesterol-fed rats. *J. Agric. Food Chem.* **2008**, *56*, 2630–2636. [CrossRef] [PubMed]

62. Jemai, H.; El Feki, A.; Sayadi, S. Antidiabetic and antioxidant effects of hydroxytyrosol and oleuropein from olive leaves in alloxan-diabetic rats. *J. Agric. Food Chem.* **2009**, *57*, 8798–8804. [CrossRef] [PubMed]

63. Giordano, E.; Dávalos, A.; Visioli, F. Chronic hydroxytyrosol feeding modulates glutathione-mediated oxido-reduction pathways in adipose tissue: A nutrigenomic study. *Nutr. Metab. Cardiovasc. Dis.* **2014**, *24*, 1144–1150. [CrossRef] [PubMed]

64. Hmimed, S.; Belarbi, M.; Visioli, F. Hydroxytyrosol augments the redox status of high fat diet-fed rats. *PharmaNutrition* **2016**, *4*, 139–142. [CrossRef]

65. Cao, K.; Xu, J.; Zou, X.; Li, Y.; Chen, C.; Zheng, A.; Li, H.; Li, H.; Szeto, I.M.-Y.; Shi, Y.; et al. Hydroxytyrosol prevents diet-induced metabolic syndrome and attenuates mitochondrial abnormalities in obese mice. *Free Radic. Biol. Med.* **2014**, *67*, 396–407. [CrossRef] [PubMed]

66. Drira, R.; Chen, S.; Sakamoto, K. Oleuropein and hydroxytyrosol inhibit adipocyte differentiation in 3 T3-L1 cells. *Life Sci.* **2011**, *89*, 708–716. [CrossRef] [PubMed]

67. Warnke, I.; Goralczyk, R.; Fuhrer, E.; Schwager, J. Dietary constituents reduce lipid accumulation in murine C3H10 T1/2 adipocytes: A novel fluorescent method to quantify fat droplets. *Nutr. Metab.* **2011**, *8*, 30. [CrossRef] [PubMed]

68. Hao, J.; Shen, W.; Yu, G.; Jia, H.; Li, X.; Feng, Z.; Wang, Y.; Weber, P.; Wertz, K.; Sharman, E.; et al. Hydroxytyrosol promotes mitochondrial biogenesis and mitochondrial function in 3T3-L1 adipocytes. *J. Nutr. Biochem.* **2010**, *21*, 634–644. [CrossRef] [PubMed]

69. Drira, R.; Sakamoto, K. Modulation of adipogenesis, lipolysis and glucose consumption in 3T3-L1 adipocytes and C2C12 myotubes by hydroxytyrosol acetate: A comparative study. *Biochem. Biophys. Res. Commun.* **2013**, *440*, 576–581. [CrossRef] [PubMed]

70. Pirozzi, C.; Lama, A.; Simeoli, R.; Paciello, O.; Pagano, T.B.; Mollica, M.P.; Di Guida, F.; Russo, R.; Magliocca, S.; Canani, R.B.; et al. Hydroxytyrosol prevents metabolic impairment reducing hepatic inflammation and restoring duodenal integrity in a rat model of NAFLD. *J. Nutr. Biochem.* **2016**, *30*, 108–115. [CrossRef] [PubMed]

71. Acín, S.; Navarro, M.A.; Arbonés-Mainar, J.M.; Guillén, N.; Sarría, A.J.; Carnicer, R.; Surra, J.C.; Orman, I.; Segovia, J.C.; de la Torre, R.; et al. Hydroxytyrosol administration enhances atherosclerotic lesion development in apo E deficient mice. *J. Biochem.* **2006**, *140*, 383–391. [CrossRef] [PubMed]

72. Violi, F.; Loffredo, L.; Pignatelli, P.; Angelico, F.; Bartimoccia, S.; Nocella, C.; Cangemi, R.; Petruccioli, A.; Monticolo, R.; Pastori, D.; et al. Extra virgin olive oil use is associated with improved post-prandial blood glucose and LDL cholesterol in healthy subjects. *Nutr. Diabetes* **2015**, *5*, e172. [CrossRef] [PubMed]

73. Hamden, K.; Allouche, N.; Damak, M.; Elfeki, A. Hypoglycemic and antioxidant effects of phenolic extracts and purified hydroxytyrosol from olive mill waste in vitro and in rats. *Chem. Biol. Interact.* **2009**, *180*, 421–432. [CrossRef] [PubMed]

74. Tabernero, M.; Sarriá, B.; Largo, C.; Martínez-López, S.; Madrona, A.; Espartero, J.L.; Bravo, L.; Mateos, R. Comparative evaluation of the metabolic effects of hydroxytyrosol and its lipophilic derivatives (hydroxytyrosyl acetate and ethyl hydroxytyrosyl ether) in hypercholesterolemic rats. *Food Funct.* **2014**, *5*, 1556–1563. [CrossRef] [PubMed]

75. Ruiz-Gutiérrez, V.; Pérez-Espinosa, A.; Vázquez, C.M.; Santa-María, C. Effects of dietary fats (fish, olive and high-oleic-acid sunflower oils) on lipid composition and antioxidant enzymes in rat liver. *Br. J. Nutr.* **1999**, *82*, 233–241. [PubMed]

76. Salas, J.; López Miranda, J.; Jansen, S.; Zambrana, J.L.; Castro, P.; Paniagua, J.A.; Blanco, A.; López Segura, F.; Jiménez Perepérez, J.A.; Pérez Jiménez, F.; et al. The diet rich in monounsaturated fat modifies in a beneficial way carbohydrate metabolism and arterial pressure. *Med. Clínica* **1999**, *113*, 765–769.

77. Ferrara, L.A.; Raimondi, A.S.; d'Episcopo, L.; Guida, L.; Dello Russo, A.; Marotta, T. Olive oil and reduced need for antihypertensive medications. *Arch. Intern. Med.* **2000**, *160*, 837–842. [CrossRef] [PubMed]

78. Thomsen, C.; Storm, H.; Holst, J.J.; Hermansen, K. Differential effects of saturated and monounsaturated fats on postprandial lipemia and glucagon-like peptide 1 responses in patients with type 2 diabetes. *Am. J. Clin. Nutr.* **2003**, *77*, 605–611. [PubMed]

79. Ruano, J.; Lopez-Miranda, J.; Fuentes, F.; Moreno, J.A.; Bellido, C.; Perez-Martinez, P.; Lozano, A.; Gómez, P.; Jiménez, Y.; Pérez Jiménez, F. Phenolic content of virgin olive oil improves ischemic reactive hyperemia in hypercholesterolemic patients. *J. Am. Coll. Cardiol.* **2005**, *46*, 1864–1868. [CrossRef] [PubMed]

80. Valls, R.-M.; Farràs, M.; Suárez, M.; Fernández-Castillejo, S.; Fitó, M.; Konstantinidou, V.; Fuentes, F.; López-Miranda, J.; Giralt, M.; Covas, M.-I.; et al. Effects of functional olive oil enriched with its own phenolic compounds on endothelial function in hypertensive patients. A randomised controlled trial. *Food Chem.* **2015**, *167*, 30–35. [CrossRef] [PubMed]

81. Ruíz-Gutiérrez, V.; Muriana, F.J.; Guerrero, A.; Cert, A.M.; Villar, J. Plasma lipids, erythrocyte membrane lipids and blood pressure of hypertensive women after ingestion of dietary oleic acid from two different sources. *J. Hypertens.* **1996**, *14*, 1483–1490. [CrossRef] [PubMed]

82. Lockyer, S.; Rowland, I.; Spencer, J.P.E.; Yaqoob, P.; Stonehouse, W. Impact of phenolic-rich olive leaf extract on blood pressure, plasma lipids and inflammatory markers: A randomised controlled trial. *Eur. J. Nutr.* **2016**. [CrossRef] [PubMed]

83. Romero, M.; Toral, M.; Gómez-Guzmán, M.; Jiménez, R.; Galindo, P.; Sánchez, M.; Olivares, M.; Gálvez, J.; Duarte, J. Antihypertensive effects of oleuropein-enriched olive leaf extract in spontaneously hypertensive rats. *Food Funct.* **2016**, *7*, 584–593. [CrossRef] [PubMed]

84. López-Villodres, J.A.; Abdel-Karim, M.; De La Cruz, J.P.; Rodríguez-Pérez, M.D.; Reyes, J.J.; Guzmán-Moscoso, R.; Rodriguez-Gutierrez, G.; Fernández-Bolaños, J.; González-Correa, J.A. Effects of hydroxytyrosol on cardiovascular biomarkers in experimental diabetes mellitus. *J. Nutr. Biochem.* **2016**, *37*, 94–100. [CrossRef] [PubMed]

85. Storniolo, C.E.; Roselló-Catafau, J.; Pintó, X.; Mitjavila, M.T.; Moreno, J.J. Polyphenol fraction of extra virgin olive oil protects against endothelial dysfunction induced by high glucose and free fatty acids through modulation of nitric oxide and endothelin-1. *Redox Biol.* **2014**, *2*, 971–977. [CrossRef] [PubMed]

86. De la Torre-Carbot, K.; Chávez-Servín, J.L.; Jaúregui, O.; Castellote, A.I.; Lamuela-Raventós, R.M.; Nurmi, T.; Poulsen, H.E.; Gaddi, A.V.; Kaikkonen, J.; Zunft, H.-F.; et al. Elevated circulating LDL phenol levels in men who consumed virgin rather than refined olive oil are associated with less oxidation of plasma LDL. *J. Nutr.* **2010**, *140*, 501–508. [CrossRef] [PubMed]

87. Castañer, O.; Covas, M.-I.; Khymenets, O.; Nyyssonen, K.; Konstantinidou, V.; Zunft, H.-F.; de la Torre, R.; Muñoz-Aguayo, D.; Vila, J.; Fitó, M. Protection of LDL from oxidation by olive oil polyphenols is associated with a downregulation of CD40-ligand expression and its downstream products in vivo in humans. *Am. J. Clin. Nutr.* **2012**, *95*, 1238–1244. [CrossRef] [PubMed]

88. Reaven, P.; Parthasarathy, S.; Grasse, B.J.; Miller, E.; Steinberg, D.; Witztum, J.L. Effects of oleate-rich and linoleate-rich diets on the susceptibility of low density lipoprotein to oxidative modification in mildly hypercholesterolemic subjects. *J. Clin. Investig.* **1993**, *91*, 668–676. [CrossRef] [PubMed]

89. Vázquez-Velasco, M.; Esperanza Díaz, L.; Lucas, R.; Gómez-Martínez, S.; Bastida, S.; Marcos, A.; Sánchez-Muniz, F.J. Effects of hydroxytyrosol-enriched sunflower oil consumption on CVD risk factors. *Br. J. Nutr.* **2011**, *105*, 1448–1452. [CrossRef] [PubMed]

90. Fki, I.; Sahnoun, Z.; Sayadi, S. Hypocholesterolemic effects of phenolic extracts and purified hydroxytyrosol recovered from olive mill wastewater in rats fed a cholesterol-rich diet. *J. Agric. Food Chem.* **2007**, *55*, 624–631. [CrossRef] [PubMed]

91. Visioli, F.; Bellomo, G.; Montedoro, G.; Galli, C. Low density lipoprotein oxidation is inhibited in vitro by olive oil constituents. *Atherosclerosis* **1995**, *117*, 25–32. [CrossRef]

92. Fitó, M.; Covas, M.I.; Lamuela-Raventós, R.M.; Vila, J.; Torrents, L.; de la Torre, C.; Marrugat, J. Protective effect of olive oil and its phenolic compounds against low density lipoprotein oxidation. *Lipids* **2000**, *35*, 633–638. [CrossRef] [PubMed]

93. Covas, M.-I.; de la Torre, K.; Farré-Albaladejo, M.; Kaikkonen, J.; Fitó, M.; López-Sabater, C.; Pujadas-Bastardes, M.A.; Joglar, J.; Weinbrenner, T.; Lamuela-Raventós, R.M.; et al. Postprandial LDL phenolic content and LDL oxidation are modulated by olive oil phenolic compounds in humans. *Free Radic. Biol. Med.* **2006**, *40*, 608–616. [CrossRef] [PubMed]

94. González-Santiago, M.; Fonollá, J.; Lopez-Huertas, E. Human absorption of a supplement containing purified hydroxytyrosol, a natural antioxidant from olive oil, and evidence for its transient association with low-density lipoproteins. *Pharmacol. Res.* **2010**, *61*, 364–370. [CrossRef] [PubMed]

95. Mateos, R.; Martínez-López, S.; Baeza Arévalo, G.; Amigo-Benavent, M.; Sarriá, B.; Bravo-Clemente, L. Hydroxytyrosol in functional hydroxytyrosol-enriched biscuits is highly bioavailable and decreases oxidised low density lipoprotein levels in humans. *Food Chem.* **2016**, *205*, 248–256. [CrossRef] [PubMed]

96. Mackness, M.I.; Arrol, S.; Abbott, C.; Durrington, P.N. Protection of low-density lipoprotein against oxidative modification by high-density lipoprotein associated paraoxonase. *Atherosclerosis* **1993**, *104*, 129–135. [CrossRef]

97. Mackness, M.I.; Durrington, P.N. HDL, its enzymes and its potential to influence lipid peroxidation. *Atherosclerosis* **1995**, *115*, 243–253. [CrossRef]

98. Rietjens, S.J.; Bast, A.; de Vente, J.; Haenen, G.R.M.M. The olive oil antioxidant hydroxytyrosol efficiently protects against the oxidative stress-induced impairment of the NObullet response of isolated rat aorta. *Am. J. Physiol. Heart Circ. Physiol.* **2007**, *292*, H1931–H1936. [CrossRef] [PubMed]

99. Khymenets, O.; Fitó, M.; Touriño, S.; Muñoz-Aguayo, D.; Pujadas, M.; Torres, J.L.; Joglar, J.; Farré, M.; Covas, M.-I.; de la Torre, R. Antioxidant activities of hydroxytyrosol main metabolites do not contribute to beneficial health effects after olive oil ingestion. *Drug Metab. Dispos.* **2010**, *38*, 1417–1421. [CrossRef] [PubMed]

100. Briante, R.; Febbraio, F.; Nucci, R. Antioxidant/prooxidant effects of dietary non-flavonoid phenols on the Cu2+-induced oxidation of human low-density lipoprotein (LDL). *Chem. Biodivers.* **2004**, *1*, 1716–1729. [CrossRef] [PubMed]

101. Petersen, K.F.; Befroy, D.; Dufour, S.; Dziura, J.; Ariyan, C.; Rothman, D.L.; DiPietro, L.; Cline, G.W.; Shulman, G.I. Mitochondrial dysfunction in the elderly: Possible role in insulin resistance. *Science* **2003**, *300*, 1140–1142. [CrossRef] [PubMed]

102. Stump, C.S.; Short, K.R.; Bigelow, M.L.; Schimke, J.M.; Nair, K.S. Effect of insulin on human skeletal muscle mitochondrial ATP production, protein synthesis, and mRNA transcripts. *Proc. Natl. Acad. Sci. USA* **2003**, *100*, 7996–8001. [CrossRef] [PubMed]

103. Ritz, P.; Berrut, G. Mitochondrial function, energy expenditure, aging and insulin resistance. *Diabetes Metab.* **2005**, *31*, 5S67–5S73. [CrossRef]

104. Morino, K.; Petersen, K.F.; Dufour, S.; Befroy, D.; Frattini, J.; Shatzkes, N.; Neschen, S.; White, M.F.; Bilz, S.; Sono, S.; et al. Reduced mitochondrial density and increased IRS-1 serine phosphorylation in muscle of insulin-resistant offspring of type 2 diabetic parents. *J. Clin. Investig.* **2005**, *115*, 3587–3593. [CrossRef] [PubMed]

105. Zheng, A.; Li, H.; Xu, J.; Cao, K.; Li, H.; Pu, W.; Yang, Z.; Peng, Y.; Long, J.; Liu, J.; et al. Hydroxytyrosol improves mitochondrial function and reduces oxidative stress in the brain of db/db mice: Role of AMP-activated protein kinase activation. *Br. J. Nutr.* **2015**, *113*, 1667–1676. [CrossRef] [PubMed]

106. Granados-Principal, S.; El-Azem, N.; Pamplona, R.; Ramirez-Tortosa, C.; Pulido-Moran, M.; Vera-Ramirez, L.; Quiles, J.L.; Sanchez-Rovira, P.; Naudí, A.; Portero-Otin, M.; et al. Hydroxytyrosol ameliorates oxidative stress and mitochondrial dysfunction in doxorubicin-induced cardiotoxicity in rats with breast cancer. *Biochem. Pharmacol.* **2014**, *90*, 25–33. [CrossRef] [PubMed]

107. Zhu, L.; Liu, Z.; Feng, Z.; Hao, J.; Shen, W.; Li, X.; Sun, L.; Sharman, E.; Wang, Y.; Wertz, K.; et al. Hydroxytyrosol protects against oxidative damage by simultaneous activation of mitochondrial biogenesis and phase II detoxifying enzyme systems in retinal pigment epithelial cells. *J. Nutr. Biochem.* **2010**, *21*, 1089–1098. [CrossRef] [PubMed]

108. Zheng, A.; Li, H.; Cao, K.; Xu, J.; Zou, X.; Li, Y.; Chen, C.; Liu, J.; Feng, Z. Maternal hydroxytyrosol administration improves neurogenesis and cognitive function in prenatally stressed offspring. *J. Nutr. Biochem.* **2015**, *26*, 190–199. [CrossRef] [PubMed]

109. Bali, E.B.; Ergin, V.; Rackova, L.; Bayraktar, O.; Küçükboyaci, N.; Karasu, Ç. Olive leaf extracts protect cardiomyocytes against 4-hydroxynonenal-induced toxicity in vitro: Comparison with oleuropein, hydroxytyrosol, and quercetin. *Planta Med.* **2014**, *80*, 984–992. [CrossRef] [PubMed]

110. Martín, M.A.; Ramos, S.; Granado-Serrano, A.B.; Rodríguez-Ramiro, I.; Trujillo, M.; Bravo, L.; Goya, L. Hydroxytyrosol induces antioxidant/detoxificant enzymes and Nrf2 translocation via extracellular regulated kinases and phosphatidylinositol-3-kinase/protein kinase B pathways in HepG2 cells. *Mol. Nutr. Food Res.* **2010**, *54*, 956–966. [CrossRef] [PubMed]

111. Zrelli, H.; Matsuoka, M.; Kitazaki, S.; Zarrouk, M.; Miyazaki, H. Hydroxytyrosol reduces intracellular reactive oxygen species levels in vascular endothelial cells by upregulating catalase expression through the AMPK-FOXO3a pathway. *Eur. J. Pharmacol.* **2011**, *660*, 275–282. [CrossRef] [PubMed]
112. Deiana, M.; Incani, A.; Rosa, A.; Atzeri, A.; Loru, D.; Cabboi, B.; Paola Melis, M.; Lucas, R.; Morales, J.C.; Assunta Dessì, M. Hydroxytyrosol glucuronides protect renal tubular epithelial cells against H(2)O(2) induced oxidative damage. *Chem. Biol. Interact.* **2011**, *193*, 232–239. [CrossRef] [PubMed]
113. Paiva-Martins, F.; Silva, A.; Almeida, V.; Carvalheira, M.; Serra, C.; Rodrígues-Borges, J.E.; Fernandes, J.; Belo, L.; Santos-Silva, A. Protective activity of hydroxytyrosol metabolites on erythrocyte oxidative-induced hemolysis. *J. Agric. Food Chem.* **2013**, *61*, 6636–6642. [CrossRef] [PubMed]
114. Deiana, M.; Aruoma, O.I.; Bianchi, M.L.; Spencer, J.P.; Kaur, H.; Halliwell, B.; Aeschbach, R.; Banni, S.; Dessi, M.A.; Corongiu, F.P. Inhibition of peroxynitrite dependent DNA base modification and tyrosine nitration by the extra virgin olive oil-derived antioxidant hydroxytyrosol. *Free Radic. Biol. Med.* **1999**, *26*, 762–769. [CrossRef]
115. De la Puerta, R.; Martínez Domínguez, M.E.; Ruíz-Gutíerrez, V.; Flavill, J.A.; Hoult, J.R. Effects of virgin olive oil phenolics on scavenging of reactive nitrogen species and upon nitrergic neurotransmission. *Life Sci.* **2001**, *69*, 1213–1222. [CrossRef]
116. O'Dowd, Y.; Driss, F.; Dang, P.M.-C.; Elbim, C.; Gougerot-Pocidalo, M.-A.; Pasquier, C.; El-Benna, J. Antioxidant effect of hydroxytyrosol, a polyphenol from olive oil: Scavenging of hydrogen peroxide but not superoxide anion produced by human neutrophils. *Biochem. Pharmacol.* **2004**, *68*, 2003–2008. [CrossRef] [PubMed]
117. Manna, C.; Galletti, P.; Cucciolla, V.; Montedoro, G.; Zappia, V. Olive oil hydroxytyrosol protects human erythrocytes against oxidative damages. *J. Nutr. Biochem.* **1999**, *10*, 159–165. [CrossRef]
118. Manna, C.; Napoli, D.; Cacciapuoti, G.; Porcelli, M.; Zappia, V. Olive oil phenolic compounds inhibit homocysteine-induced endothelial cell adhesion regardless of their different antioxidant activity. *J. Agric. Food Chem.* **2009**, *57*, 3478–3482. [CrossRef] [PubMed]
119. Goya, L.; Mateos, R.; Bravo, L. Effect of the olive oil phenol hydroxytyrosol on human hepatoma HepG2 cells. Protection against oxidative stress induced by tert-butylhydroperoxide. *Eur. J. Nutr.* **2007**, *46*, 70–78. [CrossRef] [PubMed]
120. Gutierrez, V.R.; de la Puerta, R.; Catalá, A. The effect of tyrosol, hydroxytyrosol and oleuropein on the non-enzymatic lipid peroxidation of rat liver microsomes. *Mol. Cell. Biochem.* **2001**, *217*, 35–41. [CrossRef] [PubMed]
121. Crespo, M.C.; Tomé-Carneiro, J.; Burgos-Ramos, E.; Loria Kohen, V.; Espinosa, M.I.; Herranz, J.; Visioli, F. One-week administration of hydroxytyrosol to humans does not activate Phase II enzymes. *Pharmacol. Res.* **2015**, *95*, 132–137. [CrossRef] [PubMed]
122. Takeda, Y.; Bui, V.N.; Iwasaki, K.; Kobayashi, T.; Ogawa, H.; Imai, K. Influence of olive-derived hydroxytyrosol on the toll-like receptor 4-dependent inflammatory response of mouse peritoneal macrophages. *Biochem. Biophys. Res. Commun.* **2014**, *446*, 1225–1230. [CrossRef] [PubMed]
123. Carito, V.; Ciafrè, S.; Tarani, L.; Ceccanti, M.; Natella, F.; Iannitelli, A.; Tirassa, P.; Chaldakov, G.N.; Ceccanti, M.; Boccardo, C.; et al. TNF-α and IL-10 modulation induced by polyphenols extracted by olive pomace in a mouse model of paw inflammation. *Ann. DellIstituto Super. Sanità* **2015**, *51*, 382–386.
124. Sánchez-Fidalgo, S.; Sánchez de Ibargüen, L.; Cárdeno, A.; Alarcón de la Lastra, C. Influence of extra virgin olive oil diet enriched with hydroxytyrosol in a chronic DSS colitis model. *Eur. J. Nutr.* **2012**, *51*, 497–506. [CrossRef] [PubMed]
125. Silva, S.; Sepodes, B.; Rocha, J.; Direito, R.; Fernandes, A.; Brites, D.; Freitas, M.; Fernandes, E.; Bronze, M.R.; Figueira, M.E. Protective effects of hydroxytyrosol-supplemented refined olive oil in animal models of acute inflammation and rheumatoid arthritis. *J. Nutr. Biochem.* **2015**, *26*, 360–368. [CrossRef] [PubMed]
126. Gong, D.; Geng, C.; Jiang, L.; Cao, J.; Yoshimura, H.; Zhong, L. Effects of hydroxytyrosol-20 on carrageenan-induced acute inflammation and hyperalgesia in rats. *Phytother. Res. PTR* **2009**, *23*, 646–650. [CrossRef] [PubMed]
127. Scoditti, E.; Massaro, M.; Carluccio, M.A.; Pellegrino, M.; Wabitsch, M.; Calabriso, N.; Storelli, C.; De Caterina, R. Additive regulation of adiponectin expression by the mediterranean diet olive oil components oleic Acid and hydroxytyrosol in human adipocytes. *PLoS ONE* **2015**, *10*, e0128218. [CrossRef] [PubMed]

128. Zhang, X.; Cao, J.; Zhong, L. Hydroxytyrosol inhibits pro-inflammatory cytokines, iNOS, and COX-2 expression in human monocytic cells. *Naunyn. Schmiedebergs Arch. Pharmacol.* **2009**, *379*, 581–586. [CrossRef] [PubMed]

129. Zhang, X.; Cao, J.; Jiang, L.; Zhong, L. Suppressive effects of hydroxytyrosol on oxidative stress and nuclear Factor-kappaB activation in THP-1 cells. *Biol. Pharm. Bull.* **2009**, *32*, 578–582. [CrossRef] [PubMed]

130. Scoditti, E.; Nestola, A.; Massaro, M.; Calabriso, N.; Storelli, C.; De Caterina, R.; Carluccio, M.A. Hydroxytyrosol suppresses MMP-9 and COX-2 activity and expression in activated human monocytes via PKCα and PKCβ1 inhibition. *Atherosclerosis* **2014**, *232*, 17–24. [CrossRef] [PubMed]

131. Parkinson, L.; Cicerale, S. The Health Benefiting Mechanisms of Virgin Olive Oil Phenolic Compounds. *Mol. Basel Switz.* **2016**, *21*, 1734. [CrossRef] [PubMed]

132. Rigacci, S.; Stefani, M. Nutraceutical Properties of Olive Oil Polyphenols. An Itinerary from Cultured Cells through Animal Models to Humans. *Int. J. Mol. Sci.* **2016**, *17*, 843. [CrossRef] [PubMed]

133. Dell'Agli, M.; Fagnani, R.; Mitro, N.; Scurati, S.; Masciadri, M.; Mussoni, L.; Galli, G.V.; Bosisio, E.; Crestani, M.; De Fabiani, E.; et al. Minor components of olive oil modulate proatherogenic adhesion molecules involved in endothelial activation. *J. Agric. Food Chem.* **2006**, *54*, 3259–3264. [CrossRef] [PubMed]

134. Schmitt, C.A.; Handler, N.; Heiss, E.H.; Erker, T.; Dirsch, V.M. No evidence for modulation of endothelial nitric oxide synthase by the olive oil polyphenol hydroxytyrosol in human endothelial cells. *Atherosclerosis* **2007**, *195*, e58–e64. [CrossRef] [PubMed]

135. Zrelli, H.; Wu, C.W.; Zghonda, N.; Shimizu, H.; Miyazaki, H. Combined treatment of hydroxytyrosol with carbon monoxide-releasing molecule-2 prevents TNF α-induced vascular endothelial cell dysfunction through NO production with subsequent NFκB inactivation. *BioMed Res. Int.* **2013**, *2013*, 912431. [CrossRef] [PubMed]

136. Bayram, B.; Ozcelik, B.; Grimm, S.; Roeder, T.; Schrader, C.; Ernst, I.M.A.; Wagner, A.E.; Grune, T.; Frank, J.; Rimbach, G. A diet rich in olive oil phenolics reduces oxidative stress in the heart of SAMP8 mice by induction of Nrf2-dependent gene expression. *Rejuvenation Res.* **2012**, *15*, 71–81. [CrossRef] [PubMed]

137. Mnafgui, K.; Hajji, R.; Derbali, F.; Khlif, I.; Kraiem, F.; Ellefi, H.; Elfeki, A.; Allouche, N.; Gharsallah, N. Protective Effect of Hydroxytyrosol Against Cardiac Remodeling After Isoproterenol-Induced Myocardial Infarction in Rat. *Cardiovasc. Toxicol.* **2016**, *16*, 147–155. [CrossRef] [PubMed]

138. López de las Hazas, M.-C.; Rubió, L.; Kotronoulas, A.; de la Torre, R.; Solà, R.; Motilva, M.-J. Dose effect on the uptake and accumulation of hydroxytyrosol and its metabolites in target tissues in rats. *Mol. Nutr. Food Res.* **2015**, *59*, 1395–1399. [CrossRef] [PubMed]

139. Cofrades, S.; Salcedo Sandoval, L.; Delgado-Pando, G.; López-López, I.; Ruiz-Capillas, C.; Jiménez-Colmenero, F. Antioxidant activity of hydroxytyrosol in frankfurters enriched with *n*-3 polyunsaturated fatty acids. *Food Chem.* **2011**, *129*, 429–436. [CrossRef]

140. Nieto, G.; Martínez, L.; Ros, G. Hydroxytyrosol extracts, olive oil and walnuts as functional components in chicken sausages. *J. Sci. Food Agric.* **2017**. [CrossRef] [PubMed]

141. Long, L.H.; Hoi, A.; Halliwell, B. Instability of, and generation of hydrogen peroxide by, phenolic compounds in cell culture media. *Arch. Biochem. Biophys.* **2010**, *501*, 162–169. [CrossRef] [PubMed]

142. Sung, M.M.; Kim, T.T.; Denou, E.; Soltys, C.-L.M.; Hamza, S.M.; Byrne, N.J.; Masson, G.; Park, H.; Wishart, D.S.; Madsen, K.L.; et al. Improved Glucose Homeostasis in Obese Mice Treated With Resveratrol Is Associated With Alterations in the Gut Microbiome. *Diabetes* **2017**, *66*, 418–425. [CrossRef] [PubMed]

143. Côté, C.D.; Rasmussen, B.A.; Duca, F.A.; Zadeh-Tahmasebi, M.; Baur, J.A.; Daljeet, M.; Breen, D.M.; Filippi, B.M.; Lam, T.K.T. Resveratrol activates duodenal Sirt1 to reverse insulin resistance in rats through a neuronal network. *Nat. Med.* **2015**, *21*, 498–505. [CrossRef] [PubMed]

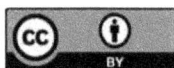

nutrients

MDPI

Article

Are miRNA-103, miRNA-107 and miRNA-122 Involved in the Prevention of Liver Steatosis Induced by Resveratrol?

Ana Gracia [1,2], Alfredo Fernández-Quintela [1,2,*], Jonatan Miranda [1,2], Itziar Eseberri [1,2], Marcela González [3] and María P. Portillo [1,2]

[1] Nutrition and Obesity Group, Department of Nutrition and Food Science, University of the Basque Country (UPV/EHU) and Lucio Lascaray Research Institute, Vitoria 01006, Spain; anajadraque@gmail.com (A.G.); jonatan.miranda@ehu.eus (J.M.); itziareseberri@hotmail.com (I.E.); mariapuy.portillo@ehu.eus (M.P.P.)

[2] CIBERobn Physiopathology of Obesity and Nutrition, Institute of Health Carlos III, Madrid 28029, Spain

[3] Nutrition and Food Science, Faculty of Biochemistry and Biological Sciences, National University of Litoral, Santa Fe 3000, Argentina; maidagon@fbcb.unl.edu.ar

* Correspondence: alfredo.fernandez@ehu.eus; Tel.: +34-945-013-066; Fax: +34-945-013-014

Received: 25 February 2017; Accepted: 1 April 2017; Published: 4 April 2017

Abstract: The aim of the present study was to determine whether the reduction in liver fat previously observed in our laboratory in a cohort of rats which had been fed an obesogenic diet was mediated by changes in the expression of microRNA (miRNA)-103-3p, miRNA-107-3p and miRNA-122-5p, which represent 70% of total miRNAs in the liver, as well as in their target genes. The expression of the three analysed miRNAs was reduced in rats treated with resveratrol. A reduction in sterol-regulatory element binding protein 1 (SREBP1) and an increase in carnitine palmitoyltransferase 1a (CPT1a) were observed in resveratrol-treated rats. No changes were found in fatty acid synthase (FAS). In cultured hepatocytes, SREBP1 protein was increased after the transfection of each miRNA. FAS protein expression was decreased after the transfection of miRNA-122-5p, and CPT1a protein was down-regulated by the over-expression of miRNA-107-3p. This study provides new evidences which show that *srebf1* is a target gene for miRNA-103-3p and miRNA-107-3p, *fasn* a target gene for miRNA-122-5p and *cpt1a* a target gene for miRNA-107-3p. Moreover, the reduction in liver steatosis induced by resveratrol in rats fed an obesegenic diet is mediated, at least in part, by the increase in CPT1a protein expression and activity, via a decrease in miRNA-107-3p expression.

Keywords: miRNA-103; miRNA-107; miRNA-122; steatosis; liver; resveratrol; rat

1. Introduction

Excessive fat accumulation in liver is known as hepatic steatosis, which is the most benign form of non-alcoholic fatty liver disease (NAFLD). It is a major cause of chronic liver disease in Western societies. It encompasses a disease spectrum ranging from simple triglyceride accumulation in hepatocytes (hepatic steatosis; NAFL) to hepatic steatosis with inflammation (non-alcoholic steatohepatitis, NASH) [1]. This disorder is closely associated with obesity and insulin resistance [2]. Although the current treatment of liver steatosis is based on dietary energy restriction and physical activity [3,4], a great deal of attention has been paid in recent years to bioactive molecules, such as phenolic compounds present in foods and plants, which can represent complementary tools.

One of the most widely studied molecules is resveratrol (*trans*-3,5,4′-trihydroxystilbene), a phytoalexin occurring naturally in grapes, berries and peanuts [5,6]. Several studies on rats and mice have shown that resveratrol is able to reduce liver fat accumulation [7,8]. Some authors have also found this effect in human beings [9,10].

The mechanisms of action of resveratrol underlying its effect on liver steatosis are mainly a reduction in lipogenesis and/or an increase in fatty acid oxidation, very commonly associated with enhanced mitochondriogenesis [11]. However, little is known concerning the potential involvement of microRNAs (miRNAs) on changes induced by resveratrol in these metabolic pathways.

MiRNAs are short double stranded RNAs (approximately 22 nucleotides) encoded in the genome that act post-transcriptionally to regulate protein expression. These non-coding RNAs can act directly on target mRNA transcripts binding to complementary target sites in 3' untranslated regions (3' UTR) of messenger RNAs (mRNAs), causing translational repression and/or mRNA destabilization. They can also act indirectly by regulating intermediate components, such as transcripts that encode transcription factors which, in turn, control the expression of downstream genes. A single miRNA can have multiple targets, acting simultaneously to regulate the post-transcriptional expression of various genes and physiological processes. Furthermore, each gene can be regulated by several miRNAs [12,13]. What is more, the expression of these miRNAs can be modified by changes induced either directly in the enzymes involved in their biogenesis process or in miRNA epigenetic modifications, or indirectly via lipoprotein-mediated miRNA delivery to cells, among others [14,15].

It has been reported in the literature that different types of polyphenols, such as proanthocyanidins or a mixture extracted from *Hibiscus sabdariffa*, are able to modify the expression of miRNA-122-5p (a liver specific miRNA and the most abundant one) and the paralogs miRNA-103-3p and miRNA-107-3p in liver [16–19].

In a previous study carried out by our group using this precise cohort of animals, resveratrol treatment did not reduce final body weight or liver weight. No changes were observed in food intake. By contrast, resveratrol treatment induced a significant decrease in hepatic triacylglycerol content. Moreover, when the activity of several enzymes involved in hepatic lipid metabolism was measured, no changes in fatty acid synthase (FAS) activity and an increase in carnitine palmitoyltransferase 1 (CPT1) activity were found, suggesting that the delipidating effect was due, at least in part, to increased fatty acid β-oxidation, which reduces the availability of fatty acids for triacylglycerol synthesis [20].

In this context, the aim of the present study was to determine whether, as in the case of other polyphenols, this reduction in liver fat was mediated by changes in the expression of miRNA-122-5p, miRNA-103-3p and miRNA-107-3p, which represent more than 75% of total miRNAs in the liver [19,21–25], as well as in their target genes.

2. Material and Methods

2.1. Animals and Experimental Design

The experiment was conducted with 16 male Sprague-Dawley rats purchased from Harlan Ibérica (Barcelona, Spain) and took place in accordance with the institution's guide for the care and use of laboratory animals (CUEID CEBA/30/2010). The rats were individually housed in polycarbonate metabolic cages (Techniplast Gazzada, Guguggiate, Italy) and placed in an air-conditioned room (22 ± 2 °C) with a 12 h light-dark cycle. After a 6-day adaptation period, rats were randomly divided into two dietary groups of eight animals each, namely a control group (Control) and a group treated with resveratrol (Resveratrol), both fed a commercial obesogenic diet (4.6 kcal/g; 44.8% energy from fat, 36.2% from carbohydrates and 19.0% from proteins) supplied by Harlan Ibérica (TD. 06415) for 6 weeks (Figure S1). Resveratrol, supplied by Monteloeder (Elche, Spain), was added to the diet as previously reported [6]. Briefly, the phenolic compound was dissolved in an ethanolic solution (5 mg/mL) and poured on the surface of the diet. Rats started eating immediately once the diet was daily replaced, and thus they ate all the resveratrol added before it started to degrade (3 h). In order to ensure a dose of 30 mg resveratrol/kg body weight/day, the amounts of resveratrol to be included in the diet for each animal were calculated daily based on their individual body weight. This dose was selected for this experiment because in a previous study we observed that, under our experimental conditions, 30 mg/kg body weight/day was the most effective of the following: 6, 15, 30 and 60 mg/kg body weight/day. Diet for control animals was added with the same amount of ethanolic solution without resveratrol. All animals had free access to food and water. Food intake and body weight were measured daily. This cohort of animals had been previously used in another study reported by our group [20,26].

At the end of the experimental period, animals were sacrificed under anaesthesia by intraperitoneally administering 400 mg chloral hydrate/kg body weight, by cardiac exsanguination, after a 12-h fasting period. The liver was dissected, weighed and immediately frozen at −80 °C.

2.2. Cell Culture

AML12 (Alpha Mouse Liver 12) hepatocytes, supplied by ATCC (ATCC CRL-2254), were cultured in 1:1 DMEM/HAM'S F12 glutamax medium containing 10% fetal bovine serum (FBS), 0.005 mg/mL insulin, 0.005 mg/mL transferrin, 5 ng/mL selenium, 40 ng/mL dexamethasone and 1% Penicillin/Streptomycin (10,000 U/mL). This medium was changed every two days. Cells were maintained at 37 °C in a humidified 5% CO_2 atmosphere.

2.3. MicroRNA Expression Analysis

Total miRNAs were extracted using E.Z.N.A. miRNA kit (R7034-02; Omega Bio-Tek, Norcross, GA, USA) according to the manufacturer's instructions. Total RNA (9 ng) was reverse-transcribed using the TaqMan MicroRNA Reverse Transcription kit (Applied Biosystems, Foster City, CA, USA), as previously reported in Gracia et al. [27]. The targeted miRNA assay sequences were as follows (source miRBase):

rno-miRNA-103-3p: 5′-AGCAGCAUUGUACAGGGCUAUGA-3′
rno-miRNA-107-3p: 5′-AGCAGCAUUGUACAGGGCUAUCA-3′
rno-miRNA-122-5p: 5′-UGGAGUGUGACAAUGGUGUUUG-3′

PCR was performed in an iCycler™–MyiQ™ Real-time PCR Detection System (Applied Biosystems, Foster City, CA, USA). Amplification was performed at 95 °C for 10 min, followed by 40 cycles of 95 °C for 15 s and 60 °C for 1 min. U6 small nuclear RNA was used as an endogenous control. All mRNA levels were normalized to the values of U6 snRNA. The results were expressed as fold changes of threshold cycle (Ct) value relative to controls using the $2^{-\Delta\Delta Ct}$ method [28].

2.4. Target Genes for miRNAs

In order to obtain the predicted and validated target genes for these miRNAs, a comparative analysis was carried out in miRecords. This database is an integrated resource for animal miRNA-target interactions, which stores predicted miRNA targets produced by 11 established miRNA target predicted programs [29]. No validated target genes were found. Among the predicted target genes, only those involved in hepatic lipid metabolism (*srebf1, fasn, cpt1a*) were selected (Table 1). *Fasn* codifies for fatty acid synthase, a key enzyme involved in de novo lipogenesis, *srebf1* is the transcription factor that regulates this enzyme, and *cpt1a* codifies for carnitine palmitoyltransferase, a key enzyme involved in the fatty acid oxidation. In addition, we reviewed the literature and found that several authors had proposed *srebf1* and *fasn* as target genes for miR-122-5p and miR-107-3p, respectively (Table 1).

Table 1. Predicted target genes and validated genes reported in the literature related to triacylglycerol metabolism of the miRNAs studied.

miRNA	Predicted Target Genes (miRecords)	Data from the Literature
rno-miR-103-3p	*Srebf1* *Cpt1a*	
rno-miR-107-3p	*Srebf1* *Cpt1a*	*Fasn*: Bhatia et al. [30]
rno-miR-122-5p	*Fasn*	*Srebf1*: Shibata et al. [31] *Srebf1*: Iliopoulos et al. [32]

Srebf1: sterol regulatory element binding factor 1; *Cpt1a*: carnitine palmitoyltransferase 1a; *Fasn*: fatty acid synthase.

2.5. miRNA Transfection

Hepatocytes in a confluence status of approximately 90%, were transfected with Lipofectamine RNAiMAX (Applied Biosystems, Foster City, CA, USA) prepared following the manufacturer's protocol, with mirVana miRNA mimics of mmu-miRNA-103-3p, mmu-miRNA-107-3p and mmu-miRNA-122-5p (homologous to rno-miRNA-103-3p, rno-miRNA-107-3p and rno-miRNA-122-5p respectively) (Applied Biosystems, Foster City, CA, USA). Each mimic was transfected for 48 h in a final concentration of 25 nM per well. Optimal transfection conditions were determined in previous experiments, and transfection efficiency was assessed using miRNA probes and fluorescent transfection controls. To rule out unspecific effects, control cells were transfected with negative controls.

2.6. Western Blot Analysis

2.6.1. Liver Protein Expression of Fatty Acid Synthase, Sterol Regulatory Element-Binding Protein 1 and Carnitine Palmitoyltransferase 1a

Fatty acid synthase (FAS) and sterol regulatory element-binding protein 1 (SREBP1) protein extraction was carried out with 100 mg of liver as previously described [33]. The protein concentration was measured by bicinchoninic acid (BCA) protein assay kit (Thermo Scientific, Wilmington, DE, USA).

Immunoblot analyses were performed in all tissue samples using 80 μg of protein for FAS and 40 μg of protein for SREBP1. Protein were separated by electrophoresis in a 7.5% sodium dodecyl sulfate (SDS)-polyacrylamide gel and transferred to polyvinylidene difluoride (PVDF) membranes. Equal loading of proteins was confirmed by staining the membranes with Coomassie Blue or incubating these membranes with polyclonal mouse β-actin antibody. The membranes of the two assays were blocked with casein phosphate buffered saline (PBS)-Tween buffer for 2 h. These membranes were incubated overnight at 4 °C with mouse origin FAS immunoglobulin G (IgG) (1:1000) and SREBP1 IgG monoclonal antibodies (1:1000) (Santa Cruz Biotechnology, Santa Cruz, CA, USA). Afterwards, in both cases, new incubation with goat- anti-mouse IgG-Horseradish Peroxidase (HRP) antibody (1:5000) (Sigma, St. Louis, MO, USA) was carried out for 2 h at room temperature. Antibodies were visualized by using a chemiluminescent substrate (Thermo Scientific, Wilmington, DE, USA) and quantified by a ChemiDoc MP imaging system (BioRad, Hercules, CA, USA). After stripping, FAS protein-containing membranes were incubated with a polyclonal mouse β-actin antibody (1:5000) followed by goat- anti-mouse IgG-HRP antibody (1:5000) (Sigma, St. Louis, MO, USA), and measured again. The FAS protein measurements were normalized by β-actin.

For carnitine palmitoyltransferase 1a (CPT1a), 100 mg of liver were homogenized in a PBS buffer with protease inhibitors (pH 7.4) and centrifuged (14,000× *g*, 1 min, 4 °C). The pellet was resuspended in 100 μL of radioimmunoprecipitation assay buffer (RIPA buffer). The homogenates were centrifuged at 36,000× *g* for 10 min at 4 °C. The protein concentration was measured by BCA protein assay kit (Thermo Scientific, Wilmington, DE, USA).

Immunoblotting was performed after immunoprecipitation. A total of 250 μg of liver extracts were diluted with three volumes of PBS (with added protease inhibitors). CPT1a was immunoprecipitated with 1 μL of monoclonal mouse anti-CPT1a antibody (ABCAM, Cambridge, MS, USA) in constant rotation, at 4 °C, overnight. Afterwards, 20 μL Protein G Agarose (Santa Cruz Biotech, Santa Cruz, CA, USA) was added to each sample, and these were rotated for 3 h at 4 °C. The immunoprecipitated tissue samples were then washed three times with 500 μL PBS buffer. A total of 30 μg of extracts were separated by electrophoresis in a 7.5% SDS–polyacrylamide gel and then transferred to a PVDF membrane. The membranes were incubated overnight at room temperature with mouse anti-CPT1a antibody (1:1000) (ABCAM, Cambridge, MS, USA). Afterwards, polyclonal goat- anti-mouse IgG-HRP antibody (1:2500) (Sigma, St. Louis, MO, USA) was incubated for 2 h at room temperature. Antibody was visualized by using a chemiluminescent substrate (Thermo Scientific, Wilmington, DE, USA) and quantified by a ChemiDoc MP imaging system (BioRad, Hercules, CA, USA).

2.6.2. SREBP1, FAS and CPT1a Protein Expression after Over-Expression in AML12

In the case of AML12 cells, total protein was extracted with 200 μL of lysis buffer as previously reported [27]. Protein concentration was measured by BCA protein assay kit (Thermo Scientific, Wilmington, DE, USA).

For FAS protein, 65 μg of cell protein extract were used to perform the immunoblotting. Protein were separated by electrophoresis in a 7.5% SDS-polyacrylamide gel and transferred to PVDF membranes. The membranes were blocked with casein PBS-Tween buffer for 2 h. These membranes were incubated overnight at 4 °C with mouse origin FAS IgG (1:1000) (Santa Cruz Biotechnology, Santa Cruz, CA, USA). Afterwards, new incubation with goat- anti-mouse IgG-HRP antibody (1:5000) (Sigma, St. Louis, MO, USA) was carried out for 2 h at room temperature. Antibodies were visualized by using a chemiluminescent substrate (Thermo Scientific, Wilmington, DE, USA) and quantified by a ChemiDoc MP imaging system (BioRad, Hercules, CA, USA). Coomassie Blue staining of membranes was used as protein loading control. In case of CPT1a and SREBP1, immunoblotting after immunoprecipitation was performed. A total of 40 μg for CPT1a and 70 μg for SREBP1 of cell extracts were immunoprecipitated. The total amount of protein was used for immunoblotting in both cases and following the same conditions as described above.

2.7. Statistical Analysis

Results are presented as median ± standard deviation. Statistical analysis was performed using IBM SPSS Statistics 24.0 (SPSS Inc., Chicago, IL, USA). All of the parameters are normally distributed according to the Shapiro-Wilk's test. Student's *t*-test was used for comparisons between both experimental groups. Significance was assessed at the $p < 0.05$ value.

3. Results

3.1. Cell Culture Studies

MiRNA-103-3p, miRNA-107-3p and miRNA-122-5p were individually over-expressed in AML12 hepatocytes. Over-expressions were confirmed by measuring each miRNA expression. Protein expression of SREBP1 was significantly increased after transfection of each miRNA ($p < 0.05$) (Figure 1A). In the case of FAS, protein expression was significantly decreased after transfection of miRNA-122-5p ($p < 0.001$) (Figure 1B). Finally, CPT1a protein expression was down-regulated by the over-expression of miRNA-107-3p ($p < 0.001$) (Figure 2).

3.2. In Vivo Study

Body weight gain in rats treated with resveratrol was similar to that observed in control animals (data previously reported in Alberdi et al. 2011 [34]). Similarly, no significant differences were observed in liver weight, expressed as a percentage of final body weight (3.4 ± 0.1 in Control group and 3.5 ± 0.2 in Resveratrol group).

In the present study, we observed that the expression of the three miRNA analysed (miRNA-103-3p, miRNA-107-3p and miRNA-122-5p) was significantly reduced in the liver of rats treated with resveratrol (Table 2). When protein expression of the target genes for these miRNAs was measured, we observed a significant reduction in SREBP1 ($p < 0.05$) and a significant increase in CPT1a ($p < 0.05$) in resveratrol-treated rats (Figures 3A and 4). No changes were found in FAS protein levels (Figure 3B).

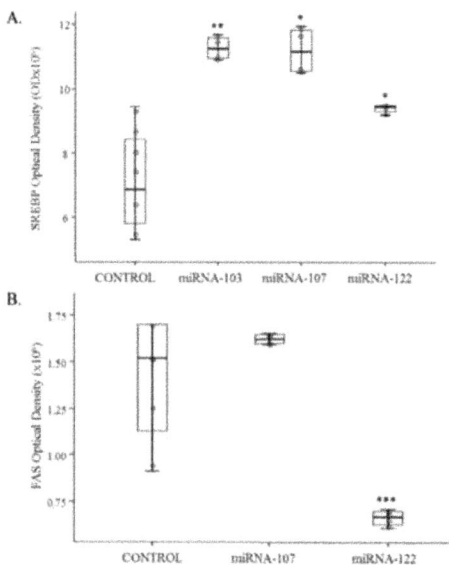

Figure 1. Protein expression of SREBP1 (**A**) and FAS (**B**) in AML12 control cells ($n = 6$) and AML12 cells over-expressing mmu-miRNA-103-3p, mmu-miRNA-107-3p and mmu-miR-122-5p ($n = 6$). Scatter dot plots including median and standard deviation were expressed as optical density. Comparisons between each treatment and the controls were analysed by Student's *t*-test * $p < 0.05$, ** $p < 0.01$, *** $p < 0.001$. SREBP1: sterol regulatory element-binding protein 1, FAS: fatty acid synthase; AML12: alpha mouse liver 12.

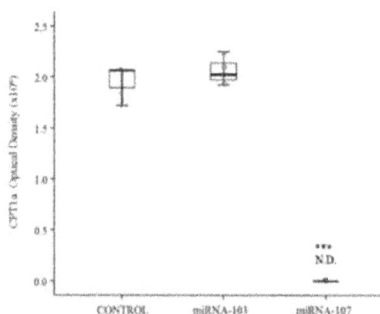

Figure 2. Protein expression of CPT1a in AML12 control cells ($n = 6$) and AML12 cells over-expressing mmu-miRNA-103-3p and mmu-miRNA-107-3p ($n = 6$). Scatter dot plots including median and standard deviation were expressed as optical density. Comparisons between each treatment and the controls were analysed by Student's *t*-test. Coomassie Blue staining was used as protein loading control. ND: not detectable. CPT1a: carnitine palmitoyltransferase 1a; AML12: alpha mouse liver 12.

Table 2. The gene expression fold change of miRNA-103, miRNA-107 and miRNA-122 in the liver of rats fed an obesogenic diet supplemented with resveratrol (Resveratrol group) or not (Control group) for 6 weeks ($n = 8$).

miRNA	Fold Change (Resveratrol vs. Control)	p
miR-103	−2.49	<0.01
miR-107	−2.08	<0.05
miR-122	−2.59	<0.01

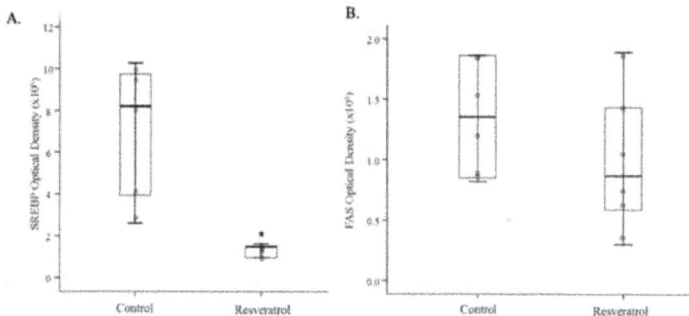

Figure 3. Protein expression of SREBP1 (**A**) and FAS (**B**) in the liver of rats fed an obesogenic diet supplemented with resveratrol (Resveratrol group) or not (Control group) for 6 weeks ($n = 8$). Scatter dot plots including median and standard deviation were expressed as optical density. * $p < 0.05$. Coomassie Blue staining was used as protein loading control for SREBP1 and β-actin for FAS. SREBP1: sterol regulatory element-binding protein 1, FAS: fatty acid synthase.

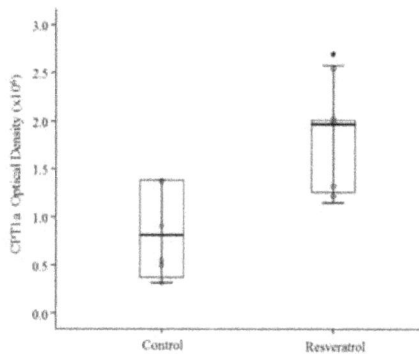

Figure 4. Protein expression of CPT1a in the liver of rats fed an obesogenic diet supplemented with resveratrol (Resveratrol group) or not (Control group) for 6 weeks ($n = 8$). Scatter dot plots including median and standard deviation were expressed as optical density. * $p < 0.05$. Coomassie Blue staining was used as protein loading control. CPT1a: carnitine palmitoyltransferase 1a

4. Discussion

As indicated in the Introduction, in a previous study we had observed that resveratrol was able to partially prevent liver steatosis induced by an obesogenic diet. We found a significant increase in the activity of CPT1a, a rate-limiting enzyme in fatty acid oxidation, in the liver of rats treated with resveratrol, without changes in FAS activity [20]. The present study helps us to gain more insight into the effect of resveratrol on the regulation of these two enzymes.

As far as the lipogenic pathway is concerned, miRecords data base showed that *srebf1* was a predicted target gene for miRNA-103-3p and miRNA-107-3p and *fasn* for miRNA-122-5p. In addition, Iliopoulos et al. [32] showed that the up-regulation of miRNA-122 induced the increased protein expression of SREBP1. Taking into account that miRNA are negative regulators of protein translation and that no miRNA-122-5p binding sites are found in the 3'UTR or the coding region of this gene, the authors suggested that miRNA-122 could regulate other genes that, in turn, could affect the transcription of *srebf1*. They concluded that *srebf1* was an indirect target gene for miRNA-122, but they did not describe the intermediate steps in the signaling cascade that led to the up-regulation of SREBP1. Later on, Shibata et al. [31] reported that silencing miRNA-122 led to decreased SOCS3 expression, which in turn increased STAT3 expression. Therefore, SREBP1 was negatively regulated by STAT3 and, consequently, a decrease in miRNA-122 induced a reduction in SREBP1 expression. In order to obtain more scientific support concerning the involvement of these three miRNAs in SREBP1 regulation, in the present study we over-expressed these miRNAs in AML12 hepatocytes. In all the three cases we observed a significant increase in SREBP1 protein expression.

In rats treated with resveratrol, we found a significantly decreased expression of miRNA-103-3p, miRNA-107-3p and miRNA-122-5p, which was paralleled by a significant decrease in SREBP1 protein expression. As far as miRNA-122-5p is concerned, taking into account the results of our transfection study, and bearing in mind the results reported by Iliopoulos et al. and Shibata et al. [31,32], it can be proposed that resveratrol decreases the protein expression of the transcription factor SREBP1 indirectly via miRNA-122-5p.

With regard to miRNA-103-3p and miRNA-107-3p, as indicated before in the Discussion section, computational analysis (miRecords) revealed complementarity between these miRNAs and the 3'UTR region of *srebf1*, suggesting that it can be a direct target gene. Usually, miRNAs regulate gene transcription in a negative way, which is to say that they inhibit this process. However, in some cases, the transcription of the RNAs is positively regulated and thus, the up-regulation of some miRNAs increases mRNA levels of their targets [35]. In our in vitro study, the over-expression of miRNA-103-3p and miRNA-107-3p in hepatocytes led to an increased expression of SREBP1, suggesting that in fact they were positive regulators. In the in vivo study, resveratrol induced the down-regulation of miRNA-103-3p and miRNA-107-3p in the liver, which was accompanied by a reduced expression of SREBP1. Taking all that into account, it may be said that miRNA-103-3p and miRNA-107-3p are involved as positive regulators in the effects of this polyphenol on SREBP protein expression [35].

As shown in Table 1, *fasn* was a predicted target gene only for miRNA-122-5p. Bhatia et al. [30] transfected HepG2 hepatocytes with miRNA-107 at various doses and they observed that, using the most common dose in transfection studies (25 nM), no changes in FAS protein expression were observed. When we measured FAS protein expression, we found no change in resveratrol-treated rats. This result is in good accordance with the lack of change in FAS activity observed in our previous study addressed to this cohort of rats. However, it was somewhat surprising because *fasn* is, according to the miRecords data base, a predicted target gene for miRNA-122-5p, which was reduced by resveratrol, and in fact our transfection experiment showed that the over-expression of miRNA-122-5p induced a significant reduction in FAS protein expression. Consequently, increased FAS expression should be expected. On the other hand, SREBP1, which is a transcription factor that regulates FAS, was reduced in resveratrol-treated rats. Thus, it could be hypothesized that the increase in FAS protein expression expected as a consequence of miRNA-122-5p down-regulation could be compensated by the decrease expected due to the reduction in SREBP1.

According to the miRecords data base, *cpt1a* is a predicted target gene for miRNA-103-3p and miRNA-107-3p. In cultured hepatocytes, we observed that only those over-expressing miRNA-107-3p showed the down-regulation of CPT1a protein expression, suggesting that in fact *cpt1a* is a real target gene for miRNA-107-3p, but not for miRNA-103-3p. In our in vivo experiment, rats treated with resveratrol showed decreased miRNA-107-3p expression and increased CPT1a protein expression. All in all, these results suggest that the increase induced by resveratrol in CPT1a protein expression, which is involved in the liver delipidating effects of this polyphenol, was mediated by a reduction in miRNA-107-3p expression.

5. Conclusions

The present study provides new evidence showing that *srebf1* is a target gene for miRNA-103-3p and miRNA-107-3p and *cpt1a* a target gene for miRNA-107-3p. Furthermore, the reduction in liver steatosis induced by resveratrol under our experimental conditions is mediated, at least in part, by increased CPT1a protein expression and activity, via a decrease in miRNA-107-3p expression.

Supplementary Materials: The following are available online at www.mdpi.com/2072-6643/9/4/360/s1, Figure S1: Diagram of the work-plan for the in vivo study.

Acknowledgments: This study was supported by grants from the Ministerio de Economía y Competitividad (AGL-2015-65719-FEDER-UE), Instituto de Salud Carlos III (CIBERobn), Government of the Basque Country (IT-572-13) and University of the Basque Country (UPV/EHU) (ELDUNANOTEK UFI11/32). A. Gracia is a PhD fellowship from the Ministerio de Economía y Competitividad.

Author Contributions: A.G., J.M. and M.G. revised the literature. A.G. (PhD student) measured microRNA expressions and revised the miRecords database. AG and IE performed the in vitro experiments. A.G. and J.M. carried out the Western blot analysis in in vivo and in vitro samples. A.F.Q. and M.P.P. designed the experiment. M.P.P. wrote the manuscript. All authors revised and approved the final manuscript.

Conflicts of Interest: The authors declare no competing financial interest.

Abbreviations

3′UTR	3′ untraslated regions
BCA	bicinchoninic acid
CPT1a	carnitine palmitoyltransferase 1a
FAS	fatty acid synthase
FBS	fetal bovine serum
miRNA	microRNA
mRNA	messenger RNA
SREBF1	sterol regulatory element binding factor 1
SREBP1	sterol regulatory element binding protein 1

References

1. Browning, J.D.; Szczepaniak, L.S.; Dobbins, R.; Nuremberg, P.; Horton, J.D.; Cohen, J.C.; Grundy, S.M.; Hobbs, H.H. Prevalence of hepatic steatosis in an urban population in the united states: Impact of ethnicity. *Hepatology* **2004**, *40*, 1387–1395. [CrossRef] [PubMed]
2. Bhatt, H.B.; Smith, R.J. Fatty liver disease in diabetes mellitus. *Hepatobiliary Surg. Nutr.* **2015**, *4*, 101–108. [PubMed]
3. Zivkovic, A.M.; German, J.B.; Sanyal, A.J. Comparative review of diets for the metabolic syndrome: Implications for nonalcoholic fatty liver disease. *Am. J. Clin. Nutr.* **2007**, *86*, 285–300. [PubMed]
4. Papandreou, D.; Andreou, E. Role of diet on non-alcoholic fatty liver disease: An updated narrative review. *World J. Hepatol.* **2015**, *7*, 575–582. [CrossRef] [PubMed]
5. Langcake, P.; Pryce, R.J. The production of resveratrol by vitis vinifera and other members of the vitaceae as a response to infection or injury. *Physiol. Plant Pathol.* **1976**, *9*, 77–86. [CrossRef]
6. Macarulla, M.T.; Alberdi, G.; Gómez, S.; Tueros, I.; Bald, C.; Rodríguez, V.M.; Martínez, J.A.; Portillo, M.P. Effects of different doses of resveratrol on body fat and serum parameters in rats fed a hypercaloric diet. *J. Physiol. Biochem.* **2009**, *65*, 369–376. [CrossRef] [PubMed]
7. Aguirre, L.; Portillo, M.P.; Hijona, E.; Bujanda, L. Effects of resveratrol and other polyphenols in hepatic steatosis. *World J. Gastroenterol.* **2014**, *20*, 7366–7380. [CrossRef] [PubMed]
8. Arias, N.; Macarulla, M.T.; Aguirre, L.; Miranda, J.; Portillo, M.P. Liver delipidating effect of a combination of resveratrol and quercetin in rats fed an obesogenic diet. *J. Physiol. Biochem.* **2015**, *71*, 569–576. [CrossRef]

9. Timmers, S.; Konings, E.; Bilet, L.; Houtkooper, R.H.; van de Weijer, T.; Goossens, G.H.; Hoeks, J.; van der Krieken, S.; Ryu, D.; Kersten, S.; et al. Calorie restriction-like effects of 30 days of resveratrol supplementation on energy metabolism and metabolic profile in obese humans. *Cell Metab.* **2011**, *14*, 612–622. [CrossRef] [PubMed]

10. Faghihzadeh, F.; Adibi, P.; Rafiei, R.; Hekmatdoost, A. Resveratrol supplementation improves inflammatory biomarkers in patients with nonalcoholic fatty liver disease. *Nutr. Res.* **2014**, *34*, 837–843. [CrossRef] [PubMed]

11. Baur, J.A.; Sinclair, D.A. Therapeutic potential of resveratrol: The in vivo evidence. *Nat. Rev. Drug Discov.* **2006**, *5*, 493–506. [CrossRef] [PubMed]

12. Fernández-Hernando, C.; Suárez, Y.; Rayner, K.J.; Moore, K.J. Micrornas in lipid metabolism. *Curr. Opin. Lipidol.* **2011**, *22*, 86–92. [CrossRef] [PubMed]

13. Arner, P.; Kulyté, A. Microrna regulatory networks in human adipose tissue and obesity. *Nat. Rev. Endocrinol.* **2015**, *11*, 276–288. [CrossRef] [PubMed]

14. Ha, M.; Kim, V.N. Regulation of microrna biogenesis. *Nat. Rev. Mol. Cell Biol.* **2014**, *15*, 509–524. [CrossRef] [PubMed]

15. Vickers, K.C.; Palmisano, B.T.; Shoucri, B.M.; Shamburek, R.D.; Remaley, A.T. Micrornas are transported in plasma and delivered to recipient cells by high-density lipoproteins. *Nat. Cell Biol.* **2011**, *13*, 423–433. [CrossRef] [PubMed]

16. Baselga-Escudero, L.; Arola-Arnal, A.; Pascual-Serrano, A.; Ribas-Latre, A.; Casanova, E.; Salvadó, M.J.; Arola, L.; Blade, C. Chronic administration of proanthocyanidins or docosahexaenoic acid reverses the increase of miR-33a and miR-122 in dyslipidemic obese rats. *PLoS ONE* **2013**, *8*, e69817. [CrossRef] [PubMed]

17. Baselga-Escudero, L.; Blade, C.; Ribas-Latre, A.; Casanova, E.; Suárez, M.; Torres, J.L.; Salvadó, M.J.; Arola, L.; Arola-Arnal, A. Resveratrol and egcg bind directly and distinctively to miR-33a and miR-122 and modulate divergently their levels in hepatic cells. *Nucleic Acids Res.* **2014**, *42*, 882–892. [CrossRef] [PubMed]

18. Baselga-Escudero, L.; Pascual-Serrano, A.; Ribas-Latre, A.; Casanova, E.; Salvadó, M.J.; Arola, L.; Arola-Arnal, A.; Bladé, C. Long-term supplementation with a low dose of proanthocyanidins normalized liver miR-33a and miR-122 levels in high-fat diet-induced obese rats. *Nutr. Res.* **2015**, *35*, 337–345. [CrossRef] [PubMed]

19. Joven, J.; Espinel, E.; Rull, A.; Aragonès, G.; Rodríguez-Gallego, E.; Camps, J.; Micol, V.; Herranz-López, M.; Menéndez, J.A.; Borrás, I.; et al. Plant-derived polyphenols regulate expression of mirna paralogs miR-103/107 and miR-122 and prevent diet-induced fatty liver disease in hyperlipidemic mice. *Biochim. Biophys. Acta* **2012**, *1820*, 894–899. [CrossRef] [PubMed]

20. Alberdi, G.; Rodríguez, V.M.; Macarulla, M.T.; Miranda, J.; Churruca, I.; Portillo, M.P. Hepatic lipid metabolic pathways modified by resveratrol in rats fed an obesogenic diet. *Nutrition* **2013**, *29*, 562–567. [CrossRef] [PubMed]

21. Heneghan, H.M.; Miller, N.; Kerin, M.J. Role of micrornas in obesity and the metabolic syndrome. *Obes. Rev.* **2010**, *11*, 354–361. [CrossRef] [PubMed]

22. Wilfred, B.R.; Wang, W.X.; Nelson, P.T. Energizing mirna research: A review of the role of mirnas in lipid metabolism, with a prediction that miR-103/107 regulates human metabolic pathways. *Mol. Genet. Metab.* **2007**, *91*, 209–217. [CrossRef] [PubMed]

23. Trajkovski, M.; Hausser, J.; Soutschek, J.; Bhat, B.; Akin, A.; Zavolan, M.; Heim, M.H.; Stoffel, M. MicroRNAs 103 and 107 regulate insulin sensitivity. *Nature* **2011**, *474*, 649–653. [CrossRef] [PubMed]

24. Park, J.H.; Ahn, J.; Kim, S.; Kwon, D.Y.; Ha, T.Y. Murine hepatic mirnas expression and regulation of gene expression in diet-induced obese mice. *Mol. Cells* **2011**, *31*, 33–38. [CrossRef] [PubMed]

25. Esau, C.; Davis, S.; Murray, S.F.; Yu, X.X.; Pandey, S.K.; Pear, M.; Watts, L.; Booten, S.L.; Graham, M.; McKay, R.; et al. MiR-122 regulation of lipid metabolism revealed by in vivo antisense targeting. *Cell Metab.* **2006**, *3*, 87–98. [CrossRef] [PubMed]

26. Miranda, J.; Portillo, M.P.; Madrid, J.A.; Arias, N.; Macarulla, M.T.; Garaulet, M. Effects of resveratrol on changes induced by high-fat feeding on clock genes in rats. *Br. J. Nutr.* **2013**, *110*, 1421–1428. [CrossRef] [PubMed]

27. Gracia, A.; Miranda, J.; Fernández-Quintela, A.; Eseberri, I.; Garcia-Lacarte, M.; Milagro, F.I.; Martínez, J.A.; Aguirre, L.; Portillo, M.P. Involvement of miR-539-5p in the inhibition of de novo lipogenesis induced by resveratrol in white adipose tissue. *Food Funct.* **2016**, *7*, 1680–1688. [CrossRef] [PubMed]

28. Livak, K.J.; Schmittgen, T.D. Analysis of relative gene expression data using real-time quantitative PCR and the $2^{-\Delta\Delta CT}$ method. *Methods* **2001**, *25*, 402–408. [CrossRef] [PubMed]

29. Xiao, F.; Zuo, Z.; Cai, G.; Kang, S.; Gao, X.; Li, T. Mirecords: An integrated resource for microRNA-target interactions. *Nucleic Acids Res.* **2009**, *37*, D105–D110. [CrossRef] [PubMed]

30. Bhatia, H.; Verma, G.; Datta, M. MiR-107 orchestrates er stress induction and lipid accumulation by post-transcriptional regulation of fatty acid synthase in hepatocytes. *Biochim. Biophys. Acta* **2014**, *1839*, 334–343. [CrossRef] [PubMed]

31. Shibata, C.; Kishikawa, T.; Otsuka, M.; Ohno, M.; Yoshikawa, T.; Takata, A.; Yoshida, H.; Koike, K. Inhibition of microRNA122 decreases SREBP1 expression by modulating suppressor of cytokine signaling 3 expression. *Biochem. Biophys. Res. Commun.* **2013**, *438*, 230–235. [CrossRef] [PubMed]

32. Iliopoulos, D.; Drosatos, K.; Hiyama, Y.; Goldberg, I.J.; Zannis, V.I. MicroRNA-370 controls the expression of microRNA-122 and cpt1alpha and affects lipid metabolism. *J. Lipid Res.* **2010**, *51*, 1513–1523. [CrossRef] [PubMed]

33. Aguirre, L.; Hijona, E.; Macarulla, M.T.; Gracia, A.; Larrechi, I.; Bujanda, L.; Hijona, L.; Portillo, M.P. Several statins increase body and liver fat accumulation in a model of metabolic syndrome. *J. Physiol. Pharmacol.* **2013**, *64*, 281–288. [PubMed]

34. Alberdi, G.; Rodríguez, V.M.; Miranda, J.; Macarulla, M.T.; Arias, N.; Andrés-Lacueva, C.; Portillo, M.P. Changes in white adipose tissue metabolism induced by resveratrol in rats. *Nutr. Metab.* **2011**, *8*, 29. [CrossRef] [PubMed]

35. Lin, X.; Luo, J.; Zhang, L.; Zhu, J. Micrornas synergistically regulate milk fat synthesis in mammary gland epithelial cells of dairy goats. *Gene Expr.* **2013**, *16*, 1–13. [CrossRef] [PubMed]

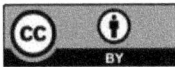

nutrients

MDPI

Article

Genistein Supplementation and Cardiac Function in Postmenopausal Women with Metabolic Syndrome: Results from a Pilot Strain-Echo Study

Cesare de Gregorio [1], Herbert Marini [1], Angela Alibrandi [2], Antonino Di Benedetto [1], Alessandra Bitto [1], Elena Bianca Adamo [3], Domenica Altavilla [4], Concetta Irace [5], Giacoma Di Vieste [1], Diego Pancaldo [6], Roberta Granese [4], Marco Atteritano [1], Salvatore Corrao [7,8], Giuseppe Licata [7], Francesco Squadrito [1] and Vincenzo Arcoraci [1,*]

[1]   Department of Clinical and Experimental Medicine, University of Messina, 98100 Messina, Italy; cdegregorio@unime.it (C.d.G.); hrmarini@unime.it (H.M.); adibenedetto@unime.it (A.D.B.); abitto@unime.it (A.B.); jackydv@hotmail.it (G.D.V.); matteritano@unime.it (M.A.); fsquadrito@unime.it (F.S.)
[2]   Department of Economics, Business, Environmental Science and Quantitative Methodologies, University of Messina, 98100 Messina, Italy; aalibrandi@unime.it
[3]   Department of Experimental, Specialized Medical and Surgical and Odonto-stomatological Sciences, University of Messina, 98100 Messina, Italy; elenabianca.adamo@unime.it
[4]   Department of Pediatric, Gynecological, Microbiological, and Biomedical Sciences, University of Messina, 98100 Messina, Italy; daltavilla@unime.it (D.A.); roberta.granese@unime.it (R.G.)
[5]   Department of Clinical and Experimental Medicine, University Magna Græcia, 88100 Catanzaro, Italy; irace@unicz.it
[6]   Department of Cardiology, SS. Annunziata Hospital, 12038 Savigliano (CN), Italy; pancaldodiego@libero.it
[7]   Centre of Research for Effectiveness and Appropriateness in Medicine (C.R.E.A.M.), Di.Bi.M.I.S., University of Palermo, 90127 Palermo, Italy; s.corrao@tiscali.it (S.C.); licatag@unipa.it (G.L.)
[8]   Department of Internal Medicine, National Relevance and High Specialization Hospital Trust ARNAS Civico, Di Cristina, Benfratelli, 90127 Palermo, Italy
*   Correspondence: Vincenzo.Arcoraci@unime.it; Tel.: +39-90-221-3994

Received: 21 April 2017; Accepted: 31 May 2017; Published: 7 June 2017

Abstract: Genistein, a soy-derived isoflavone, may improve cardiovascular risk profile in postmenopausal women with metabolic syndrome (MetS), but few literature data on its cardiac effects in humans are available. The aim of this sub-study of a randomized double-blind case-control study was to analyze the effect on cardiac function of one-year genistein dietary supplementation in 22 post-menopausal patients with MetS. Participants received 54 mg/day of genistein ($n = 11$) or placebo ($n = 11$) in combination with a Mediterranean-style diet and regular exercise. Left ventricular (LV) systolic function was assessed as the primary endpoint, according to conventional and strain-echocardiography measurements. Also, left atrial (LA) morphofunctional indices were investigated at baseline and at the final visit. Results were expressed as median with interquartile range (IQ). A significant improvement of LV ejection fraction (20.3 (IQ 12.5) vs. −1.67 (IQ 24.8); $p = 0.040$)), and LA area fractional change (11.1 (IQ 22.6) vs. 2.8 (9.5); $p = 0.034$)) were observed in genistein patients compared to the controls, following 12 months of treatment. In addition, body surface area indexed LA systolic volume and peak LA longitudinal strain significantly changed from basal to the end of the study in genistein-treated patients. One-year supplementation with 54 mg/day of pure genistein improved both LV ejection fraction and LA remodeling and function in postmenopausal women with MetS.

Keywords: genistein; metabolic syndrome; menopause; cardiac function; echocardiography

1. Introduction

Estrogen favorably influences calcium homeostasis, serum lipid levels, blood pressure control, inflammatory status, and vascular reactivity in women [1–5]. Data from Italian and other European registries indicate that postmenopausal women presenting with traits of metabolic syndrome (MetS), mostly diabetes mellitus (DM) and hyperlipemia, are at high risk of cardiovascular (CV) events [1,6,7]. Moreover, the use of lipid-lowering therapy is strongly influenced by reimbursement criteria revision, and the female gender was identified as a patient-related predictor of low adherence [8–10]. The advantages of estrogen supplementation are preserved in early menopause, failing to maintain cardiovascular protection, thus further therapeutic options continue to be studied [11–13]. Genistein aglycone (hereinafter referred to as genistein) is a soy isoflavone, which has progressively gained clinical consideration for the management of postmenopausal symptoms. Its molecular structure resembles that of 17β–estradiol and binds the same estrogen-receptors in a dose-dependent manner. Regular supplementation in combination with a Mediterranean-style diet, regular exercise, and medical therapy improve CV risk, endothelial function, and vascular reactivity in MetS women, although, to date, very little data are available concerning the effect of genistein on heart function [12,14–18].

The aim of this study was therefore to investigate whether genistein therapy might influence heart function in postmenopausal patients with MetS.

2. Materials and Methods

2.1. Design and Setting

A group of postmenopausal women, affected by type-2 DM and free from previous CV events, was enrolled from the population of postmenopausal women referred to the Department of Clinical and Experimental Medicine (University Hospital, Messina, Italy) for MetS. All patients were of Caucasian origin. This study was planned as a sub-study aimed to investigate the influence of genistein on heart function, from the original randomized multicenter clinical trial (clinicaltrials.gov registration NCT00541710) managed in collaboration with the University of Palermo (Palermo, Italy) and the University of Magna Graecia (Catanzaro, Italy) [16]. All patients gave written informed consent and the Ethical Committee of the University Hospital of Palermo approved the protocol of this study (approval number: RODA-12254).

Diagnosis of MetS was made considering the presence of at least three criteria among those provided by the modified US National Cholesterol Education Program Adult Treatment Panel III [19], as follows: (a) waist circumference >88 cm; (b) triglycerides >8.3 mmol/L or on drug treatment for elevated triglycerides; (c) high-density lipoprotein cholesterol (HDL-C) <2.8 mmol/L or on drug treatment for reduced HDL-C; (d) type-2 DM, according to current guidelines [20]; (e) blood pressure >130/90 mm Hg or on anti-hypertensive therapy. Criteria for menopause included: absence of menstrual period in the preceding year, follicle-stimulating hormone level >50 IU/L, and 17β-estradiol serum level ≤100 pmol/L (≤27 pg/mL) [2,3].

Family history, physical examination, measurement of body surface area (BSA, m^2), waist circumference (cm) and body mass index (BMI, kg/m^2), routine laboratory sampling (fasting glucose, total cholesterol, HDL-C, low-density lipoprotein cholesterol (LDL-C), triglyceride levels), fasting serum insulin, and the insulin resistance index by the homeostasis model assessment for insulin resistance (HOMA-IR) were carried out at baseline, 6 months, and 12 months of therapy. Visfatin, adiponectin, and homocysteine (HCY) serum levels were also evaluated, as previously described [16].

Patients with a previous or current cardiovascular event, renal or hepatic failure, coagulopathy, cancer, use of sex hormones or estrogen receptor modulators, steroids, long term treatment with non-steroidal anti-inflammatory drugs, alcohol abuse, or those who smoked more than two cigarettes per day were excluded from the study.

Hypoglycaemic and/or anti-hypertensive drugs were continued during the study period, if required. Fasting glucose target <8.3 mmol/L and blood pressure ≤135/85 mm Hg were recommended to be achieved in all study participants.

Left ventricular (left ventricle, LV) systolic function was evaluated as the primary endpoint to analyze the effect of genistein on cardiac function. In particular, LV systolic function and left atrial (left atrium, LA) morphofunctional indices were investigated according to high-resolution strain-echocardiography imaging measurements.

2.2. Randomization

Patients from the original trial were assigned by using a computer–generated double–blind randomization sequence to receive genistein (genistein group) or placebo (control group) twice a day. Both tablets were supplied by Mastelli srl (Sanremo, Italy). The genistein daily dose was 54 mg and tablets were identical to the placebo in appearance and taste. Genistein serum levels were measured both at baseline and the final visit, as previously described [16,21]. Only the first 11 patients of each group underwent ultrasound studies, due to a budget reduction from the original proposal (Figure 1). Patients were enrolled according to the computer–generated double–blind randomization sequence, using the first randomization numbers for each group and maintaining the blinding of researchers directly involved in the study. Genistein and placebo were given for 12 months.

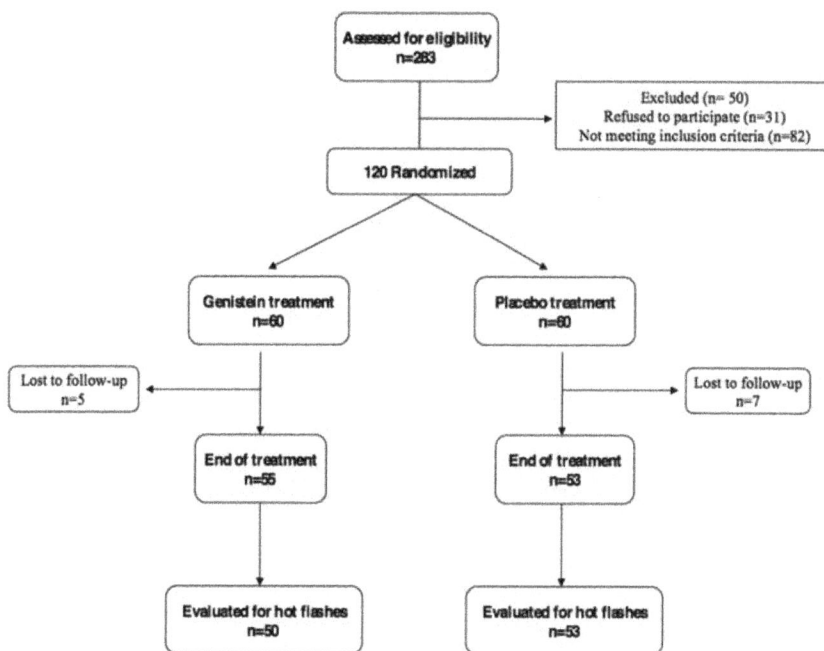

Figure 1. CONSORT diagram (Consolidated Standards of Reporting Trials diagram). The first 11 patients of each arm underwent ultrasound study.

Sample size was calculated in the parent study to provide 80% power to detect an expected absolute between-group difference in HOMA-IR of 20% after one year of treatment, assuming a two-tailed level of 0.05 as significant [16].

2.3. Diet and Exercise

Patients were all recommended to follow a Mediterranean-style dietary regimen (25–30% fat, less than 10% saturated fatty acids, 55–60% carbohydrates, and 15% protein), but further intake of soy products or supplements was discouraged.

Regular exercise, such as walking or biking for 80 to 100 min per week, was also suggested to participants and was recorded weekly for each patient. Dietary and treatment adherence was recorded at each visit.

2.4. Electrocardiogram and Echocardiogram

After performing a conventional 12-lead electrocardiogram (ECG), ultrasound study was carried out with a commercially available station (Esaote Mylab 30, Florence, Italy), equipped with an M–mode, two–dimensional color–Doppler and strain-feature analysis. Imaging was achieved by the conventional five trans-thoracic views (parasternal long-axis and short-axis, apical 2, 4, and 5 chambers). Quantitative findings were measured as the mean value of three consecutive beats. Simultaneous ECG monitoring was carried out in each patient. Left ventricular diameters, wall thickness, mass, systolic and diastolic volumes, ejection fraction (Simpson's rule biplane method), LA area and fractional area change [(systolic area minus diastolic area)/systolic area %], as well as LA and LV longitudinal shortening, were calculated according to recommendations of both the American and European Societies of Echocardiography [22]. Cardiac chamber volumes and mass were indexed to body surface area.

Left ventricular systolic function strongly related to ejection fraction. Moreover, LV shape, LV strain analysis, mitral annulus posterior systolic excursion (MAPSE), and longitudinal function (tissue S' velocity) were also evaluated.

We also investigated LV diastolic function by PW-Doppler, sampling the mitral inflow early and late diastolic velocities (E–wave and A–wave, respectively, and E/A ratio) and tissue–Doppler velocity both at basal septum level and lateral mitral annulus (E' velocity, A' velocity and E/E' ratio).

A dedicated strain software package (X–Strain TM by Esaote, Florence, Italy) was used for both LA and LV longitudinal strain [23]. Good quality imaging with an adequate frame rate (50–70 frames per second) was needed for this purpose. Data were digitally stored and analyzed by a Fourier equation that warrants heart motion periodicity–based accuracy. Strain curves were generated by a feature–tracking mode (Figure 2). Strain measurements were generated by processing the region of interest (several endocardial points from either parasternal short axis or apical 4-chamber view). Left ventricular longitudinal and circumferential strains are negative, whereas radial strain and peak atrial longitudinal strain (PALS) are positive values.

2.5. Statistical Analysis

Descriptive statistical analyses were performed to evaluate basal demographic and clinical characteristics. All results were expressed as medians with interquartile range (IQ) for continuous variables, and absolute and percentage frequencies for categorical variables.

All variables were evaluated at basal time and after 12 months of treatment, and percentage changes from baseline were evaluated at the end of the treatment in both genistein and placebo patients to determine the differences between groups.

The Kolmogorov-Smirnov test for normality was performed to evaluate normal distribution. Since some of the numerical variables were not normally distributed and the low sample number did not guarantee valid asymptotic results, a non-parametric approach was used.

The U Mann–Whitney test for independent values was applied to compare characteristics of the randomized subjects, according to treatment group. In addition, differences within group for paired measurements were tested by the Wilcoxon signed-rank test analysis.

Statistical analyses were performed using Statistical Package for Social Science (SPSS Statistics 17.0, Chicago, IL, USA) software for Windows package. $p < 0.05$ was considered statistically significant.

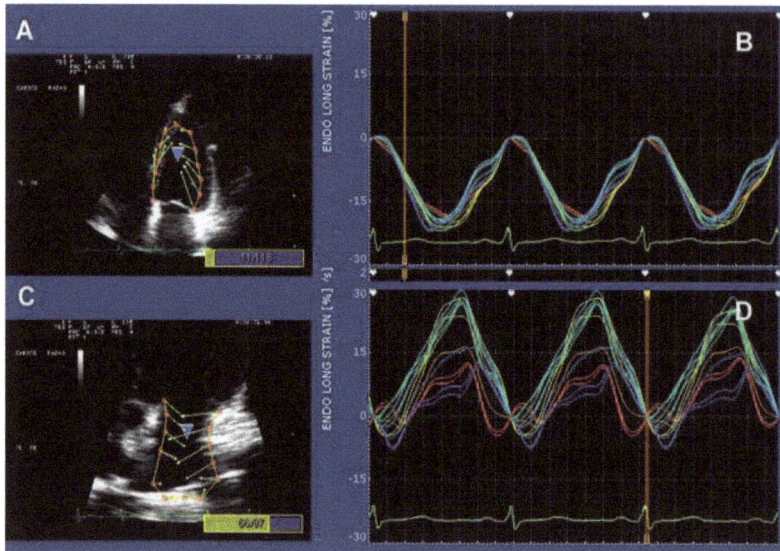

Figure 2. Strain–featured processing from the four–chamber apical view in a genistein patient. Vectors and curves are generated by processing 13 endocardial points on either the left ventricular (panels (**A**) and (**B**)) or the left atrial wall (panels (**C**) and (**D**)).

3. Results

3.1. Baseline Characteristics

A total of 22 patients, aged 55 (IQ 6) years, were enrolled from the main randomized controlled trial: 11 from the genistein and 11 from the control group, respectively. No differences in clinical, laboratory, or morphofunctional values between groups were shown at basal. Adherence to diet and exercise was similar between groups. All patients met the criteria for MetS diagnosis. Eighteen patients (82%), nine in each group, showed mild to moderate systemic hypertension with no differences in systolic-diastolic mean pressure between groups. Waist circumference >88 cm was measured in eight (73%) genistein patients and nine (82%) controls (ns). Five (45%) and six (54%) patients were obese in the genistein and placebo groups, respectively. The characteristics of patients in each group at basal and after 12 months are described in Table 1. Resting ECG was normal in all patients. None of patients were treated with glitazones. Beta blockers users were one in the genistein and two in the placebo group. Angiotensin-converting enzyme inhibitors or Angiotensin II receptor antagonist users were nine in the genistein and 10 in the placebo group.

3.2. Clinical and Laboratory Results at Follow-Up

All patients completed the study. Genistein levels increased from 15 nmol/L (95%CI 7.3–22.6) at baseline to 780 nmol/L (95%CI 741.7–818.3) at 12 months in treated subjects. BMI and waist values were similar at the end of follow-up in both groups. Resting blood pressure was on target in the majority of patients (90%) and no differences from basal to the end of follow-up or between groups were observed. Fasting glucose and insulin levels were similar at the beginning and at the end of follow-up in both groups. After 12 months of treatment, HOMA-IR ($p = 0.007$), visfatin ($p = 0.016$), and homocysteine (*p* = 0.034) significantly decreased in the genistein group compared to the controls. Conversely, serum adiponectin increased in the genistein, but not significantly, compared to the control group at the end of the treatment (Table 2). Changes in total cholesterol, LDL cholesterol, HDL cholesterol, and triglycerides at the end of the treatment were similar between groups.

Table 1. Clinical, laboratory, and morphofunctional values measured at baseline and after 12 months, stratified by treatment groups.

Parameters	Genistein			Controls		
	Basal Median (IQ)	12 Month Median (IQ)	# *p* Value	Basal Median (IQ)	12 Month Median (IQ)	# *p* Value
Body mass index (kg/m^2)	30.3 (5.0)	31.5 (7.0)	0.167	30.4 (11.2)	29.9 (10.8)	0.593
Waist circumference (cm)	105.0 (16.0)	104.0 (25.0)	0.798	99.0 (19.0)	98.0 (17.0)	0.438
Systolic blood pressure (mm Hg)	130.0 (38.0)	120.0 (40.0)	0.075	130.0 (30.0)	130.0 (20.0)	0.320
Diastolic blood pressure (mm Hg)	80.0 (15.0)	70.0 (30.0)	0.085	80.0 (10.0)	80.0 (0.0)	0.496
Fasting glucose (mmol/L)	7.1 (2.7)	7.0 (0.9)	0.099	7.8 (2.2)	6.5 (4.3)	0.959
Total cholesterol (mmol/L)	4.9 (1.4)	4.2 (0.7)	0.003	4.9 (1.1)	4.4 (1.1)	0.051
LDL-cholesterol (mmol/L)	2.9 (1.1)	1.6 (0.8)	0.009	2.8 (1.3)	2.5 (0.6)	0.120
HDL-cholesterol (mmol/L)	1.3 (0.7)	1.5 (0.6)	0.093	1.3 (0.4)	1.4 (0.6)	0.798
Triglycerides (mmol/L)	1.5 (0.9)	1.2 (0.8)	0.008	1.4 (0.8)	1.2 (0.7)	0.075
Insulin levels (nUI/L)	9.7 (7.8)	8.5 (5.3)	0.050	12.2 (12.3)	13.4 (17.9)	0.477
HOMA-IR	3.4 (1.5)	3.0 (1.7)	0.010	3.7 (4.8)	4.7 (5.2)	0.110
Visfatin (ng/mL)	3.1 (2.0)	1.3 (0.7)	0.016	2.1 (2.2)	2.4 (1.3)	0.477
Adiponectin (µg/mL)	6.2 (1.1)	8.0 (5.9)	0.003	5.3 (2.6)	6.2 (2.6)	0.021
Homocysteine (µmol/L)	13.3 (15.3)	10.0 (2.2)	0.003	17.5 (10.8)	14.2 (7.7)	0.091
Left Ventricle						
End-diastolic diameter (mm)	47.4 (9.2)	46.2 (8.2)	0.929	45.8 (7.7)	44.2 (5.1)	0.859
BSA-index mass (g/m^2)	82.9 (33.7)	73.0 (27.8)	0.657	78.6 (15.3)	84.7 (19.9)	1.000
Height-indexed mass (g/m$^{2.7}$)	38.0 (27.7)	44.6 (16.9)	0.328	41.1 (7.9)	39.2 (11.6)	0.859
End-diastolic volume (mL)	67.0 (14.9)	65.0 (26.0)	0.533	72.0 (23.0)	70.0 (28.0)	0.894
BSA-index end-diastolic vol. (mL/m^2)	40.3 (13.9)	37.9 (10.5)	0.328	37.2 (10.9)	39.2 (15.1)	0.790
End-diastolic shape	0.6 (0.09)	0.6 (0.1)	0.241	0.6 (0.08)	0.6 (0.1)	0.859
Ejection fraction	0.6 (0.04)	0.7 (0.05)	0.009	0.7 (0.11)	0.7 (0.10)	0.790
MAPSE (mm)	15.8 (4.1)	16.5 (1.3)	0.182	16.3 (4.8)	16.0 (4.9)	0.790
TDV Septal S'-wave (cm/s)	10.0 (3.0)	10.0 (2.0)	0.764	8.0 (4.0)	8.0 (3.0)	0.258
TDV Lateral S'-wave (cm/s)	10.0 (1.0)	12.0 (2.0)	0.022	10.0 (2.0)	11.0 (3.0)	0.305
Left Ventricular Diastolic Indices						
Mitral E/A velocity ratio	1.0 (0.23)	0.8 (0.33)	0.449	0.8 (0.44)	0.9 (0.28)	0.965
Mitral E-wave DT (ms)	204.0 (16.0)	216.0 (13.0)	0.075	223.0 (24.0)	242.0 (27.0)	0.059
E/E' velocity ratio	6.8 (1.0)	7.5 (2.6)	0.533	7.2 (3.5)	7.8 (3.3)	0.859
Left Ventricular Global Strain Measurements						
Radial Strain (%)	32.0 (10.9)	30.0 (15.0)	0.789	36.0 (9.5)	27.9 (12.3)	0.110
Circumferential Strain (%)	−21.0 (7.7)	−22.5 (4.9)	1.000	−23.5 (9.2)	−25.3 (5.0)	0.594
Longitudinal Strain (%)	−17.5 (1.5)	−17.3 (1.6)	0.328	−15.8 (4.7)	−18.8 (4.9)	0.213
Left Atrium						
BSA-indexed ES volume (mL/m^2)	29.5 (4.2)	22.6 (11.0)	0.041	32.3 (10.2)	27.5 (7.2)	0.248
Fractional area change (%)	37.0 (6.0)	41.0 (6.0)	0.035	35.0 (2.0)	35.0 (5.0)	0.510
PALS (%)	25.5 (5.8)	31.0 (8.5)	0.021	23.6 (10.2)	24.0 (6.5)	0.929

Values are expressed as medians with interquartile range (IQ); BSA, body surface area; DT, deceleration time; E/A, early/late diastolic velocity through the mitral inflow; E/E' velocity ratio, ratio between mitral E velocity and tissue E velocity; ES, end-systolic; HDL high-density lipoprotein; HOMA-IR, homeostasis model assessment for insulin resistance; LDL, low-density lipoprotein; MAPSE, mitral annular posterior systolic excursion; PALS, peak atrial longitudinal strain; S', tissue systolic velocity; TDV, tissue Doppler velocity; # *p*-values were calculated using the Wilcoxon rank test for each group, from baseline to the end of the treatment (12 months) as well as within-group comparisons.

3.3. Cardiac Morphofunctional Indices

Adequate ultrasound imaging was attained from each patient. Changes in cardiac morphology and function are described in Tables 1 and 2. Both LV ejection fraction (*p* = 0.040) and LA fractional area change (*p* = 0.034) significantly increased in the genistein patients compared the to controls during the treatment.

Additionally, LV ejection fraction ($p = 0.009$), tissue systolic wave velocity at lateral mitral annulus ($p = 0.022$), LA volume ($p = 0.041$), LA fractional area change ($p = 0.035$), and PALS ($p = 0.021$) also significantly improved in genistein-treated patients compared to basal, whereas no differences were shown in the control group. Advanced echo-strain analysis showed no relevant changes in LV radial, circumferential, and longitudinal global deformation (Table 2). No advanced LV diastolic dysfunction was observed. Grade 1–2 diastolic dysfunction was present at enrollment in two genistein patients and one control. However, at the end of follow-up, just one patient in the genistein group and four in the placebo group showed diastolic anomalies.

Table 2. Variations of clinical, laboratory values, and morphofunctional findings at Doppler echocardiography after 12 months of treatment: between groups comparison.

Parameters	Percentage Changes from Baseline after 12 Months Treatment		
	Genistein Median (IQ)	Controls Median (IQ)	# *p* Value
Body mass index (kg/m^2)	1.6 (5.7)	0.9 (4.5)	0.171
Waist circumference (cm)	0.0 (4.9)	0.0 (4.4)	0.898
Systolic blood pressure (mm Hg)	0.0 (11.8)	0.0 (12.2)	0.076
Diastolic blood pressure (mm Hg)	−8.3 (12.5)	0.0 (6.7)	0.057
Fasting glucose (mmol/L)	−7.1 (23.5)	−0.9 (18.3)	0.332
Total cholesterol (mmol/L)	−12.4 (14.9)	−15.5 (23.3)	0.748
LDL-cholesterol (mmol/L)	−18.1 (45.1)	−16.8 (43.2)	0.270
HDL-cholesterol (mmol/L)	16.3 (27.6)	−2.1 (15.6)	0.243
Triglycerides (mmol/L)	−12.5 (13.8)	−21.5 (56.6)	0.898
Insulin levels (nUI/L)	−21.5 (27.9)	1.7 (81.0)	0.193
HOMA-IR	−19.7 (39.0)	18.0 (71.2)	0.007
Visfatin (ng/mL)	−50.9 (73.2)	−7.0 (32.2)	0.016
Adiponectin (µg/mL)	29.4 (62.8)	12.6 (38.6)	0.088
Homocysteine (µmol/L)	−24.3 (34.4)	−8.1 (50.1)	0.034
Left Ventricle			
End-diastolic diameter (mm)	3.2 (14.7)	0.2 (26.5)	0.949
BSA-index mass (g/m^2)	2.9 (30.4)	10.5 (41.6)	0.748
Height-indexed mass (g/m$^{2.7}$)	16.3 (22.2)	−5.4 (45.1)	0.519
End-diastolic volume (mL)	−1.3 (45.5)	−7.8 (67.8)	0.898
BSA-index end-diastolic vol. (mL/m^2)	−0.4 (49.1)	7.0 (48.5)	1.000
End-diastolic shape	3.2 (5.8)	−1.6 (7.6)	0.606
Ejection fraction	20.3 (12.5)	−1.7 (24.8)	0.040
MAPSE (mm)	4.4 (38.0)	0.6 (26.4)	0.606
TDV Septal S′-wave (cm/s)	0.0 (26.5)	−12.5 (48.1)	0.332
TDV Lateral S′-wave (cm/s)	10.0 (9.1)	9.1 (31.3)	0.606
Left Ventricular Diastolic Indices			
Mitral E/A velocity ratio	−9.8 (34.8)	6.0 (56.8)	0.652
Mitral E-wave DT (ms)	10.0 (12.4)	6.0 (11.9)	0.748
E/E′ velocity ratio	6.4 (72.6)	3.9 (49.9)	0.748
Left Ventricular Global Strain Measurements			
Radial Strain (%)	12.6 (44.3)	−13.4 (35.1)	0.133
Circumferential Strain (%)	0.9 (30.9)	3.7 (38.9)	0.797
Longitudinal Strain (%)	−2.8 (11.3)	4.3 (24.9)	0.243
Left Atrium			
BSA-indexed ES volume (mL/m^2)	−22.6 (47.7)	−20.8 (61.1)	0.151
Fractional area change (%)	11.1 (22.6)	2.8 (9.5)	0.034
PALS (%)	13.3 (25.4)	−11.2 (51.3)	0.270

Values are expressed as medians with interquartile range (IQ); BSA, body surface area; DT, deceleration time; E/A, early/late diastolic velocity through the mitral inflow; E/E′ velocity ratio, ratio between mitral E velocity and tissue E velocity; ES, end-systolic; HDL high-density lipoprotein; HOMA-IR, homeostasis model assessment for insulin resistance; LDL, low-density lipoprotein; MAPSE, mitral annular posterior systolic excursion; PALS, peak atrial longitudinal strain; S′, tissue systolic velocity; TDV, tissue Doppler velocity; # *p*-values were calculated using the Wilcoxon rank test for each group, from baseline to the end of the treatment (12 months) as well as within-group comparisons.

3.4. Adverse Events and Side-Effects

No clinically relevant side effects, flushing, or palpitations were reported. Nobody experienced serious arrhythmias or cardiac symptoms.

4. Discussion

Recent findings indicate that approximately 25% of the USA population shows traits of MetS, and the constellation of symptoms becomes of clinical concern particularly in postmenopausal patients with DM and hyperlipemia, whose CV risk is higher than that in the general population. Moreover, low adherence to treatment with lipid-lowering drugs is particularly high in female patients, strongly influenced by reimbursement criteria revision, and educational programs in primary care result in challenging efficacy in reaching the clinical targets. [8,9,24,25]. As a consequence, the increasing prevalence of MetS over the last decade hinders the efforts of physicians to improve the CV risk profile through better glycaemic homeostasis [1,2,6,26].

Our group has previously recognized an improvement in the HOMA-IR and several markers of CV risk of MetS postmenopausal patients treated with genistein [14–16]. Furthermore, the present findings suggest an interesting impact of genistein treatment on cardiac function in this clinical setting [12].

Using the strain deformation analysis, the most advanced technique to discover early and subclinical LV impairment at the present time [23], our results suggest that one year of treatment with genistein at the dose of 54 mg/day did not worsen LV chamber size or function. On the contrary, genistein treatment improved LV ejection fraction. Such a gain in LV systolic function cannot be exclusively attributed to a direct genistein effect on myocardium, but could rather depend on several factors, including the improvement in adipokine serum levels. In addition, the lack of improvement in the control group emphasizes the efficacy of the treatment with genistein. Similarly, the improvement in the LA size and function has been limited to the genistein group. These patients showed a decrease in LA systolic volume index together with a raise in fractional area change and PALS, without changes in systo-diastolic blood pressure. This finding is particularly interesting since patients with DM and hypertension, or MetS, have an increased risk of atrial fibrillation and heart failure [27–29].

Therefore, the present study suggests that genistein could also reduce the LA afterload and potential dysfunction. In fact, hypertensive, diabetic, and overweight patients have an increased risk of atrial dysfunction. Significant changes in LA volume and longitudinal deformation might contribute to the reduction of LA dilatation, fibrosis, and the occurrence of atrial fibrillation, regardless of the loading conditions at the time of examination [27,28].

The cardioprotective effects of genistein could be partially justified by the improvement in the adipokine profile. Adiponectin increased significantly over the 12 months in both groups and the change was not significantly different between groups. Adiponectin promotes insulin-sensitizing effects and peripheral glucose use, as previously reported [16]. Low circulating levels of adiponectin were found in obese patients with type-2 DM, as well as in postmenopausal MetS women [30–33]. Adiponectin is a modulator of vascular remodeling, and low serum adiponectin levels are predictors of atherosclerosis and myocardial infarction, and are associated with higher incidence of cardiovascular events [34]. These effects are probably related to the anti-inflammatory action of adiponectin, in fact, it reduces the production of inflammatory cytokines and adhesion molecules in endothelial cells [35].

On the contrary, the pro-inflammatory visfatin was reduced by genistein after one year of treatment. Visfatin increase in type-2 DM patients was related to heart failure and acute coronary syndromes [36–39]; visfatin appears to mediate vascular endothelial inflammation by inducing the expression of adhesion molecules (VCAM-1 and ICAM-1) and pro-inflammatory cytokines such as IL-1β, IL-6, and TNF-α [40]. These effects on adipokines might explain the observed protective effect on myocardium. Genistein, by reducing HOMA-IR, may also decrease glucose–mediated cardiotoxicity, lowering glycated proteins and reactive oxygen species, which are involved in the pathogenesis of interstitial fibrosis in diabetic cardiomyopathy [41,42].

Among the pro-inflammatory factors, homocysteine, which has been suggested as an independent risk factor for endothelial dysfunction and atherosclerosis [43], was also reduced by genistein. Since homocysteine could indirectly impact cardiac function in women with MetS, its reduction in genistein-treated patients confirms our previous data obtained in healthy postmenopausal subjects [16] regarding the possible cardioprotective role of this isoflavone.

Despite the intriguing present results, some limitations of the study should be taken into account. Our results were obtained from a population without signs of cardiac dysfunction and all women were of Caucasian origin, thus we do not know if the same effects could be reproduced in different ethnic groups. The small sample size is a limitation of the present study and no definitive conclusions can be drawn from our proof of concept study. However, this study was able to demonstrate, for the first time, that genistein significantly improved cardiovascular function in postmenopausal women with metabolic syndrome. Accordingly, using this preliminary information, a future larger study expressly designed to evaluate the effect of genistein on cardiac function is encouraged.

In conclusion, our preliminary data suggest that a daily supplementation with 54 mg of pure genistein improves both LA remodeling and LV function in postmenopausal women with MetS.

Acknowledgments: This study was funded by Italian Ministry of University and Research (grant number 20073XZSR3).

Author Contributions: V.A., C.D.G., H.M., G.L., F.S. conceived and designed the experiments; C.D.G., H.M., A.D.B., C.I., G.D.V., S.C. performed the experiments; V.A., A.A., S.C. analyzed the data; M.A., R.G., E.A., D.P., A.B., D.A. contributed reagents/materials/analysis tools; V.A., C.D.G., F.S., A.B. wrote the paper. All authors approved the final version of the manuscript.

Conflicts of Interest: The authors declare no conflict of interest.

References

1. Giampaoli, S.; Stamler, J.; Donfrancesco, C.; Panico, S.; Vanuzzo, D.; Cesana, G.; Mancia, G.; Pilotto, L.; Mattiello, A.; Chiodini, P.; et al. The metabolic syndrome: A critical appraisal based on the cuore epidemiologic study. *Prev. Med.* **2009**, *48*, 525–531. [CrossRef] [PubMed]
2. Janssen, I.; Powell, L.H.; Crawford, S.; Lasley, B.; Sutton-Tyrrell, K. Menopause and the metabolic syndrome: The study of women's health across the nation. *Arch. Intern. Med.* **2008**, *168*, 1568–1575. [CrossRef] [PubMed]
3. Xing, D.; Nozell, S.; Chen, Y.F.; Hage, F.; Oparil, S. Estrogen and mechanisms of vascular protection. *Arterioscler. Thromb. Vasc. Biol.* **2009**, *29*, 289–295. [CrossRef] [PubMed]
4. Yang, X.P.; Reckelhoff, J.F. Estrogen, hormonal replacement therapy and cardiovascular disease. *Curr. Opin. Nephrol. Hypertens.* **2011**, *20*, 133–138. [CrossRef] [PubMed]
5. Caputi, A.P.; Arcoraci, V.; Benvenuti, C. Soy isoflavones, lactobacilli, vitamin d3 and calcium. Observational study in menopause. *G. Ital. Ostet. Ginecol.* **2006**, *28*, 212–221.
6. Bonora, E.; Targher, G.; Formentini, G.; Calcaterra, F.; Lombardi, S.; Marini, F.; Zenari, L.; Saggiani, F.; Poli, M.; Perbellini, S.; et al. The metabolic syndrome is an independent predictor of cardiovascular disease in type 2 diabetic subjects. Prospective data from the verona diabetes complications study. *Diabet. Med. J. Br. Diabet. Assoc.* **2004**, *21*, 52–58. [CrossRef]
7. Rexrode, K.M.; Manson, J.E.; Lee, I.M.; Ridker, P.M.; Sluss, P.M.; Cook, N.R.; Buring, J.E. Sex hormone levels and risk of cardiovascular events in postmenopausal women. *Circulation* **2003**, *108*, 1688–1693. [CrossRef] [PubMed]
8. Ferrajolo, C.; Arcoraci, V.; Sullo, M.G.; Rafaniello, C.; Sportiello, L.; Ferrara, R.; Cannata, A.; Pagliaro, C.; Tari, M.G.; Caputi, A.P.; et al. Pattern of statin use in southern italian primary care: Can prescription databases be used for monitoring long-term adherence to the treatment? *PLoS ONE* **2014**, *9*, e102146. [CrossRef] [PubMed]
9. Trifiro, G.; Alacqua, M.; Corrao, S.; Moretti, S.; Tari, D.U.; Galdo, M.; Caputi, A.P.; Arcoraci, V. Lipid-lowering drug use in italian primary care: Effects of reimbursement criteria revision. *Eur. J. Clin. Pharmacol.* **2008**, *64*, 619–625. [CrossRef] [PubMed]
10. Trifiro, G.; Alacqua, M.; Corrao, S.; Tari, M.; Arcoraci, V. Statins for the primary prevention of cardiovascular events in elderly patients: A picture from clinical practice without strong evidence from clinical trials. *J. Am. Geriatr. Soc.* **2008**, *56*, 175–177. [CrossRef] [PubMed]
11. Nilsson, S.; Gustafsson, J.A. Estrogen receptors: Therapies targeted to receptor subtypes. *Clin. Pharmacol. Ther.* **2011**, *89*, 44–55. [CrossRef] [PubMed]

12. Sbarouni, E.; Iliodromitis, E.K.; Zoga, A.; Vlachou, G.; Andreadou, I.; Kremastinos, D.T. The effect of the phytoestrogen genistein on myocardial protection, preconditioning and oxidative stress. *Cardiovasc. Drugs Ther. Spons. Int. Soc. Cardiovasc. Pharmacother.* **2006**, *20*, 253–258. [CrossRef] [PubMed]

13. Taylor, H.S.; Manson, J.E. Update in hormone therapy use in menopause. *J. Clin. Endocrinol. Metab.* **2011**, *96*, 255–264. [CrossRef] [PubMed]

14. Irace, C.; Marini, H.; Bitto, A.; Altavilla, D.; Polito, F.; Adamo, E.B.; Arcoraci, V.; Minutoli, L.; Di Benedetto, A.; Di Vieste, G.; et al. Genistein and endothelial function in postmenopausal women with metabolic syndrome. *Eur. J. Clin. Investig.* **2013**, *43*, 1025–1031. [CrossRef] [PubMed]

15. Marini, H.; Bitto, A.; Altavilla, D.; Burnett, B.P.; Polito, F.; Di Stefano, V.; Minutoli, L.; Atteritano, M.; Levy, R.M.; Frisina, N.; et al. Efficacy of genistein aglycone on some cardiovascular risk factors and homocysteine levels: A follow-up study. *Nutr. Metab. Cardiovasc. Dis. NMCD* **2010**, *20*, 332–340. [CrossRef] [PubMed]

16. Squadrito, F.; Marini, H.; Bitto, A.; Altavilla, D.; Polito, F.; Adamo, E.B.; D'Anna, R.; Arcoraci, V.; Burnett, B.P.; Minutoli, L.; et al. Genistein in the metabolic syndrome: Results of a randomized clinical trial. *J. Clin. Endocrinol. Metab.* **2013**, *98*, 3366–3374. [CrossRef] [PubMed]

17. Arcoraci, V.; Atteritano, M.; Squadrito, F.; D'Anna, R.; Marini, H.; Santoro, D.; Minutoli, L.; Messina, S.; Altavilla, D.; Bitto, A. Antiosteoporotic activity of genistein aglycone in postmenopausal women: Evidence from a post-hoc analysis of a multicenter randomized controlled trial. *Nutrients* **2017**, *9*. [CrossRef] [PubMed]

18. Bitto, A.; Granese, R.; Triolo, O.; Villari, D.; Maisano, D.; Giordano, D.; Altavilla, D.; Marini, H.; Adamo, E.B.; Nicotina, P.A.; et al. Genistein aglycone: A new therapeutic approach to reduce endometrial hyperplasia. *Phytomedicine* **2010**, *17*, 844–850. [CrossRef] [PubMed]

19. Grundy, S.M.; Cleeman, J.I.; Daniels, S.R.; Donato, K.A.; Eckel, R.H.; Franklin, B.A.; Gordon, D.J.; Krauss, R.M.; Savage, P.J.; Smith, S.C., Jr.; et al. Diagnosis and management of the metabolic syndrome: An american heart association/national heart, lung, and blood institute scientific statement. *Circulation* **2005**, *112*, 2735–2752. [CrossRef] [PubMed]

20. Task Force, M.; Ryden, L.; Grant, P.J.; Anker, S.D.; Berne, C.; Cosentino, F.; Danchin, N.; Deaton, C.; Escaned, J.; Hammes, H.P.; et al. Esc guidelines on diabetes, pre-diabetes, and cardiovascular diseases developed in collaboration with the easd: The task force on diabetes, pre-diabetes, and cardiovascular diseases of the european society of cardiology (esc) and developed in collaboration with the european association for the study of diabetes (easd). *Eur. Heart J.* **2013**, *34*, 3035–3087.

21. Bitto, A.; Burnett, B.P.; Polito, F.; Russo, S.; D'Anna, R.; Pillai, L.; Squadrito, F.; Altavilla, D.; Levy, R.M. The steady-state serum concentration of genistein aglycone is affected by formulation: A bioequivalence study of bone products. *Biomed. Res. Int.* **2013**, *2013*, 273498. [CrossRef] [PubMed]

22. Lang, R.M.; Bierig, M.; Devereux, R.B.; Flachskampf, F.A.; Foster, E.; Pellikka, P.A.; Picard, M.H.; Roman, M.J.; Seward, J.; Shanewise, J.; et al. Recommendations for chamber quantification. *Eur. J. Echocardiogr. J. Work. Group Echocardiogr. Eur. Soc. Cardiol.* **2006**, *7*, 79–108. [CrossRef] [PubMed]

23. Mor-Avi, V.; Lang, R.M.; Badano, L.P.; Belohlavek, M.; Cardim, N.M.; Derumeaux, G.; Galderisi, M.; Marwick, T.; Nagueh, S.F.; Sengupta, P.P.; et al. Current and evolving echocardiographic techniques for the quantitative evaluation of cardiac mechanics: Ase/eae consensus statement on methodology and indications endorsed by the japanese society of echocardiography. *Eur. J. Echocardiogr. J. Work. Group Echocardiogr. Eur. Soc. Cardiol.* **2011**, *12*, 167–205. [CrossRef] [PubMed]

24. Arcoraci, V.; Santoni, L.; Ferrara, R.; Furneri, G.; Cannata, A.; Sultana, J.; Moretti, S.; Di Luccio, A.; Tari, D.U.; Pagliaro, C.; et al. Effect of an educational program in primary care: The case of lipid control in cardio-cerebrovascular prevention. *Int. J. Immunopathol. Pharmacol.* **2014**, *27*, 351–363. [CrossRef] [PubMed]

25. Corrao, S.; Arcoraci, V.; Arnone, S.; Calvo, L.; Scaglione, R.; Di Bernardo, C.; Lagalla, R.; Caputi, A.P.; Licata, G. Evidence-based knowledge management: An approach to effectively promote good health-care decision-making in the information era. *Intern. Emerg. Med.* **2009**, *4*, 99–106. [CrossRef] [PubMed]

26. McCullough, A.J. Epidemiology of the metabolic syndrome in the USA. *J. Dig. Dis.* **2011**, *12*, 333–340. [CrossRef] [PubMed]

27. Li, S.H.; Yang, B.; Gong, H.P.; Tan, H.W.; Zhong, M.; Zhang, Y.; Zhang, W. Impaired atrial synchronicity in patients with metabolic syndrome associated with insulin resistance and independent of hypertension. *Hypertens. Res. Off. J. Jpn. Soc. Hypertens.* **2009**, *32*, 791–796. [CrossRef] [PubMed]

28. Lin, K.J.; Cho, S.I.; Tiwari, N.; Bergman, M.; Kizer, J.R.; Palma, E.C.; Taub, C.C. Impact of metabolic syndrome on the risk of atrial fibrillation recurrence after catheter ablation: Systematic review and meta-analysis. *J. Interv. Card. Electrophysiol. Int. J. Arrhythm. Pacing* **2014**, *39*, 211–223. [CrossRef] [PubMed]

29. Seo, J.M.; Park, T.H.; Lee, D.Y.; Cho, Y.R.; Baek, H.K.; Park, J.S.; Kim, M.H.; Kim, Y.D.; Choi, S.Y.; Lee, S.M.; et al. Subclinical myocardial dysfunction in metabolic syndrome patients without hypertension. *J. Cardiovasc. Ultrasound* **2011**, *19*, 134–139. [CrossRef] [PubMed]

30. Gil-Campos, M.; Canete, R.R.; Gil, A. Adiponectin, the missing link in insulin resistance and obesity. *Clin. Nutr.* **2004**, *23*, 963–974. [CrossRef] [PubMed]

31. Havel, P.J. Control of energy homeostasis and insulin action by adipocyte hormones: Leptin, acylation stimulating protein, and adiponectin. *Curr. Opin. Lipidol.* **2002**, *13*, 51–59. [CrossRef] [PubMed]

32. Northcott, J.M.; Yeganeh, A.; Taylor, C.G.; Zahradka, P.; Wigle, J.T. Adipokines and the cardiovascular system: Mechanisms mediating health and disease. *Can. J. Physiol. Pharmacol.* **2012**, *90*, 1029–1059. [CrossRef] [PubMed]

33. Rabe, K.; Lehrke, M.; Parhofer, K.G.; Broedl, U.C. Adipokines and insulin resistance. *Mol. Med.* **2008**, *14*, 741–751. [CrossRef] [PubMed]

34. Diaz-Melean, C.M.; Somers, V.K.; Rodriguez-Escudero, J.P.; Singh, P.; Sochor, O.; Llano, E.M.; Lopez-Jimenez, F. Mechanisms of adverse cardiometabolic consequences of obesity. *Curr. Atheroscler. Rep.* **2013**, *15*, 364. [CrossRef] [PubMed]

35. Ouchi, N.; Walsh, K. Cardiovascular and metabolic regulation by the adiponectin/c1q/tumor necrosis factor-related protein family of proteins. *Circulation* **2012**, *125*, 3066–3068. [CrossRef] [PubMed]

36. Bitto, A.; Arcoraci, V.; Alibrandi, A.; D'Anna, R.; Corrado, F.; Atteritano, M.; Minutoli, L.; Altavilla, D.; Squadrito, F. Visfatin correlates with hot flashes in postmenopausal women with metabolic syndrome: Effects of genistein. *Endocrine* **2017**, *55*, 899–906. [CrossRef] [PubMed]

37. Grzywocz, P.; Mizia-Stec, K.; Wybraniec, M.; Chudek, J. Adipokines and endothelial dysfunction in acute myocardial infarction and the risk of recurrent cardiovascular events. *J. Cardiovasc. Med.* **2015**, *16*, 37–44.

38. Romacho, T.; Sanchez-Ferrer, C.F.; Peiro, C. Visfatin/nampt: An adipokine with cardiovascular impact. *Med. Inflamm.* **2013**, *2013*, 946427. [CrossRef] [PubMed]

39. Straburzynska-Migaj, E.; Pilaczynska-Szczesniak, L.; Nowak, A.; Straburzynska-Lupa, A.; Sliwicka, E.; Grajek, S. Serum concentration of visfatin is decreased in patients with chronic heart failure. *Acta Biochim. Pol.* **2012**, *59*, 339–343. [PubMed]

40. Mattu, H.S.; Randeva, H.S. Role of adipokines in cardiovascular disease. *J. Endocrinol.* **2013**, *216*, T17–T36. [CrossRef] [PubMed]

41. Bugyei-Twum, A.; Advani, A.; Advani, S.L.; Zhang, Y.; Thai, K.; Kelly, D.J.; Connelly, K.A. High glucose induces smad activation via the transcriptional coregulator p300 and contributes to cardiac fibrosis and hypertrophy. *Cardiovasc. Diabetol.* **2014**, *13*, 89. [CrossRef] [PubMed]

42. Hintz, K.K.; Ren, J. Phytoestrogenic isoflavones daidzein and genistein reduce glucose-toxicity-induced cardiac contractile dysfunction in ventricular myocytes. *Endocr. Res.* **2004**, *30*, 215–223. [CrossRef] [PubMed]

43. Abraham, J.M.; Cho, L. The homocysteine hypothesis: Still relevant to the prevention and treatment of cardiovascular disease? *Clevel. Clin. J. Med.* **2010**, *77*, 911–918. [CrossRef] [PubMed]

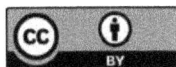

nutrients

MDPI

Article

Fruit Fiber Consumption Specifically Improves Liver Health Status in Obese Subjects under Energy Restriction

Irene Cantero [1,2], Itziar Abete [1,2,3], J. Ignacio Monreal [4,5], J. Alfredo Martinez [1,2,3,4,*] and M. Angeles Zulet [1,2,3,4]

1   Department of Nutrition, Food Science and Physiology, Faculty of Pharmacy and Nutrition,
    University of Navarra, 31008 Pamplona, Spain; icantero.1@alumni.unav.es (I.C.); iabetego@unav.es (I.A.);
    mazulet@unav.es (M.A.Z.)
2   Centre for Nutrition Research, Faculty of Pharmacy and Nutrition, University of Navarra,
    31008 Pamplona, Spain
3   CIBERObn, Physiopathology of obesity and nutrition, Instituto de Salud Carlos III, 28029 Madrid, Spain
4   Navarra Institute for Health Research (IdiSNA), 31008 Pamplona, Spain;
    jimonreal@unav.es or jimonreal@unav.es
5   Clinical Chemistry Department, University Clinic of Navarra, University of Navarra, 31008 Pamplona, Spain
*   Correspondence: jalfmtz@unav.es; Tel.: +34-948-42-56-00 (ext. 806317)

Received: 4 May 2017; Accepted: 22 June 2017; Published: 28 June 2017

Abstract: The prevalence of non-alcoholic-fatty-liver-disease (NAFLD) is associated with obesity, diabetes, and metabolic syndrome (MS). This study aimed to evaluate the influence of two energy-restricted diets on non-invasive markers and scores of liver damage in obese individuals with features of MS after six months of follow-up and to assess the role of fiber content in metabolic outcomes. Seventy obese individuals from the RESMENA (Reduction of Metabolic Syndrome in Navarra) study were evaluated at baseline and after six months of energy-restricted nutritional intervention (American Heart Association (AHA) and RESMENA dietary groups). Dietary records, anthropometrical data, body composition by dual energy X-ray absorptiometry (DXA), and routine laboratory measurements were analyzed by standardized methods. Regarding liver status, cytokeratin-18 fragments and several non-invasive scores of fatty liver were also assessed. The RESMENA strategy was a good and complementary alternative to AHA for the treatment of obesity-related comorbidities. Participants with higher insoluble fiber consumption (≥ 7.5 g/day) showed improvements in fatty liver index (FLI), hepatic steatosis index (HIS), and NAFLD liver fat score (NAFLD_LFS), while gamma-glutamyl transferase (GGT) and transaminases evidenced significant improvements as a result of fruit fiber consumption (≥ 8.8 g/day). Remarkably, a regression model evidenced a relationship between liver status and fiber from fruits. These results support the design of dietary patterns based on the consumption of insoluble fiber and fiber from fruits in the context of energy restriction for the management of obese patients suffering fatty liver disease.

Keywords: obesity; fatty liver disease; metabolic syndrome; insoluble fiber; fiber; AHA; RESMENA

1. Introduction

Non-alcoholic fatty liver disease (NAFLD) is a condition of hepatic steatosis in the absence of excessive alcohol consumption [1]. The spectrum of NAFLD ranges from simple steatosis to non-alcoholic steatohepatitis (NASH), which can lead to fibrosis and finally hepatocellular carcinoma [2]. As a consequence of the obesity epidemic, this liver pathology (NAFLD) is emerging as an important public health issue and is the most common cause of chronic liver disease in Western countries, with a prevalence of about 20–30% the general adult population [1]. The pathogenesis of

NAFLD is multifactorial and triggered by environmental factors such as unbalanced diets or/and overnutrition as well as by sedentary lifestyles [1]. Concerning the diagnosis of NAFLD, liver biopsy is considered the "gold standard" of steatosis, fibrosis, and cirrhosis. However, it is rarely performed because it is an invasive procedure with a significant degree of sampling error [2]. Thus, investigators are focusing on the design and application of non-invasive liver damage scores for the diagnosis and management of liver disease [3].

Nowadays, the treatment of NAFLD is based on lifestyle modifications, such as changes in dietary patterns [4]. Thus, weight loss, exercise, and healthy eating habits are the main strategies to reduce the incidence and prevalence of NAFLD, although the metabolic mechanisms are still poorly understood [5]. Previous studies have evidenced a role of weight loss on NAFLD management [6]. However, further investigations to elucidate the interplay between specific dietary components and fatty liver combined with weight loss are necessary [7], as the number of randomized controlled studies conducted in this area remain scarce [8]. In this context, the aim of this study was to evaluate the influence of two energy-restricted diets on non-invasive markers and scores of liver damage in obese individuals with features of metabolic syndrome after six months of follow-up and to assess the role of fiber content (quality and quantity) in metabolic outcomes.

2. Materials and Methods

2.1. Study Design

The current study included a total of 70 subjects from the RESMENA (Reduction of Metabolic Syndrome in Navarra) study, which was designed as a randomized controlled intervention trial to compare the effects of two hypocaloric dietary strategies on metabolic syndrome (MS) comorbidities after six-months of follow-up [9]. Initially, a total of 109 Caucasian adults were enrolled in the study, however, 12 did not present MS according to the International Diabetes Federation (IDF) criteria when the study began, and another four subjects decided not to start the dietary treatment after signing the written informed consent. Therefore, 93 subjects were assigned using the "random between 1 and 2" function in the Microsoft Office Excel 2003 software (Microsoft Iberica, Barcelona, Spain) to follow one of the two energy-restricted diets. After six months of weight loss intervention, twenty-three participants (11 from RESMENA and 12 from the American Heart Association (AHA) dietary group) did not complete the dietary intake questionnaire and/or were missing data regarding biomarkers of liver status at the end of the intervention. Thus, a total of 70 participants had complete information to carry out the objective of this study (Figure 1). Subjects were asked to maintain their usual physical activity (MET—metabolic equivalent of the task), which was controlled by a 24-h physical activity questionnaire administered at the beginning and at the end of the study.

The RESMENA study followed the CONSORT 2010 guidelines, except for blinding. This research was performed according to the ethical guidelines of the Declaration of Helsinki, and was appropriately registered (www.clinicaltrials.gov; NCT01087086). The study was approved by the Research Ethics Committee of the University of Navarra (ref. 065/2009). Additional aspects of this intervention trial have been detailed elsewhere [9].

2.2. Nutritional Intervention

Two hypocaloric dietary patterns (AHA vs. RESMENA)—both with the same energy restriction (−30% of the individual's requirements)—were prescribed and compared. The AHA diet was based on American Heart Association guidelines, including 3–5 meals/day, a macronutrient distribution of 55% total caloric value (TCV) from carbohydrates (whole grains were recommended, but not mandatory), 15% from proteins, and 30% from lipids. On the other hand, the RESMENA diet was designed with a higher meal frequency, consisting of seven meals/day, and a macronutrient distribution of 40% TCV from carbohydrates (whole grains were required), 30% from proteins (mainly vegetable protein), and 30% from lipids (omega-3 and extra virgin olive oil intake required).

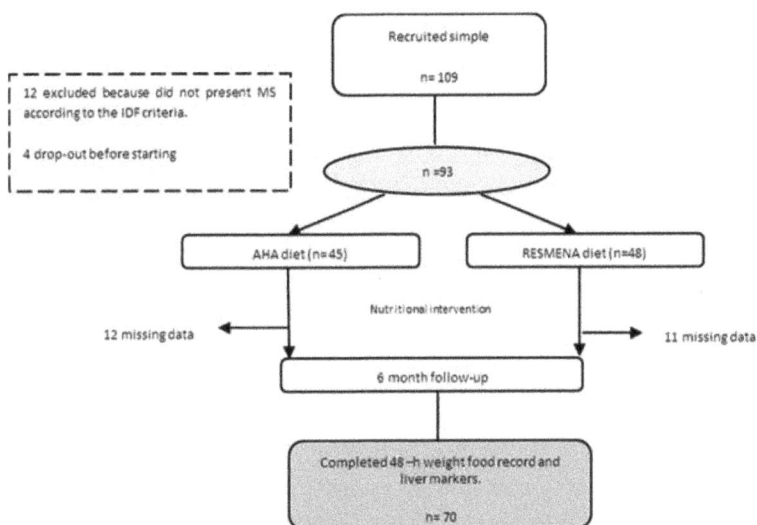

Figure 1. Study design flowchart. AHA: American Heart Association; IDF: International Diabetes Federation; MS: metabolic syndrome.

A 48-h weighed food record was collected at the beginning and at the end of the study, and was used to assess the volunteer's adherence to the prescribed diet. The energy and nutrient content of these questionnaires were determined using the DIAL software (Alce Ingenieria, Madrid, Spain), as described elsewhere [10]. This is a validated program in Spain, designed with Spanish foods, and provides information regarding grams of insoluble and soluble fiber obtained from the diet, as well as the total fiber supplied by different food groups (fiber from fruits, vegetables, or cereals, separately).

Anthropometric measurements were assessed in fasting conditions following standardized procedures, as previously reported [9]. Body weight, waist circumference (WC), and body composition as assessed by dual-energy X-ray absorptiometry (Lunar Prodigy, software version 6.0, Madison, WI, USA) were examined at baseline and at the end of the intervention using validated protocols [10]. Body mass index (BMI) was calculated as body weight divided by squared height (kg/m^2). Conicity index (CI) was calculated as the (waist circumference/(0.109 × square root of weight/height)) as published [11], where WC and height were measured in meters and weight was measured in kg. Blood glucose, total cholesterol (TC), triglycerides (TG), alanine aminotransferase (ALT), aspartate aminotransferase (AST), and gamma-glutamyl transferase (GGT) were measured on an autoanalyzer (Pentra C-200; HORIBA ABX, Madrid, Spain). Plasma concentrations of cytokeratin-18 (CK18)-fragments (M30 and M65) levels were assessed by ELISA assay (Mercodia, Uppsala, Sweden) with an autoanalyzer system (Triturus, Grifols SA, Barcelona, Spain) following the manufacturer's instructions.

The fatty liver index (FLI) is an algorithm derived from serum TG, BMI, WC, and GGT levels [12–15], and was validated in a large group of subjects with or without suspected liver disease with an accuracy of 0.84 (95% CI) in detecting fatty liver. Fatty liver index varies between 0 and 100, indicating the presence of steatosis with a score ≥ 60. The NAFLD liver fat score [16] was calculated by a complex equation, combining the following parameters: the presence of MS (according to IDF criteria), the presence of Type 2 diabetes, fasting serum insulin, aspartate amino-transferase (AST), and the aspartate–alanine aminotransferase ratio (AST/ALT ratio). This score (NAFLD_LFS) allows the prediction of steatosis, defined as a liver fat content ≥ 5.56% as assessed by ¹H-magnetic resonance spectroscopy (¹H-MRS) with good accuracy (area under the receiver operating characteristic curve

(AUROC): 0.86). The hepatic steatosis index (HSI) was also calculated for the assessment of liver steatosis. The formula includes ALT/AST ratio, diabetes, and gender [17]. A value > 36 indicates liver steatosis. Additional hepatic steatosis predictors were calculated based on the available data such as the BAAT (body mass index, age, alanine aminotransferase, triglycerides) and BARD (body mass index, aspartate aminotransferase:alanine aminotransferase, diabetes) scores which included BMI, age, alanine amino transferase (ALT), and TG; and BMI, AST/ALT ratio and presence of diabetes, respectively [18]. Finally, the visceral adiposity index (VAI) was calculated [19], given that is a simple index of visceral fat function that predicts cardiometabolic risk in general population.

2.3. Statistical Analysis

Analyses were performed using 12.0 (Stata Corp College Station, TX, USA). Fiber dietary groups were classified as total fiber consumption (total dietary fiber), insoluble fiber (total insoluble dietary fiber), soluble fiber (total soluble dietary fiber), fruit fiber (specifically fiber from fruits), vegetable fiber (specifically fiber from vegetables), and cereal fiber (specifically fiber from cereals). The median values of fiber intake were used to classify the participants into high ($\geq$50th percentile) or low (<50th percentile) fiber consumption. Normality distributions of the evaluated variables were determined by Shapiro–Wilk test. Continuous variables were compared between groups by the Student's *t*-test or the Mann–Whitney *U* test for parametric or non-parametric variables, respectively. Categorical variables were compared by the chi-squared test. The relationship between variables was assessed by the Pearson's correlation coefficient or the Spearman's rho (*p*). A linear regression model was performed to assess the influence of independent variables such as fiber from fruits, age, total energy intake, and physical activity estimations on the variability of FLI score. The linear regression model was not adjusted for weight variable, since FLI carries the BMI value in its calculation. All *p*-values presented are two-tailed, and differences were considered statistically significant at $p < 0.05$.

3. Results

The average age of participants was 49 ± 9 years, of which 50.5% were women. At the beginning of the study, no significant differences were observed between dietary groups. After 6 months, the mean of body weight loss was 7.9 ± 4.8 kg and 9.7 ± 5.4 kg in the AHA and RESMENA dietary groups, respectively (Table 1). Both nutritional treatments significantly reduced BMI, CI, WC, total and android fat mass, as well as IDF (International Diabetes Federation) of metabolic syndrome after 6 months of nutritional intervention. Likewise, the cardiometabolic risk factors (Triglycerides/glucose ratio (TyG index), waist-to-height ratio, % diabetes, % hypertension) showed significant reductions with both diets. However, the changes (baseline vs. 6 months) in the reported variables did not differ between the RESMENA and AHA dietary strategies, with the exception of high-density lipoprotein cholesterol (HDL-c) levels, which were significantly increased in AHA compared to the RESMENA group at the end of study (Table 1). Regarding dietary intake, the analysis of weighed dietary records showed that total fiber intake was higher during the intervention period than the intake before starting the nutritional program (baseline) in both dietary groups, while participants from the RESMENA dietary group showed a significantly higher intake of insoluble fiber after six months (Table 1).

Table 1. Characteristics of the participants at baseline and after 6 months according to dietary treatment.

n = 70	AHA (*n* = 33)		RESMENA (*n* = 37)		Δ*p*-Value
	Baseline	6 Months	Baseline	6 Months	
Body composition					
Weight (kg)	99.2 (19)	91.8 (17) **	100.4 (16)	92.6 (16) **	0.155
BMI	35.8 (4)	32.9 (4) **	35.7 (4)	32.2 (4) **	0.153
Conicity Index	1.3	1.2 **	1.3	1.2 **	0.083
WC (cm)	110.2 (13)	103.3 (13) **	111.8 (12)	102.4 (2) **	0.441
Total Fat Mass (%)	41.7 (6)	38.5 (7) **	42.3 (6)	38.2 (7) **	0.191
Android FM (kg)	4.5 (1.3)	3.9 (1.8)	4.8 (1.2)	3.6 (1) **	0.151
IDF criteria					
Glucose (mg/dL)	121.5 (33)	115.4 (24) **	123.8 (37)	111.7 (29) **	0.559
TG (mg/dL)	175.3 (90)	139.6 (87) *	194.2(122)	145.4 (83) **	0.863
SBP (mmHg)	150 (17)	137 (13) **	147 (21)	135 (15) **	0.654
DBP (mmHg)	85 (9)	78 (10) *	84 (9)	78 (10) **	0.436
HDL-c (mg/dL)	46.3 (9)	51.5 (11) **	43.3 (9)	46.2 (10)	0.042
LDL-c (mg/dL)	140.4 (36)	140.1(36) **	136.7 (41)	136.3 (41) *	0.570
TC (mg/dL)	221.8 (39)	226.5 (40)	218.5 (47)	213.3 (39)	0.332
Homa-index	4.6 (3.7)	2.6 (2.9) **	4.4 (3.0)	2.3 (1.7) **	0.820
Cardiometabolic risk factors					
TyG index	9.1 (0.5)	8.8 (0.5) *	9.1 (0.7)	8.8 (0.6) **	0.487
Waist to height ratio	0.6 (0.0)	0.6 (0.1) **	0.6 (0.1)	0.6 (0.1) **	0.095
LDL-c/HDL-c	3.0 (1.0)	3.5 (0.7)	3.1(0.9)	3.7 (0.8)	0.432
Diabetes %	74.4	65.7	74.4	52.7 *	0.389
Hypertension %	93	43	82.9	52 *	0.323
Macronutrient intake					
Total Energy (kcal)	2102 (450)	1529 (316) **	2276 (565)	1548 (381) **	0.527
Carbohydrate (g)	186.5 (58)	140.4 (45) **	201.3 (65)	138.2 (37) **	0.098
Proteins (g)	93.7 (21)	66.6 (18) **	95.7 (20)	78.2 (17) **	0.198
Lipids (g)	97.1 (27)	69.4(17) **	101.3 (29)	66.5 (20) **	0.231
Fiber consumption (g/1000 kcal)					
Total fiber	18.7 (10)	20.7 (8) *	21.8 (7)	26.0 (7) *	0.585
Soluble fiber	2.1 (0.9)	2.1 (0.8)	2.0 (0.6)	2.5 (0.9)	0.657
Insoluble fiber	4.3 (3.2)	4.5 (2.1)	3.2 (1)	5.6 (1.5) *	0.190

(Mean ± SD); Paired and Unpaired *t*-tests were carried out. * $p < 0.05$, comparison within each dietary group (baseline and after 6 months); ** $p < 0.001$, within each dietary group (baseline and after 6 months). Δ*p*-value, comparison of the changes (baseline and 6 months) between dietary groups (AHA vs. RESMENA); BMI: body mass index; FM: fat mass; SBP: Systolic blood pressure; DPB: Diastolic blood pressure; HDL-c: high-density lipoprotein cholesterol; IDF, International Diabetes Federation; LDL-c: low-density lipoprotein cholesterol; TC: total cholesterol; TG: triglycerides; WC: waist circumference; TyG: Triglycerides/glucose ratio.

In relation to liver health, a significant decrease was observed in ALT, GGT, and M30 levels as well as NAFLD_LF score, FLI, HSI, VAI and BAAT scores with both dietary strategies (AHA and RESMENA) after 6 months of follow-up (Table 2). Given that transaminases showed significant difference at baseline between dietary groups, the analyses concerning transaminases were adjusted by ALT and AST values at baseline. AST values only showed a significant reduction in the RESMENA group. In contrast, fragments of M65 only obtained significant improvements in the AHA group. In addition, the BARD score did not show relevant improvements either dietary group. It is important to note that the changes (baseline vs. 6 months) in the reported variables were not different between dietary strategies (Table 2). Thus, both dietary strategies were equally effective regarding liver status. Consequently and based on previous investigations [20,21], both dietary groups were merged for the analysis of fiber consumption because they produced similar outcomes for all relevant variables and markers.

Table 2. Non-invasive markers of liver damage at baseline and after 6 months according to dietary treatment.

n = 70	AHA (*n* = 33)		RESMENA (*n* = 37)		Δ*p*-Value
	Baseline	6 Months	Baseline	6 Months	
Hepatic measurements					
ALT (U/L)	37.4 (21)	25.2 (8) *	29.4 (11)	22.8 (8) **	0.642 #
AST (U/L)	25.1 (10)	23.3 (6)	21.7 (6)	20.2 (4) **	0.126 #
GGT (U/L)	40.2 (24)	30.3 (17) *	41.4 (26)	27.1 (14) **	0.135
M65 (U/L)	307.8 (198)	217.6 (108) **	259.4 (135)	230.9 (91)	0.125
M30 (U/L)	200.3 (125)	128.7 (51) *	156.1 (99)	103.5 (35) *	0.304
NAFLD_LFS	2.2 (2.6)	0.4 (2.2) **	1.9 (1.9)	−0.09 (1.9) **	0.429
FLI	84.6 (17)	68.4 (25) **	85.2 (16)	69.4 (25) **	0.793
HSI	49.2 (6)	44.1 (5) **	48.4 (5)	43.1 (5) **	0.759
VAI	2.8 (1.9)	2.0 (1.7) **	3.6 (2.9)	2.3 (15) **	0.920
BARD	2.5 (0.9)	2.8 (1.1)	2.6 (1.2)	2.8 (1)	0.713
BAAT	2.1 (0.7)	1.6 (0.7) **	2.0 (0.6)	1.7 (0.7) **	0.265

(Mean ± SD); M30 and M65: cytokeratin-18 (CK18) fragments; ALT: alanine aminotransferase; AST: aspartate aminotransferase; GGT: gamma-glutamyl transferase; FLI: fatty liver index; HSI: hepatic steatosis index; VAI: visceral adipose index; NAFLD_LFS: non-alcoholic fatty liver disease liver fat score; BARD score; BAAT score; Paired and unpaired *t*-tests were carried out. * $p < 0.05$, comparison within each dietary group baseline vs. after 6 months. ** $p < 0.001$, within each dietary group baseline vs. after 6 months; Δ*p*-value, comparison changes (baseline and 6 months) between dietary groups. # Adjusted by baseline value.

We analyzed the potential role of dietary macronutrients (carbohydrates, fat, and proteins) on liver status (FLI), and no significant associations were observed: carbohydrates ($\beta = 0.011$; $p = 0.751$; $R = 0.0017$), lipids ($\beta = 0.126$; $p = 0.084$; $R = 0.049$), saturated fatty acids ($\beta = -0.017$; $p = 0.431$, $R = 0.009$), monounsaturated fatty acids ($\beta = -0.031$, $p = 0.390$, $R = 0.001$), polyunsaturated fatty acids ($\beta = -0.198$; $p = 0.209$; $R = 0.208$), omega-3 fatty acids ($\beta = -0.930$; $p = 0.288$; $R = 0.051$), and proteins $\beta = -0.66$; $p = 0.480$; $R = 0.008$). In order to analyze the specific role of fiber on liver health, the predictors of liver damage according to high and low (<50th percentile vs. ≥50th percentile) consumption of different types of fiber were assessed at the end of the study (Table 3). Insoluble fiber and fiber from fruits showed interesting results, since participants with higher consumption of these types of fiber reduced markers of liver status associated with fatty liver. It is important to highlight that a high consumption of insoluble fiber resulted in improvements in FLI, HSI, NAFLD_LFS, while significant improvements in GGT and transaminases (AST and ALT) were observed as a result of fruit fiber consumption.

Table 3. Non-invasive markers of liver damage categorized according to the median of fiber consumption after 6 months.

n = 70	Total Fiber (g/Day)		Insoluble Fiber (g/Day)		Soluble Fiber (g/Day)		Fruit Fiber (g/Day)	
	<39.1	≥39.1	<7.5	≥7.5	<3.2	≥3.2	<8.8	≥8.8
ALT (U/L)	26.3 (9)	23.3 (8)	26.2 (9)	23.4 (8)	26.4 (9)	23.5 (7)	27.2 (8)	22.4 (8) #
AST (U/L)	21.5 (6)	21. 6(6)	22.8 (5)	21.6 (6)	22.6 (5)	21.4 (6)	23.8 (5)	19.3 (5) #
GGT (U/L)	29.4 (17)	28.2 (15)	28.1 (14)	29.5 (18)	28.1 (16)	28.2 (17)	34.1 (18)	23.5 (11) *
M65 (U/L)	218.6 (83)	232.1 (118)	223.1 (14)	227.4 (20)	231.4 (15)	220.6 (20)	236.5 (22)	213.4 (12)
M30 (U/L)	120.2 (50)	109.4 (45)	123.2 (9)	107.5 (7)	124.3 (9)	107.4 (6)	121.2 (8)	113.6 (7)
FLI	75.3 (17)	57.2 (29)	74. 4 (21)	60.6 (27) *	71.1 (25)	62.2 (25)	72.4 (23)	65.8 (26)
HSI	45.2 (5)	42.4 (6)	4.27 (3)	41.2 (4) *	44.6 (5)	42.7 (6)	43.6 (6)	44.1 (5)
VAI	0.5 (2)	−0.1 (1)	2.4 (1)	1.7 (1)	2.1 (1.8)	1.9 (1.4)	2.4 (2.1)	1.9 (1.1)
NAFLD_LFS	2.6 (1)	2.8 (1)	0.9 (2)	−0.5 (1) *	0.2 (2.4)	0.1 (1.7)	0.8 (2.2)	−0.3 (1.7)

* $p < 0.05$ indicates differences between values above and below the median. # $p < 0.05$. Adjusted by baseline values; Cut off mean values: Total fiber (41.0 g); Insoluble fiber (3.1 g); Soluble fiber (1.6 g); Fruit fiber (3.4 g). ALT: alanine aminotransferase; AST: aspartate aminotransferase; GGT: gamma-glutamyl transferase; FLI: fatty liver index; HSI: hepatic steatosis index; VAI: visceral adipose index; NAFLD_LFS: non-alcoholic fatty liver disease liver fat score.

Reinforcing this idea, a linear regression analysis was carried out to assess the influence of changes in the consumption of different types of fiber in changes in the FLI. Fiber from fruits demonstrated a positive relationship (*R*-adjusted: 0.049; *p* = 0.048; Figure 2). The effect of each fiber group was also analyzed: vegetables (β = 0.287; *p* = 0.138, *R* = 0.037), cereals (β = −0.295; *p* = 0.608, *R* = 0.004), insoluble (β = 0.491; *p* = 0.159, *R* = 0.033), soluble (β = −0.472; *p* = 0.545, *R* = 0.002). The linear regression model was adjusted by age, total energy (kcal), and physical activity (metabolic equivalent of the task, MET) changes (Table 4). When these variables were jointly considered, the predictors of the model explained up to 11.6% of the variation of changes in the FLI (adjusted R^2 = 0.116; P_{model} < 0.026).

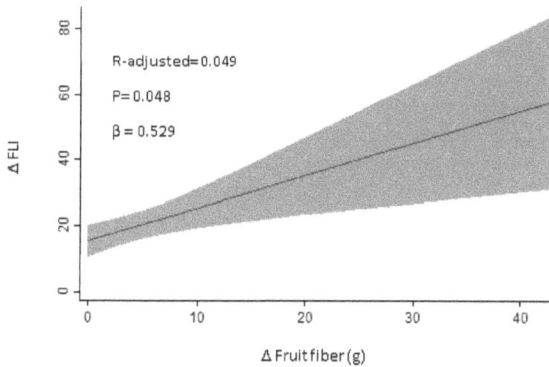

Figure 2. Regression analysis with changes in FLI and fruit fiber.

Table 4. Regression analysis with changes in fatty liver index and changes in the consumption of fiber from fruits at 6 months.

Δ Fatty Liver Index	β	*p*	P_{model}	*R*-Adjusted
Δ Fiber Fruits	0.5769	0.025	0.0265	0.1168
Age	−0.4860	0.03	-	-
Δ Total energy (kcal)	−0.0691	0.149	-	-
Δ MET	0.0003	0.461	-	-

MET, metabolic equivalent of the task.

4. Discussion

The design of new dietary strategies for NAFLD prevention and for the reduction of causal factors is needed [22]. Increasing rates of obesity and MS are having an important impact on the rising incidence and prevalence of liver diseases such as NAFLD; thus, well-designed dietary interventions are necessary [22]. In this context, the present study compared the effects of two energy-restricted dietary strategies on anthropometric, biochemical, and non-invasive markers of liver status in obese individuals with MS features after 6 months of follow-up. Regarding weight loss, body composition, IDF criteria, and cardiometabolic risk, both dietary regimens had equal effect on most metabolic markers. HDL-c concentrations were increased in both dietary groups, but only reached significance in the AHA group. This outcome might be expected, since the AHA diet is specifically based on the AHA guidelines [23], which focus on cardiovascular care and therefore on lipid profile management. Interestingly, the RESMENA diet had a positive effect on body weight by reducing android fat mass—a body region which has been commonly associated with hepatic steatosis [24]. On the other hand, current research has focused on identifying biomarkers to predict NASH or NAFLD [25,26]. In this context, Bedogni et al. (2006) designed a simple scoring system named FLI which includes TG, GGT, BMI, and WC, and it is easily calculated [12]. FLI was developed for the prediction of fatty liver disease and shows a good area under the curve of 0.84 [26]. The accuracy of FLI in comparison with the ultrasonography method for detection and quantification of hepatic steatosis has been validated in several countries [12,27]. Furthermore, previous studies [17,28–30] have demonstrated and validated other non-invasive markers of liver status that were used in this study (CK18-fragments, HSI, VAI, BARD and BAAT score, NAFLD_LFS) in addition to GGT and transaminases. By employing these non-invasive biomarkers and scores to assess liver status, we showed that energy-restriction within both dietary patterns produced similar and significant beneficial effects on liver status, as shown in other dietary studies [31]. The BARD score did not indicate improvements after either of the nutritional interventions, which might be due to the fact that the BARD score is used to exclude advanced fibrosis in NAFLD, and other authors have noted that its sensitivity is low [30,32]. Considering the global results presented in this study, particularly improvements in android fat and liver status, we propose RESMENA as a novel dietary strategy to be explored in subjects with obesity and fatty liver.

Energy restriction is a key factor for the management of NAFLD [33]. Indeed, the American Association for the Study of Liver Diseases (AASLD) recommends a loss of at least 3–5% of body weight to improve steatosis and a greater weight loss (up to 10%) to improve necroinflammation [34]. Other investigations have also demonstrated that weight loss interventions are effective in reducing NAFLD severity [6]. However, not only is the amount of energy a key component to be considered, but also the quality of the diet. In relation to fatty acids, diets rich in saturated fat and cholesterol and low in polyunsaturated fat have been associated with NASH [6], while omega-3 fatty acids have been proposed for the treatment of NAFLD or NASH [34,35]. In fact, the Mediterranean diet can reduce liver fat even in the absence of weight loss, and is the most recommended dietary pattern for NAFLD [36,37]. The Mediterranean diet is characterized by reduced carbohydrate intake (especially sugars and refined carbohydrates), and an increased intake of monounsaturated and omega-3 fatty acids. In the present study, both dietary patterns (AHA and RESMENA) included the same energy restriction (−30% E) and were designed taking into account the effect of a different distribution of macronutrients as well as the beneficial role of specific dietary components. In the present work, energy restriction was a key factor involved in the improvement of liver health; however, other dietary components—particularly fiber—may also be involved in the management of steatosis. Several studies have reported that fiber may play an important role in obesity and related diseases such as insulin resistance and liver diseases [38]. To our knowledge, this is the first study evaluating the association between types of fiber and liver status in subjects with obesity and metabolic syndrome following an energy-restricted diet. Although adherence to the dietary strategies was similar, resulting in no differences in macronutrient distribution, a variety of hepatic damage markers were lower in those individuals who had a higher fiber intake. In particular, fiber derived from fruit had a beneficial impact, suggesting that not only energy restriction but also other dietary components positively influence liver health.

In this context, Zelber-Sagi et al., 2011 suggested that the consumption of diets higher in fiber could have a preventive role in hepatic disease [39]. Fiber contains components which are not classified as essential nutrients, but could be important mediators in human health. In fact, a pilot study of seven patients with NASH reported a significant decrease in aspartate aminotransferase levels compared to a placebo after 8 weeks of supplementation with oligofructose at 16 g/day [40]. Another study providing 10 g/day of psyllium fiber to 12 patients over the course of three months found a normalization of transaminases and GGT levels [41]. Dietary fiber can be divided in two groups—soluble and insoluble—based on physical, chemical, and functional characteristics [42]. Insoluble fibers are insoluble in water and gastric fluids. Soluble fiber dissolves in water and can resist gastrointestinal enzymatic digestion; therefore, soluble fiber can pass the small intestine to reach the colon where it can be fermented by intestinal microbiota [43]. This suggests that both soluble and insoluble fibers could have different roles in gastrointestinal health [44]. For this reason, different fiber types were investigated in the present study. Interestingly, we found two important fiber groups that could have a major effect on the reduction of predictors of liver heath: insoluble fiber and fiber from fruits. Although increasing dietary fiber has a favorable effect on body weight [45], and several studies suggest that fermentation activities of the gut microbiota may be a possible contributor to NAFLD [46], data regarding the effect of different types of fiber remain unclear [47]. Therefore, current research is warranted to determine the optimal dietary fibers for prevention and reduction of fatty liver disease accompanying obesity.

A limitation of this study is that NAFLD was evaluated using non-invasive markers instead of imaging techniques and/or liver biopsies. However, the design of the current trial is based on validated non-invasive and affordable markers, which makes them an optimal form of diagnosis in clinical practice. In relation to improvements in liver status, other components occurring in the dietary pattern such us antioxidants, vitamins, fatty acids, energy restriction etc., may also explain the observed benefits on liver health, as they could work synergistically with fiber. In addition, comparisons involving means or regression analyses showed the same trend, although the statistical outcomes were more confirmatory when adjusted by age, total energy, and MET, which is in agreement with the expectations. The discordance between the results obtained with different analysis merits attention before concluding that all observed results are due to fruit fiber. On the other hand, one of the main strengths of the present research is that it is a randomized controlled trial, considered the gold standard in the hierarchy of research designs for evaluating the efficacy and safety of a nutritional intervention. Moreover, the fact that every dietary pattern has been personally designed for each patient, taking into account sex, height, initial body weight, and physical activity, should also be highlighted. Finally, it is important to point out that a well-recognized healthy dietary pattern (AHA) was used as reference, which demonstrates that the positive results obtained with the RESMENA diet are of significance.

5. Conclusions

These data support that the RESMENA diet may be a valid strategy to counteract MS features and liver damage accompanying obesity. In addition, this study reveals that the type of dietary fiber differentially impacts liver health status in obese subjects under energy restriction. However, these results should be interpreted with caution, since other components contained in fruits, in addition to fruit fiber, could be involved in the observed benefits.

Acknowledgments: The authors are grateful to the volunteers of the study as well as to the physician Blanca E. Martínez de Morentín, the nurse Salomé Pérez, the technician Verónica Ciaurriz and the dietitians Rocio de la Iglesia, Patricia Lopez-Legarrea and Aurora Pérez-Cornago for the contribution to RESMENA project. The pre-doctoral research grant to Irene Cantero from the Centre for Nutrition Research of the University of Navarra is gratefully acknowledged. Finally, we want to thank to the Health Department of the Government of Navarra (48/2009), The Linea Especial about Nutrition, Obesity and Health (University of Navarra LE/97), CIBERobn (Physiopathology of Obesity and Nutrition) and RETICS for their support. **Funding:** Health Department of the Government of Navarra (48/2009), University of Navarra LE/97, CIBERObn and RETICS for their support. We acknowledge Cassondra Saande (native English speaker) for reviewing the final version of the manuscript.

Author Contributions: M.A.Z. and J.A.M. were responsible for the global design and coordination of the project, and financial management. I.C., I.A., J.I.M., J.A.M. and M.A.Z. conceived, designed, and wrote the article. All the authors actively participated in the manuscript preparation, as well as read and approved the final manuscript.

Conflicts of Interest: The authors declare no conflict of interest.

References

1. Thoma, C.; Day, C.P.; Trenell, M.I. Lifestyle interventions for the treatment of non-alcoholic fatty liver disease in adults: A systematic review. *J. Hepatol.* **2012**, *56*, 255–266. [CrossRef] [PubMed]
2. Loomba, R.; Sanyal, A.J. The global NAFLD epidemic. *Nat. Rev. Gastroenterol. Hepatol.* **2013**, *10*, 686–690. [CrossRef] [PubMed]
3. Pais, R.; Charlotte, F.; Fedchuk, L.; Bedossa, P.; Lebray, P.; Poynard, T.; Ratziu, V.; LIDO Study Group. A systematic review of follow-up biopsies reveals disease progression in patients with non-alcoholic fatty liver. *J. Hepatol.* **2013**, *59*, 550–556. [CrossRef] [PubMed]

4. Kobayashi, Y.; Tatsumi, H.; Hattori, M.; Sugiyama, H.; Wada, S.; Kuwahata, M.; Tanaka, S.; Kanemasa, K.; Sumida, Y.; Naito, Y.; et al. Comparisons of dietary intake in japanese with non-alcoholic fatty liver disease and type 2 diabetes mellitus. *J. Clin. Biochem. Nutr.* **2016**, *59*, 215–219. [CrossRef] [PubMed]

5. Katsagoni, C.N.; Georgoulis, M.; Papatheodoridis, G.V.; Panagiotakos, D.B.; Kontogianni, M.D. Effects of lifestyle interventions on clinical characteristics of patients with non-alcoholic fatty liver disease: A meta-analysis. *Metabolism* **2017**, *68*, 119–132. [CrossRef] [PubMed]

6. Razavi Zade, M.; Telkabadi, M.H.; Bahmani, F.; Salehi, B.; Farshbaf, S.; Asemi, Z. The effects of dash diet on weight loss and metabolic status in adults with non-alcoholic fatty liver disease: A randomized clinical trial. *Liver Int.* **2016**, *36*, 563–571. [CrossRef] [PubMed]

7. Africa, J.A.; Newton, K.P.; Schwimmer, J.B. Lifestyle interventions including nutrition, exercise, and supplements for nonalcoholic fatty liver disease in children. *Dig. Dis. Sci.* **2016**, *61*, 1375–1386. [CrossRef] [PubMed]

8. Guo, X.F.; Yang, B.; Tang, J.; Li, D. Fatty acid and non-alcoholic fatty liver disease: Meta-analyses of case-control and randomized controlled trials. *Clin. Nutr.* **2017**, *16*. [CrossRef] [PubMed]

9. Perez-Cornago, A.; Lopez-Legarrea, P.; de la Iglesia, R.; Lahortiga, F.; Martinez, J.A.; Zulet, M.A. Longitudinal relationship of diet and oxidative stress with depressive symptoms in patients with metabolic syndrome after following a weight loss treatment: The resmena project. *Clin. Nutr.* **2014**, *33*, 1061–1067. [CrossRef] [PubMed]

10. Zulet, M.A.; Bondia-Pons, I.; Abete, I.; de la Iglesia, R.; López-Legarrea, P.; Forga, L.; Navas-Carretero, S.; Martínez, J.A. The reduction of the metabolyc syndrome in navarra-spain (resmena-s) study: A multidisciplinary strategy based on chrononutrition and nutritional education, together with dietetic and psychological control. *Nutr. Hosp.* **2011**, *26*, 16–26. [PubMed]

11. Kissebah, A.H.; Krakower, G.R. Regional adiposity and morbidity. *Physiol. Rev.* **1994**, *74*, 761–811. [PubMed]

12. Bedogni, G.; Bellentani, S.; Miglioli, L.; Masutti, F.; Passalacqua, M.; Castiglione, A.; Tiribelli, C. The fatty liver index: A simple and accurate predictor of hepatic steatosis in the general population. *BMC Gastroenterol.* **2006**, *6*, 33. [CrossRef] [PubMed]

13. Bonnet, F.; Gastaldelli, A.; Pihan-Le Bars, F.; Natali, A.; Roussel, R.; Petrie, J.; Tichet, J.; Marre, M.; Fromenty, B.; Balkau, B.; et al. Gamma-glutamyltransferase, fatty liver index and hepatic insulin resistance are associated with incident hypertension in two longitudinal studies. *J. Hypertens.* **2017**, *35*, 493–500. [CrossRef] [PubMed]

14. Yang, K.C.; Hung, H.F.; Lu, C.W.; Chang, H.H.; Lee, L.T.; Huang, K.C. Association of non-alcoholic fatty liver disease with metabolic syndrome independently of central obesity and insulin resistance. *Sci. Rep.* **2016**, *6*. [CrossRef] [PubMed]

15. Silaghi, C.A.; Silaghi, H.; Colosi, H.A.; Craciun, A.E.; Farcas, A.; Cosma, D.T.; Hancu, N.; Pais, R.; Georgescu, C.E. Prevalence and predictors of non-alcoholic fatty liver disease as defined by the fatty liver index in a type 2 diabetes population. *Clujul Med.* **2016**, *89*, 82–88. [CrossRef] [PubMed]

16. Kotronen, A.; Peltonen, M.; Hakkarainen, A.; Sevastianova, K.; Bergholm, R.; Johansson, L.M.; Lundbom, N.; Rissanen, A.; Ridderstråle, M.; Groop, L.; et al. Prediction of non-alcoholic fatty liver disease and liver fat using metabolic and genetic factors. *Gastroenterology* **2009**, *137*, 865–872. [CrossRef] [PubMed]

17. Lee, J.H.; Kim, D.; Kim, H.J.; Lee, C.H.; Yang, J.I.; Kim, W.; Kim, Y.J.; Yoon, J.H.; Cho, S.H.; Sung, M.W.; et al. Hepatic steatosis index: A simple screening tool reflecting nonalcoholic fatty liver disease. *Dig. Liver Dis.* **2010**, *42*, 503–508. [CrossRef] [PubMed]

18. Ratziu, V.; Giral, P.; Charlotte, F.; Bruckert, E.; Thibault, V.; Theodorou, I.; Khalil, L.; Turpin, G.; Opolon, P.; Poynard, T. Liver fibrosis in overweight patients. *Gastroenterology* **2000**, *118*, 1117–1123. [CrossRef]

19. Dai, D.; Chang, Y.; Chen, Y.; Chen, S.; Yu, S.; Guo, X.; Sun, Y. Visceral adiposity index and lipid accumulation product index: Two alternate body indices to identify chronic kidney disease among the rural population in northeast china. *Int. J. Environ. Res. Public Health* **2016**, *13*, 1231. [CrossRef] [PubMed]

20. Perez-Cornago, A.; Ramirez, M.J.; Zulet, M.A.; Martinez, J.A. Effect of dietary restriction on peripheral monoamines and anxiety symptoms in obese subjects with metabolic syndrome. *Psychoneuroendocrinology* **2014**, *47*, 98–106. [CrossRef] [PubMed]

21. Perez-Cornago, A.; Mansego, M.L.; Zulet, M.A.; Martinez, J.A. DNA hypermethylation of the serotonin receptor type-2a gene is associated with a worse response to a weight loss intervention in subjects with metabolic syndrome. *Nutrients* **2014**, *6*, 2387–2403. [CrossRef] [PubMed]

22. Lopez-Legarrea, P.; de la Iglesia, R.; Abete, I.; Bondia-Pons, I.; Navas-Carretero, S.; Forga, L.; Martínez, J.A.; Zulet, M.A. Short-term role of the dietary total antioxidant capacity in two hypocaloric regimes on obese with metabolic syndrome symptoms: The resmena randomized controlled trial. *Nutr. Metab.* **2013**, *10*, 1743–7075. [CrossRef] [PubMed]

23. Van Horn, L.; Carson, J.A.; Appel, L.J.; Burke, L.E.; Economos, C.; Karmally, W.; Lancaster, K.; Lichtenstein, A.H.; Johnson, R.K.; Thomas, R.J.; et al. Recommended dietary pattern to achieve adherence to the american heart association/american college of cardiology (aha/acc) guidelines: A scientific statement from the american heart association. *Circulation* **2016**, *134*, e505–e529. [CrossRef] [PubMed]

24. Hodson, L.; Banerjee, R.; Rial, B.; Arlt, W.; Adiels, M.; Boren, J.; Marinou, K.; Fisher, C.; Mostad, I.L.; Stratton, I.M.; et al. Menopausal status and abdominal obesity are significant determinants of hepatic lipid metabolism in women. *J. Am. Heart. Assoc.* **2015**, *4*, 002258. [CrossRef] [PubMed]

25. Kantartzis, K.; Rettig, I.; Staiger, H.; Machann, J.; Schick, F.; Scheja, L.; Gastaldelli, A.; Bugianesi, E.; Peter, A.; Schulze, M.B.; Fritsche, A.; Häring, H.U.; Stefan, N. An extended fatty liver index to predict non-alcoholic fatty liver disease. *Diabetes Metab.* **2017**, *12*, 229–239. [CrossRef] [PubMed]

26. Calori, G.; Lattuada, G.; Ragogna, F.; Garancini, M.P.; Crosignani, P.; Villa, M.; Bosi, E.; Ruotolo, G.; Piemonti, L.; Perseghin, G. Fatty liver index and mortality: The cremona study in the 15th year of follow-up. *Hepatology* **2011**, *54*, 145–152. [CrossRef] [PubMed]

27. Damms-Machado, A.; Louis, S.; Schnitzer, A.; Volynets, V.; Rings, A.; Basrai, M.; Bischoff, S.C. Gut permeability is related to body weight, fatty liver disease, and insulin resistance in obese individuals undergoing weight reduction. *Am. J. Clin. Nutr.* **2017**, *105*, 127–135. [CrossRef] [PubMed]

28. Rosso, C.; Caviglia, G.P.; Abate, M.L.; Vanni, E.; Mezzabotta, L.; Touscos, G.A.; Olivero, A.; Marengo, A. Cytokeratin 18-aspartate396 apoptotic fragment for fibrosis detection in patients with non-alcoholic fatty liver disease and chronic viral hepatitis. *Dig. Liver. Dis.* **2016**, *48*, 55–61. [CrossRef] [PubMed]

29. Zhang, S.; Du, T.; Zhang, J.; Lu, H.; Lin, X.; Xie, J.; Yang, Y.; Yu, X. The triglyceride and glucose index (tyg) is an effective biomarker to identify nonalcoholic fatty liver disease. *Lipids Health Dis.* **2017**, *16*, 017–0409. [CrossRef] [PubMed]

30. Siddiqui, M.S.; Patidar, K.R.; Boyett, S.; Luketic, V.A.; Puri, P.; Sanyal, A.J. Performance of non-invasive models of fibrosis in predicting mild to moderate fibrosis in patients with non-alcoholic fatty liver disease. *Liver Int.* **2016**, *36*, 572–579. [CrossRef] [PubMed]

31. Pimentel, C.F.; Lai, M. Nutrition interventions for chronic liver diseases and nonalcoholic fatty liver disease. *Med. Clin. N. Am.* **2016**, *100*, 1303–1327. [CrossRef] [PubMed]

32. Raszeja-Wyszomirska, J.; Szymanik, B.; Ławniczak, M.; Kajor, M.; Chwist, A.; Milkiewicz, P.; Hartleb, M. Validation of the bard scoring system in polish patients with nonalcoholic fatty liver disease (NAFLD). *BMC Gastroenterol.* **2010**, *10*, 10–67. [CrossRef] [PubMed]

33. Heymsfield, S.B.; Wadden, T.A. Mechanisms, pathophysiology, and management of obesity. *N. Engl. J. Med.* **2017**, *376*, 254–266. [CrossRef] [PubMed]

34. Chalasani, N.; Younossi, Z.; Lavine, J.E.; Diehl, A.M.; Brunt, E.M.; Cusi, K.; Charlton, M.; Sanyal, A.J. The diagnosis and management of non-alcoholic fatty liver disease: Practice guideline by the american association for the study of liver diseases, american college of gastroenterology, and the american gastroenterological association. *Hepatology* **2012**, *55*, 2005–2023. [CrossRef] [PubMed]

35. Musso, G.; Gambino, R.; De Michieli, F.; Cassader, M.; Rizzetto, M.; Durazzo, M.; Fagà, E.; Silli, B.; Pagano, G. Dietary habits and their relations to insulin resistance and postprandial lipemia in nonalcoholic steatohepatitis. *Hepatology* **2003**, *37*, 909–916. [CrossRef] [PubMed]

36. Zelber-Sagi, S.; Salomone, F.; Mlynarsky, L. The mediterranean dietary pattern as the diet of choice for non-alcoholic fatty liver disease: Evidence and plausible mechanisms. *Liver Int.* **2017**, *2*, 13435. [CrossRef] [PubMed]

37. Romero-Gomez, M.; Zelber-Sagi, S.; Trenell, M. Treatment of nafld with diet, physical activity and exercise. *J. Hepatol.* **2017**, *22*, 32052–32054. [CrossRef] [PubMed]

38. Du, H.; van der, A.D.; Boshuizen, H.C.; Forouhi, N.G.; Wareham, N.J.; Halkjaer, J.; Tjonneland, A.; Overvad, K.; Jakobsen, M.U.; Boeing, H.; et al. Dietary fiber and subsequent changes in body weight and waist circumference in european men and women. *Am. J. Clin. Nutr.* **2010**, *91*, 329–336. [CrossRef] [PubMed]

39. Zelber-Sagi, S.; Ratziu, V.; Oren, R. Nutrition and physical activity in nafld: An overview of the epidemiological evidence. *World J. Gastroenterol.* **2011**, *17*, 3377–3389. [CrossRef] [PubMed]
40. Daubioul, C.A.; Horsmans, Y.; Lambert, P.; Danse, E.; Delzenne, N.M. Effects of oligofructose on glucose and lipid metabolism in patients with nonalcoholic steatohepatitis: Results of a pilot study. *Eur. J. Clin. Nutr.* **2005**, *59*, 723–726. [CrossRef] [PubMed]
41. Rocha, R.; Cotrim, H.P.; Siqueira, A.C.; Floriano, S. Non alcoholic fatty liver disease: Treatment with soluble fibres. *Arq. Gastroenterol.* **2007**, *44*, 350–352. [CrossRef] [PubMed]
42. McCleary, B.V.; DeVries, J.W.; Rader, J.I.; Cohen, G.; Prosky, L.; Mugford, D.C.; Okuma, K. Determination of insoluble, soluble, and total dietary fiber (codex definition) by enzymatic-gravimetric method and liquid chromatography: Collaborative study. *J. AOAC Int.* **2012**, *95*, 824–844. [CrossRef] [PubMed]
43. Sawicki, C.M.; Livingston, K.A.; Obin, M.; Roberts, S.B.; Chung, M.; McKeown, N.M. Dietary fiber and the human gut microbiota: Application of evidence mapping methodology. *Nutrients* **2017**, *9*, 125. [CrossRef] [PubMed]
44. Holscher, H.D. Dietary fiber and prebiotics and the gastrointestinal microbiota. *Gut Microbes* **2017**, *6*, 1290756. [CrossRef] [PubMed]
45. Mello, V.D.; Laaksonen, D.E. Dietary fibers: Current trends and health benefits in the metabolic syndrome and type 2 diabetes. *Arq. Bras. Endocrinol. Metabol.* **2009**, *53*, 509–518. [CrossRef] [PubMed]
46. Russell, W.R.; Hoyles, L.; Flint, H.J.; Dumas, M.E. Colonic bacterial metabolites and human health. *Curr. Opin. Microbiol.* **2013**, *16*, 246–254. [CrossRef] [PubMed]
47. Zolfaghari, H.; Askari, G.; Siassi, F.; Feizi, A.; Sotoudeh, G. Intake of nutrients, fiber, and sugar in patients with nonalcoholic fatty liver disease in comparison to healthy individuals. *Int. J. Prev. Med.* **2016**, *7*, 2008–7802.

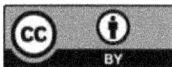

nutrients

MDPI

Article

Alterations in Circulating Amino Acid Metabolite Ratio Associated with Arginase Activity Are Potential Indicators of Metabolic Syndrome: The Korean Genome and Epidemiology Study

Jiyoung Moon [1,†], Oh Yoen Kim [2,†], Garam Jo [1] and Min-Jeong Shin [1,*]

[1] Department of Public Health Sciences, BK21PLUS Program in Embodiment: Health-Society Interaction, Graduate School, Korea University, Seoul 02841, Korea; answldud8503@naver.com (J.M.); grcho94@korea.ac.kr (G.J.)

[2] Department of Food Science and Nutrition, Dong-A University, Busan 49315, Korea; oykim@dau.ac.kr

[*] Correspondence: mjshin@korea.ac.kr; Tel.: +82-2-3290-5643; Fax: +82-2-940-2849

[†] These two authors equally contributed to the work.

Received: 30 May 2017; Accepted: 5 July 2017; Published: 12 July 2017

Abstract: Upregulated arginase activity, which competes with nitric oxide synthase (NOS), impairs nitric oxide production and has been implicated in various metabolic disorders. This study examined whether circulating amino acid metabolite ratios are associated with arginase and NOS activities and whether arginine bioavailability is associated with metabolic syndrome (MetS). Data related to arginase and NOS activities were collected from non-diabetic Koreans without cardiovascular disease ($n = 1998$) in the Ansan–Ansung cohorts (2005–2006). Subsequently, correlation and multivariate logistic regression analyses were performed. With the increase in the number of MetS risk factors, ratios of circulating amino acid metabolites, such as those of ornithine/citrulline, proline/citrulline, and ornithine/arginine, also significantly increased, whereas arginine bioavailability significantly decreased. These metabolite ratios and arginase bioavailability were also significantly correlated with MetS risk-related parameters, which remained significant after adjusting for covariates. In addition, logistic regression analysis revealed that high ratios of circulating metabolites and low arginine bioavailability, which indicated increased arginase activity, were significantly associated with a high MetS risk. This study demonstrated that altered ratios of circulating amino acid metabolites indicates increased arginase activity and decreased arginine bioavailability, both of which can be potential markers for MetS risk.

Keywords: metabolic syndrome; arginase activity; ornithine; citrulline; proline; arginine; bioavailability

1. Introduction

Metabolic syndrome (MetS) is a continuously increasing global epidemic [1] and a key pathological condition leading to the development of type 2 diabetes (T2DM), cardiovascular disease (CVD) [2–6], and nonalcoholic fatty liver disease [4,6–9].

Recently, arginase blockade has attracted a lot of interest as a promising therapeutic target for treating diabetes-induced vascular dysfunction [10–12]. Arginase inhibition has been reported to increase the availability of L-arginine to nitric oxide synthase (NOS) pathway for nitric oxide (NO) production which triggers the biological process for vasodilation by relaxing smooth muscle cells, leading to improvement of endothelial dysfunction in patients with metabolic disorders (i.e., CVD and T2DM) [10]. Our previous study has also demonstrated that arginase inhibition ameliorates obesity-induced abnormalities in hepatic lipids, endothelial function, and whole-body adiposity [11,12]. In addition, L-arginine supplementation has been reported to enhance whole-body insulin sensitivity and reduce plasma levels of fatty acids and triglycerides (TGs), indicating that it is a potentially effective treatment strategy for obesity and MetS [13–17]. Arginase catalyzes L-arginine hydrolysis into urea and L-ornithine, a proline precursor, and competes with NOS for L-arginine in combined NO and citrulline production; this regulates NOS activity and NO (Figure 1) [18,19]. The competitive nature of interaction between arginase and NOS indicates that increased arginase activity and/or arginase-mediated L-arginine depletion may lower NO bioavailability, which may potentially be associated with mechanisms underlying metabolic disorders, such as T2DM and cardiovascular dysfunction [20]. Thus, arginase and NOS activities may play a major role in regulating pathological/metabolic conditions by contributing to the alteration in arginine (substrate) bioavailability and ratios of secondary amino acid metabolites (namely those of ornithine, citrulline, and proline).

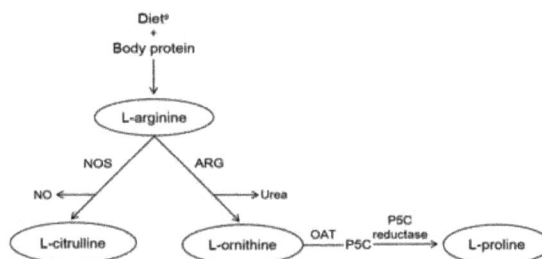

Figure 1. Arginine metabolism. ARG, arginase; NO, nitric oxide; NOS, nitric oxide synthase; OAT, ornithine aminotransferase; P5C, L-pyrroline-5-carboxylate. $^\Phi$ Major dietary sources of L-arginine are meat, poultry, fish, dairy products, nuts, etc.

In this study, therefore, we hypothesized that circulating amino acid metabolite ratios may reflect arginase and NOS activities, and arginine bioavailability is associated with MetS risk, which can be useful indicators for assessing MetS risk.

2. Materials and Methods

2.1. Study Participants

This is a cross-sectional analysis of data from an ongoing prospective cohort study which is a community-based cohort study with data collected from the Korean Genome and Epidemiology Study (KoGES). Detailed information on the study design and aims of the KoGES has been reported [21]. In brief, a total of 10,030 individuals aged 40–69 years who lived in Ansan (urban) and Ansung (rural) were recruited for a baseline in 2001–2002, aiming to establish a national genomic cohort and examine the epidemiologic characteristics in Korea. All participants visited a community clinic for questionnaire-based interviews on demographic information, lifestyle, health condition, and medical history, and for anthropometry and clinical examination, and follow-up examinations were conducted biennially. The present study was based on the data on the third follow-up examination during May 2005–November 2006. Of the 7515 participants, this study was conducted with 2580 participants whose information for metabolites was available. After we excluded subjects who had diabetes and cardiovascular diseases, a total of 1998 subjects (913 men and 1085 women aged 43–74 years) were finally included for the analysis of this study. The written informed consent was obtained from each participant, and the study protocol was approved by the Institute Review Board at the Korea University (KU-IRB-16-EX-272-A-1).

2.2. General Information, Anthropometric and Biochemical Measurements

Survey questionnaires were administered by trained interviewers to obtain demographic and behavioral information (i.e., information on age, sex, physical activity, cigarette smoking, and alcohol consumption). Smoking status and drinking status was classified into three categories: never, former, and current. Participants were asked how long they had participated in five types of activities (sedentary, very light, light, moderate, and intense physical activity). The total metabolic equivalents (METs) were calculated by summing the METs for each type of activity (1.0 for sedentary, 1.5 for very light, 2.4 for light, 5.0 for moderate, and 7.5 for intense activities) [22]. Physical activity was divided into three categories based on the total METs: low (<20), moderate (20–40), and high (≥40) level of activities. Height and body weight (kg) were measured to the nearest 0.1 cm or 0.1 kg while wearing lightweight clothes without shoes. BMI was calculated as weight in kilograms divided by height in meters squared (kg/m^2). Waist circumference (WC, cm) was measured at the midpoint between the lowest rib and the iliac crest in a standing position in 0.1 cm unit, and the average of three repeated measurements was used in the analysis. Repeated measurements of blood pressure (BP) were performed by a trained technician using a mercury sphygmomanometer. Two readings were taken on the left and right arms of subject in a lying position with a 5-min rest between readings. The measurements were recorded to the nearest 2 mmHg and its average was calculated for systolic and diastolic BPs (SBP, and DBP). The blood samples were collected after at least 8 h of fasting for assays of triglycerides (TG; mg/dL), high-density lipoprotein cholesterol (HDLC; mg/dL), fasting blood glucose (FBG; mg/dL), total cholesterol (TC; mg/dL), aspartate aminotransferase (AST; IU/L) and alanine aminotransferase (ALT; IU/L) measured using an automatic analyzer (ADVIA 1650 and 1680, Siemens, Tarrytown, NY, USA). Low-density lipoprotein cholesterol (LDLC; mg/dL) were calculated using the Friedwald equation [23]: LDLC (mg/dL) = TC (mg/dL) − HDLC (mg/dL) − (TG (mg/dL)/5) with TG levels below 400 mg/dL.

2.3. Metabolite Measurement

Targeted metabolomic measurements were performed using the Biocrates platform method using the AbsoluteIDQ^{TM} p180 Kit (BIOCRATES Life Sciences AG, Innsbruck, Austria) with stable nternal standards as reference for the calculation of all metabolite concentrations. AbsoluteIDQ^{TM} p180 Kit contains a 96-well plate with a filter plate. A total of 10 uL serum was loaded on a filter, and then extracts were analyzed by FIA-MS/MS and LC-MS/MS method. Quality assessment of the metabolite concentration measurement was performed with the MetVal^{TM} software package (BIOCRATES Life Sciences AG, Innsbruck, Austria), and quality control (QC) was performed using a calibrator and QC samples included on each plate. Finally, 139 metabolites were detected and quantification by analyzing 36 QC serum samples. For this study, four circulating amino acid metabolites including ornithine, proline, citrulline, arginine were selected and the ratios such as ornithine/citrulline, proline/citrulline, ornithine/arginine, and arginine bioavailability related to the arginase activity were tested to evaluate the association with MetS risk.

2.4. Definition of Metabolic Syndrome

MetS was defined by the guidelines of the National Cholesterol Education Program Adult Treatment panel III [24] with a combination of the World Health Organization and Asian Pacific cutoff value for WC [25]. Briefly, subjects who met at least three of the following criteria were considered as having MetS: (1) SBP ≥ 130/DBP ≥ 85 mmHg or antihypertensive drug use; (2) TG ≥ 150 mg/dL or TG-lowering medication use; (3) HDLC ≤ 40 mg/dL in men and ≤ 50mg/dL in women or HDLC-increasing drug use; (4) WC ≥ 90 cm in men and ≥ 80 cm in women; and (5) FBG ≥ 100 mg/dL or antidiabetic drug use (insulin or oral agents).

2.5. Statistical Analysis

All analyses were performed using Stata SE 12.0 (Stata Corp, College Station, TX, USA). Continuous variables measured in this study were presented as mean ± standard error (SE), and categorical variables are expressed as percentage (%). Differences between MetS people and non-MetS people were determined with Student's *t*-tests and a general linear model (GLM) with Bonferroni's multiple comparisons test considering potential confounding factors for continuous data and the chi-square test for the categorical data. The potential confounding factors included sex, age, BMI (log-transformed), smoking status (never, former, current), and drinking status (never, former, current). Because of skewed distribution, body weight, BMI, other parameters (TG, HDLC, FBG, AST, and ALT), and all metabolites (ornithine, citrulline, proline, arginine) were logarithmically transformed before analysis. General linear model (GLM) with Bonferroni's multiple comparisons test were also used to compare differences in ratios of amino acid according to MetS risk status divided into three groups based on the number of MetS risk factors (0, 1–2, ≥3), after adjusting for potential confounding valuables. Pearson correlation coefficients (*r*-values) were calculated to determine the relationship between circulating amino acids metabolites and MetS risk factors or related biochemical parameters, including TG, HDLC, FBG, SBP, DBP, TC, LDLC, AST and ALT. The partial Spearman correlations were also estimated adjusting for sex, age, BMI, and smoking/drinking status. In addition, logistic regression analyses were carried out to obtain the odds ratios (ORs) and 95% confidence intervals (CIs). We evaluated the associations of circulating amino acids metabolites levels with MetS. All statistical analyses were conducted in three models as follows: unadjusted (Model 0), adjusted for sex, age and BMI (Model 1), and additionally adjusted for smoking and drinking status (Model 2). A *p*-value < 0.05 was considered significant.

3. Results

3.1. General Characteristics of Participants According to Metabolic Syndrome

As shown in Table 1, study participants were divided into two groups: non-MetS (*n* = 1699) and MetS (*n* = 299). The MetS group had a higher proportion of females, contained older and heavier participants, consumed less alcohol, and smoked fewer cigarettes than the non-MetS group. Therefore, these parameters were controlled for further analysis. As expected, the MetS group exhibited significantly larger WCs, higher BPs, higher TG and FBG levels, and lower HDLC levels than the non-MetS group. In addition, serum levels of TC, LDLC, AST, and ALT were also higher in the MetS group than in the non-MetS group. The statistical significances were maintained after the adjustment.

Table 1. Basic population characteristics according to MetS status.

Total (*n* = 1998)	Non-MetS (*n* = 1699)	MetS (*n* = 299)	P_0	P_1	P_2
Age (years)	56.02 ± 0.22	59.92 ± 0.50	<0.001	-	-
Male (%)	48.73	28.43	<0.001	-	-
Body weight (kg) $^\Phi$	61.23 ± 0.25	65.88 ± 0.59	<0.001	-	-
BMI (kg/m^2) $^\Phi$	23.89 ± 0.07	26.82 ± 0.17	<0.001	-	-
Physical activity (%)					
Low	14.83	11.41			
Moderate	36.35	37.25	0.292	0.296	0.454
High	48.82	51.34			
Drinking status (%)					
Never	47.00	55.85			
Former	4.71	3.68	0.018	<0.001	-
Current	48.29	40.47			
Smoking status (%)					
Never	61.13	74.92			
Former	18.14	8.70	<0.001	<0.001	-
Current	20.73	16.39			
MetS risk factors					
WC (cm)	83.13 ± 0.21	93.44 ± 0.45	<0.001	-	<0.001
TG (mg/dL) $^\Phi$	121.63 ± 1.90	233.57 ± 11.31	<0.001	<0.001	<0.001
HDLC (mg/dL) $^\Phi$	45.55 ± 0.25	37.85 ± 0.40	<0.001	<0.001	<0.001
FBG (mg/dL) $^\Phi$	89.85 ± 0.25	95.97 ± 0.68	<0.001	<0.001	<0.001
SBP (mmHg)	114.20 ± 0.37	129.14 ± 0.90	<0.001	<0.001	<0.001
DBP (mmHg)	74.98 ± 0.23	84.19 ± 0.57	<0.001	<0.001	<0.001

Table 1. *Cont.*

Total (n = 1998)	Non-MetS (n = 1699)	MetS (n = 299)	P_0	P_1	P_2
Biochemical parameters					
TC (mg/dL)	191.08 ± 0.85	202.56 ± 2.24	<0.001	<0.001	<0.001
LDLC (mg/dL)	121.43 ± 0.74	125.34 ± 2.08	0.054	<0.001	<0.001
AST (IU/L) $^\Phi$	25.21 ± 0.27	27.74 ± 2.20	0.271	<0.001	<0.001
ALT (IU/L) $^\Phi$	22.49 ± 0.41	24.97 ± 1.06	0.003	<0.001	<0.001

Data are presented as mean ± standard error or percentage (%). $^\Phi$ tested after log-transformed; tested by *t*-test (unadjusted), general linear model (GLM) with Bonferroni's multiple comparisons test (adjusted), or chi square test; P_0: unadjusted *p*-value; P_1: *p*-value after adjusting for age, sex and BMI. P_2: *p*-value after adjusting for age, sex, BMI, cigarette smoking and alcohol consumption; ALT: alanine aminotransferase; AST: aspartate aminotransferase; DBP: diastolic BP; SBP: systolic BP; FBG: fasting blood glucose; HDLC: high density lipoprotein cholesterol; LDLC: low-density lipoprotein cholesterol; MetS: metabolic syndrome; TC, total cholesterol; TG, triglyceride; WC, waist circumference.

3.2. Circulating Amino Acid Metabolite Ratios Associated with Arginase and Nitric Oxide Synthase Activities According to Metabolic Syndrome Risk Status

Ratios of circulating amino acid metabolites, namely ornithine, citrulline, proline, and arginine, associated with arginase and NOS activities and arginine bioavailability, were individually measured, and subsequently, ratios of these metabolites were calculated. The ornithine to citrulline (ornithine/citrulline) and proline to citrulline (proline/citrulline) ratios indirectly indicated the arginase/NOS activity ratio, whereas the ornithine/arginine ratio directly indicated arginase activity. As shown in Figure 2, with the increase in the number of MetS risk factors, ornithine/citrulline, proline/citrulline, and ornithine/arginine ratios also significantly increased (MetS risk factor = 0, *n* = 478; MetS risk factor = 1–2, *n* = 1221; MetS risk factor ≥3, *n* = 299). On the other hand, arginine bioavailability, defined as arginine/(ornithine + citrulline), significantly decreased with the increase in the number of MetS risk factors.

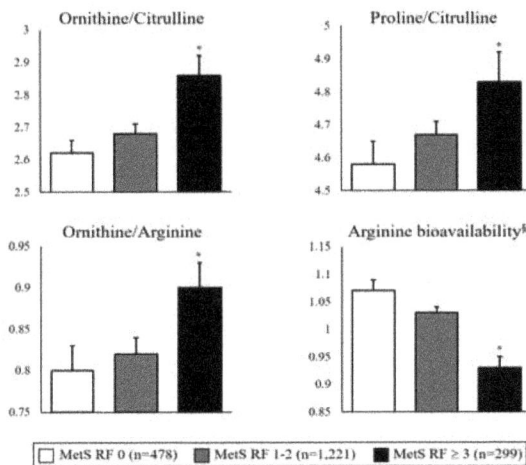

Figure 2. Association between circulating amino acids metabolites and MetS risk status. Data are presented as mean ± standard error; tested after log-transformed; tested by general linear model (GLM) with Bonferroni's multiple comparisons test (adjustment for age, sex, BMI, cigarette smoking and alcohol consumption); MetS RF: MetS risk factor. * represents significant differences in the values between Mets RF ≥ 3 group and MetS RF 0/MetS RF 1–2 groups; § Arginine bioavailability is defined as Arginine/(Ornithine + Citrulline).

3.3. Correlations between Amino Acid Metabolites and Metabolic Syndrome Risk-Related Parameters

Pearson (r_0, P_0) and partial (r_1, P_1) correlation analyses were performed to identify the relationship between the MetS risk-related metabolic parameters and the ratios of amino acid metabolites. As shown in Figure 3, WCs were positively correlated with the ornithine/citrulline ratio ($r_0 = 0.128$, $P_0 < 0.001$; $r_1 = 0.134$, $P_1 < 0.001$), proline/citrulline ratio ($r_0 = 0.146$, $P_0 < 0.001$; $r_1 = 0.202$, $P_1 < 0.001$), and ornithine/arginine ratio ($r_0 = 0.123$, $P_0 < 0.001$; $r_1 = 0.089$, $P_1 < 0.001$) but were negatively correlated with arginine bioavailability ($r_0 = -0.111$, $P_0 < 0.001$; $r_1 = -0.071$, $P_1 = 0.002$) before and after adjustments for age, sex, BMI, cigarette smoking, and alcohol consumption. In addition, after the adjustment, serum levels of TG ($r_1 = 0.062$, $P_1 < 0.05$), FBG ($r_1 = 0.051$, $p < 0.05$), AST ($r_1 = 0.114$, $P_1 < 0.05$), and ALT ($r_1 = 0.097$, $P_1 < 0.05$) were positively correlated but those of HDLC ($r_1 = -0.051$, $P_1 < 0.05$) were negatively correlated with the ornithine/citrulline ratio (Table 2). DBPs ($r = 0.035$, $p < 0.05$), TC levels ($r_1 = 0.028$, $P_1 < 0.05$), and ALT levels ($r_1 = 0.079$, $P_1 < 0.05$) were positively correlated but AST levels ($r_1 = -0.005$, $P_1 < 0.05$) were negatively correlated with the proline/citrulline ratio. Serum levels of TG ($r_1 = 0.027$, $P_1 < 0.05$) and ALT ($r_1 = 0.054$, $P_1 < 0.05$) were positively correlated but those of HDLC ($r_1 = -0.088$, $P_1 < 0.05$), and FBG ($r_1 = -0.002$, $P_1 < 0.05$) were negatively correlated with the ornithine/arginine ratio. On the other hand, arginine bioavailability was positively correlated with serum levels of HDLC ($r_1 = 0.110$, $P_1 < 0.05$), and TC ($r_1 = 0.074$, $P_1 < 0.05$) but negatively correlated with DBPs ($r_1 = -0.051$, $P_1 = 0.05$) and AST levels ($r_1 = -0.107$, $P_1 < 0.05$) (Table 2).

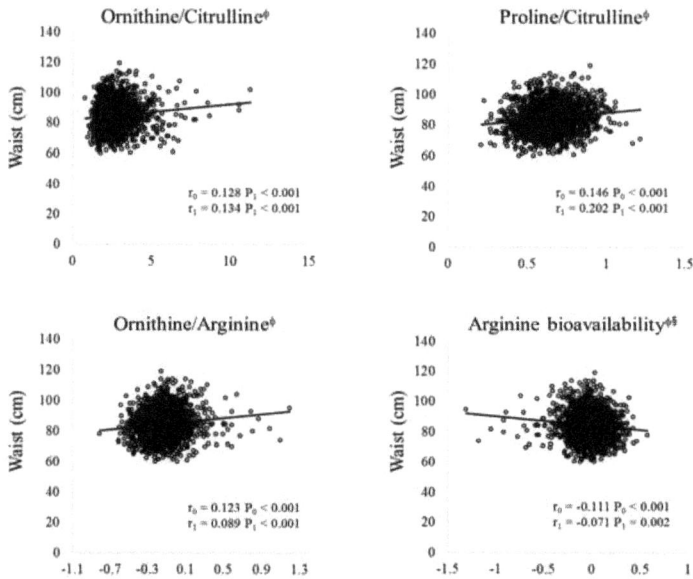

Figure 3. Relationship between circulating amino acids metabolites and waist circumference. Data are represented as mean $\pm$ standard error; *r*—correlation co-efficient, *p*: *p*-value. Data were tested by Pearson (r_0, P_0, unadjusted) and Partial (r_1, P_1: adjusted for age, sex, BMI, cigarette smoking and alcohol consumption) correlation analyses. $^\Phi$ tested after log-transformed; § Arginine bioavailability = Arginine/(Ornithine + Citrulline).

Table 2. Correlation between circulating amino acid metabolites, MetS risk factors, and related biochemical parameters.

Total (*n* = 1998)	ORN/CIT	PRO/CIT	ORN/ARG	Arginine Bioavailability [§]
TG (mg/dL) [Φ]	0.062 *	0.149	0.027 *	−0.026
HDLC (mg/dL) [Φ]	−0.051 *	−0.056	−0.088 *	0.110 *
FBG (mg/dL) [Φ]	0.051 *	0.134	−0.002 *	0.021
SBP (mmHg)	0.020	0.038	0.021	−0.029
DBP (mmHg)	0.041	0.035 *	0.054	−0.051 *
TC (mg/dL)	0.010	0.028 *	−0.048	0.074 *
LDLC (mg/dL)	−0.017	−0.022	−0.043	0.044
AST (IU/L) [Φ]	0.114 *	−0.005 *	0.170	−0.107 *
ALT (IU/L) [Φ]	0.097 *	0.079 *	0.054 *	−0.025

Correlation coefficient, tested by partial correlation analysis with adjustment for age, sex, BMI, and smoking status and alcohol consumption. [Φ] tested after log-transformed; * p-value < 0.05; [§] Arginine bioavailability = Arginine/(Ornithine + Citrulline); ALT, alanine aminotransferase; AST, aspartate aminotransferase; DBP, diastolic blood pressure; FBG, fasting blood glucose; HDLC, high-density lipoprotein cholesterol; LDLC, low-density lipoprotein cholesterol; SBP, systolic blood pressure; TC, total cholesterol; TG, triglyceride.

3.4. Association between Circulating Amino Acid Metabolite Ratios and Metabolic Syndrome Risk

Associations between amino acid metabolite ratios and MetS risk were evaluated by comparing ORs (95% CIs), which were calculated using a logistic regression model with adjustments for confounding factors (namely age, sex, BMI, cigarette smoking, and alcohol consumption) (Table 3). Study population was divided into quartile groups according to each amino acid metabolite ratio. The highest quartile group of the ornithine/citrulline ratio demonstrated higher MetS risk than the lowest quartile group before and after the adjustment (OR_0: 1.98, 95% CI: 1.39–2.82, P_0 < 0.001; OR_1: 1.75, 95% CI: 1.18–2.59, P_1 = 0.005; OR_2: 1.71, 95% CI: 1.15–2.54, P_2 = 0.008). In addition, the highest quartile group of the ornithine/arginine ratio demonstrated higher MetS risk than the lowest quartile group before and after the adjustment (OR_0: 2.89, 95% CI: 1.98–4.22, P_0 < 0.001; OR_1: 2.58, 95% CI: 1.70–3.90, P_1 < 0.001; OR_2: 2.57, 95% CI: 1.69–3.90, P_2 < 0.001). However, the proline/citrulline ratio was not significantly associated with MetS, whereas arginine bioavailability was negatively associated with MetS (OR_0: 0.38, 95% CI: 0.26–0.55, P_0 < 0.001; OR_1: 0.40, 95% CI: 0.26–0.60, P_1 < 0.001; OR_2: 0.40, 95% CI: 0.26–0.61, P_2 < 0.001). Next, multiple regression analysis was performed to identify the association of contributing factors, amino acid metabolite ratios, and arginine bioavailability with MetS risk. ORs for the association of the ornithine/citrulline ratio and arginine bioavailability with MetS were 1.33 (95% CI: 0.87–2.05, p = 0.188) and 0.45 (95% CI: 0.29–0.69, p < 0.001), respectively, after the adjustment. ORs for the association of the proline/citrulline ratio and arginine bioavailability with MetS were 1.48 (95% CI: 0.97–2.25, p = 0.070) and 0.38 (95% CI: 0.25–0.58, p < 0.001), respectively, after the adjustment. ORs for the association of the ornithine/arginine ratio and arginine bioavailability with MetS were 2.62 (95% CI: 0.92–7.44), p = 0.070) and 0.97 (95% CI: 0.34–2.78, p = 0.961), respectively, after the adjustment.

Table 3. Risk of MetS associated with circulating amino acid metabolites.

Total (*n* = 1998)	OR$_0$ (95% CI) p-Value	OR$_1$ (95% CI) p-Value	OR$_2$ (95% CI) p-Value
ORN/CIT [Φ]	1.98 (1.39, 2.82) <0.001	1.75 (1.18, 2.59) 0.005	1.71 (1.15, 2.54) 0.008
PRO/CIT [Φ]	1.29 (0.91, 1.85) 0.154	1.33 (0.88, 2.01) 0.174	1.30 (0.86, 1.97) 0.215
ORN/ARG [Φ]	2.89 (1.98, 4.22) <0.001	2.58 (1.70, 3.90) <0.001	2.57 (1.69, 3.90) <0.001
Arginine bioavailability [Φ,§]	0.38 (0.26, 0.55) <0.001	0.40 (0.26, 0.60) <0.001	0.40 (0.26, 0.61) <0.001

OR: odds ratio, CI: confidence interval, [Φ] tested after log-transformed; The association was calculated using the OR (95% CIs) of a logistic regression model (OR$_0$: unadjusted, OR$_1$: adjusted for age, sex, and BMI, OR$_2$ adjusted for age, sex, BMI and smoking status and alcohol consumption). [§] Arginine bioavailability = Arginine/(Ornithine + Citrulline); ARG, Arginine; CIT, Citrulline; ORN, Ornithine; PRO, Proline.

4. Discussion

This study demonstrated that alterations in circulating amino acid metabolite ratios, which are indicative of arginase and NOS activities, and arginine bioavailability were significantly associated with MetS risk: people with high ratios of circulating metabolites (particularly, those of ornithine/citrulline and ornithine/arginine) and low levels of arginine bioavailability demonstrated high MetS risk. These results suggested that circulating amino acid metabolite ratios, which are indicative of arginase activity and arginine bioavailability can potentially serve as biomarkers for assessing MetS risk.

Accumulating evidence has shown strong association of a group of metabolic disorders, such as obesity, insulin resistance, hyperglycemia, diabetes, CVD, and atherosclerosis [26,27], with arginase and NOS pathways of L-arginine substrate [10–12,28–39]. Arginase isoforms, which are involved in the urea cycle and are expressed in the hepatic, vascular smooth muscle, and endothelial cells, are responsible for converting L-arginine to urea and L-ornithine, and L-ornithine is further metabolized to proline by ornithine aminotransferase [18,40]. Arginases are activated by inflammatory factors and atherothrombosis mediators, including oxidized low-density lipoprotein [41] and thrombin [42], thereby inhibiting NO-mediated endothelial relaxation. The upregulated arginase activity also contributes to the lack of L-arginine for NOS pathway, which decreases NO bioavailability and leads to various metabolic complications, such as diabetes, inflammation, and cardiovascular disorders, including endothelial dysfunction, high BP, diabetic vascular disease, and atherosclerosis [20,37,43–45]. Recent studies have indicated that increased NO production can result from arginase inhibition or L-arginine supplementation, which reduces the arginase activity [10–17]. These results have demonstrated the importance of arginase inhibition in endothelial dysfunction, which occurs in several pathological states, such as atherosclerotic and vascular disease. In addition, arginase inhibition plays an important role in restoring metabolic disorders, such as T2DM [10,37], endothelial dysfunction in adjuvant arthritis [34], hypertension [32] and atherosclerosis [46]. In our previous studies, arginase inhibition not only ameliorated body fat, hepatic lipid abnormalities, and adipose tissue inflammation but also restored endothelial dysfunction in obesity-induced animals, which was mediated by increased NO production [11,12,43]. Emerging evidence has indicated that NOS-synthesized NO plays a key role in regulating energy metabolism and pathogenesis of metabolic abnormalities, indicating that NO output may be beneficial for preventing and treating obesity and insulin resistance [47]. NO bioavailability is reduced in diet-induced obese animals [48,49] and in overweight humans with insulin resistance [50]. Furthermore, increased endothelial NOS (eNOS) activity prevents the obesogenic effects of a high-fat diet, which indicates the anti-obesity effect of eNOS in regulating lipid metabolism [51]. Thus, enhanced physiological levels of NO can ameliorate all disorders in obese conditions and reduce the arginase activity [52].

To date, accumulating evidence has shown the important implications of arginase activity on MetS but has demonstrated limited information about the effect of altered amino acid metabolite ratios on arginase activity in the presence of metabolic abnormalities. Our previous study has demonstrated that arginase gene expression is significantly upregulated in overweight people and that arginase mRNA levels are closely associated with phenotype biomarkers for obesity, disturbed lipid profiles, and endothelial dysfunction [28]. In the present study, we analyzed arginine, a substrate of arginase and NOS, and the secondary products produced by these two enzymes (ornithine, citrulline, and proline) and found a significant correlation between these amino acid metabolite ratios and MetS risk-related parameters. In this study, arginine and its catabolic metabolites including ornithine, proline, and citrulline were used for the indicator of arginase and NOS since there is with no net loss of these metabolites during urea synthesis. Among these parameters, WC was significantly correlated with all amino acid metabolite ratios; it was positively correlated with ornithine/citrulline, proline/citrulline, and ornithine/arginine ratios but negatively correlated with arginine bioavailability. As stated above, ornithine/citrulline and proline/citrulline ratios indirectly indicated the arginase/NOS activity ratio, whereas the ornithine/arginine ratio directly indicated arginase activity. In this study, ornithine/citrulline, proline/citrulline, and ornithine/arginine ratios were significantly increased with the increase in the number of MetS risk factors. The increased ornithine/citrulline and proline/citrulline ratios indicated that arginase activity was higher than NOS activity. The increased ornithine/arginine ratio implied that arginase activity was upregulated but NOS activity was downregulated. On the other hand, arginine bioavailability significantly decreased with the increase in the number of MetS risk factors, which suggested that the levels of arginine available as a substrate for arginase and NOS were low in the MetS status. In addition, multiple regression analyses revealed that arginine bioavailability was more independent of risk factors than arginase and NOS activities. These data indicated that circulating amino acid metabolite ratios reflect arginase and NOS activities and may explain the potential mechanism of arginase and NOS pathways in metabolic disorders. On the other hand, it should be noted that the ratio of proline to citrulline was not associated with the ORs for MetS, possibly due to the fact that proline is not a direct metabolite of arginase.

This study has a limitation. Measurements of circulating amino acids were not repeated. This is a potential limitation because circulating enzymes in blood can occasionally change; however, because the data were collected from a relatively large population, such changes and, consequently, the limitation can be overlooked. Despite this limitation, the present study demonstrated a strong relationship between circulating amino acids and MetS-related risk parameters, suggesting that alterations in circulating amino acid metabolite ratios, which are associated with arginase and NOS activities, and arginine bioavailability are potential indicators for assessing MetS risk. These alterations may also indicate important information for deciphering the pathogenesis of disturbances in amino acid metabolism related to the arginase activity.

Acknowledgments: This study was provided with bioresources from the National Biobank of Korea and the Centers for Disease Control and Prevention, Republic of Korea (KBP-2016-062). This research was supported by the Basic Science Research Program, through the National Research Foundation of Korea (NRF), funded by the Ministry of Education, Science, and Technology (NRF-2015R1A2A1A15054758).

Author Contributions: M.-J.S. conceived the study and acquired data. J.M., O.Y.K., G.J. and M.-J.S. developed the statistical analysis plan; G.J. analyzed the data. J.M., O.Y.K. and M.-J.S. prepared the first draft of the manuscript; J.M., O.Y.K., G.J. and M.J.S. contributed to the writing of the manuscript. All authors reviewed and agreed on the final version of the manuscript.

Conflicts of Interest: The authors declare no conflict of interest.

References

1. International Diabetes Federation (IDF). *IDF Consensus Worldwide Definition of the Metabolic Syndrome*; International Diabetes Federation (IDF): Brussels, Belgium, 2006.
2. Hossain, P.; Kawar, B.; El Nahas, M. Obesity and diabetes in the developing world—A growing challenge. *N. Engl. J. Med.* **2007**, *2007*, 213–215. [CrossRef] [PubMed]
3. Mello, M.M.; Studdert, D.M.; Brennan, T.A. Obesity—The new frontier of public health law. *N. Engl. J. Med.* **2006**, *354*, 2601–2610. [CrossRef] [PubMed]
4. Kaur, J. A comprehensive review on metabolic syndrome. *Cardiol. Res. Pract.* **2014**, *2014*. [CrossRef] [PubMed]
5. Lakka, H.M.; Laaksonen, D.E.; Lakka, T.A.; Niskanen, L.K.; Kumpusalo, E.; Tuomilehto, J.; Salonen, J.T. The metabolic syndrome and total and cardiovascular disease mortality in middle-aged men. *JAMA* **2006**, *288*, 2709–2716. [CrossRef]
6. Alberti, K.; Eckel, R.; Grundy, S.; Zimmet, P.; Cleeman, J.; Donato, K. Harmonizing the metabolic syndrome. A joint interim statement of the international diabetes federation task force on epidemiology and prevention; national heart, lung and blood institute; american heart association; world heart federation; international atherosclerosis society; and international atherosclerosis for the study of obesity. *Circulation* **2009**, *120*, 1640–1645. [PubMed]
7. Williams, T. Metabolic syndrome: Nonalcoholic fatty liver disease. *FP Essent.* **2015**, *435*, 24–29. [PubMed]

8. Marchesini, G.; Brizi, M.; Morselli-Labate, A.M.; Bianchi, G.; Bugianesi, E.; McCullough, A.J.; Forlani, G.; Melchionda, N. Association of nonalcoholic fatty liver disease with insulin resistance. *Am. J. Med.* **1999**, *107*, 450–455. [CrossRef]

9. Marchesini, G.; Brizi, M.; Bianchi, G.; Tomassetti, S.; Bugianesi, E.; Lenzi, M.; McCullough, A.J.; Natale, S.; Forlani, G.; Melchionda, N. Nonalcoholic fatty liver disease. *Diabetes* **2001**, *50*, 1844–1850. [CrossRef] [PubMed]

10. Shemyakin, A.; Kövamees, O.; Rafnsson, A.; Böhm, F.; Svenarud, P.; Settergren, M.; Jung, C.; Pernow, J. Arginase inhibition improves endothelial function in patients with coronary artery disease and type 2 diabetes mellitusclinical perspective. *Circulation* **2012**, *126*, 2943–2950. [CrossRef] [PubMed]

11. Moon, J.; Do, H.J.; Cho, Y.; Shin, M.-J. Arginase inhibition ameliorates hepatic metabolic abnormalities in obese mice. *PLoS ONE* **2014**, *9*, e103048. [CrossRef] [PubMed]

12. Chung, J.H.; Moon, J.; Lee, Y.S.; Chung, H.-K.; Lee, S.-M.; Shin, M.-J. Arginase inhibition restores endothelial function in diet-induced obesity. *Biochem. Biophys. Res. Commun.* **2014**, *451*, 179–183. [CrossRef] [PubMed]

13. McKnight, J.R.; Satterfield, M.C.; Jobgen, W.S.; Smith, S.B.; Spencer, T.E.; Meininger, C.J.; McNeal, C.J.; Wu, G. Beneficial effects of L-arginine on reducing obesity: Potential mechanisms and important implications for human health. *Amino Acids* **2010**, *39*, 349–357. [CrossRef] [PubMed]

14. Jobgen, W.; Fu, W.J.; Gao, H.; Li, P.; Meininger, C.J.; Smith, S.B.; Spencer, T.E.; Wu, G. High fat feeding and dietary L-arginine supplementation differentially regulate gene expression in rat white adipose tissue. *Amino Acids* **2009**, *37*, 187–198. [CrossRef] [PubMed]

15. Clemmensen, C.; Madsen, A.N.; Smajilovic, S.; Holst, B.; Bräuner-Osborne, H. L-Arginine improves multiple physiological parameters in mice exposed to diet-induced metabolic disturbances. *Amino Acids* **2012**, *43*, 1265–1275. [CrossRef] [PubMed]

16. Jobgen, W.; Meininger, C.J.; Jobgen, S.C.; Li, P.; Lee, M.-J.; Smith, S.B.; Spencer, T.E.; Fried, S.K.; Wu, G. Dietary L-arginine supplementation reduces white fat gain and enhances skeletal muscle and brown fat masses in diet-induced obese rats. *J. Nutr.* **2008**, *139*, 230–237. [CrossRef] [PubMed]

17. Fu, W.J.; Haynes, T.E.; Kohli, R.; Hu, J.; Shi, W.; Spencer, T.E.; Carroll, R.J.; Meininger, C.J.; Wu, G. Dietary L-arginine supplementation reduces fat mass in zucker diabetic fatty rats. *J. Nutr.* **2005**, *135*, 714–721. [PubMed]

18. Caldwell, R.B.; Toque, H.A.; Narayanan, S.P.; Caldwell, R.W. Arginase: An old enzyme with new tricks. *Trends Pharmacol. Sci.* **2015**, *36*, 395–405. [CrossRef] [PubMed]

19. Vanhoutte, P.M. Arginine and arginase. *Circ. Res.* **2008**, *102*, 923–932. [CrossRef] [PubMed]

20. Pernow, J.; Jung, C. Arginase as a potential target in the treatment of cardiovascular disease: Reversal of arginine steal? *Cardiovasc. Res.* **2013**, *98*, 334–343. [CrossRef] [PubMed]

21. Cho, Y.S.; Go, M.J.; Kim, Y.J.; Heo, J.Y.; Oh, J.H.; Ban, H.J.; Yoon, D.; Lee, M.H.; Kim, D.J.; Park, M.; et al. A large-scale genome-wide association study of asian populations uncovers genetic factors influencing eight quantitative traits. *Nat. Genet.* **2009**, *41*, 527–534. [CrossRef] [PubMed]

22. Ainsworth, B.E.; Haskell, W.L.; Whitt, M.C.; Irwin, M.L.; Swartz, A.M.; Strath, S.J.; O'Brien, W.L.; Bassett, D.R., Jr.; Schmitz, K.H.; Emplaincourt, P.O.; et al. Compendium of physical activities: An update of activity codes and met intensities. *Med. Sci. Sports Exerc.* **2000**, *32*, S498–S504. [CrossRef] [PubMed]

23. Friedewald, W.T.; Levy, R.I.; Fredrickson, D.S. Estimation of the concentration of low-density lipoprotein cholesterol in plasma, without use of the preparative ultracentrifuge. *Clin. Chem.* **1972**, *18*, 499–502. [PubMed]

24. Expert Panel on Detection, Evaluation, and Treatment of High Blood Cholesterol in Adults. Executive summary of the third report of the national cholesterol education program (NCEP) expert panel on detection, evaluation, and treatment of high blood cholesterol in adults (adult treatment panel iii). *JAMA* **2001**, *285*, 2486–2497.

25. Kim, J.A.; Choi, C.J.; Yum, K.S. Cut-off values of visceral fat area and waist circumference: Diagnostic criteria for abdominal obesity in a korean population. *J. Korean Med. Sci.* **2006**, *21*, 1048–1053. [CrossRef] [PubMed]

26. Zieba, R. Obesity: A review of currently used antiobesity drugs and new compounds in clinical development. *Postep. Hig. Med. Doswiadczalnej* **2006**, *61*, 612–626.

27. Halford, J. Obesity drugs in clinical development. *Curr. Opin. Investig. Drugs* **2006**, *7*, 312–318. [PubMed]

28. Kim, O.Y.; Lee, S.-M.; Chung, J.H.; Do, H.J.; Moon, J.; Shin, M.-J. Arginase I and the very low-density lipoprotein receptor are associated with phenotypic biomarkers for obesity. *Nutrition* **2012**, *28*, 635–639. [CrossRef] [PubMed]

29. Katusic, Z.S. Mechanisms of endothelial dysfunction induced by aging. *Circ. Res.* **2007**, *101*, 640–641. [CrossRef] [PubMed]

30. Yang, Z.; Ming, X.-F. Endothelial arginase: A new target in atherosclerosis. *Curr. Hypertens. Rep.* **2006**, *8*, 54–59. [CrossRef] [PubMed]

31. Bagnost, T.; Ma, L.; Da Silva, R.F.; Rezakhaniha, R.; Houdayer, C.; Stergiopulos, N.; André, C.; Guillaume, Y.; Berthelot, A.; Demougeot, C. Cardiovascular effects of arginase inhibition in spontaneously hypertensive rats with fully developed hypertension. *Cardiovasc. Res.* **2010**, *87*, 569–577. [CrossRef] [PubMed]

32. Bagnost, T.; Berthelot, A.; Bouhaddi, M.; Laurant, P.; André, C.; Guillaume, Y.; Demougeot, C. Treatment with the arginase inhibitor Nω-hydroxy-nor-L-arginine improves vascular function and lowers blood pressure in adult spontaneously hypertensive rat. *J. Hypertens.* **2008**, *26*, 1110–1118. [CrossRef] [PubMed]

33. Prati, C.; Berthelot, A.; Wendling, D.; Demougeot, C. Endothelial dysfunction in rat adjuvant-induced arthritis: Up-regulation of the vascular arginase pathway. *Arthritis Rheum.* **2011**, *63*, 2309–2317. [CrossRef] [PubMed]

34. Prati, C.; Berthelot, A.; Kantelip, B.; Wendling, D.; Demougeot, C. Treatment with the arginase inhibitor Nw-hydroxy-nor-L-arginine restores endothelial function in rat adjuvant-induced arthritis. *Arthritis Res. Ther.* **2012**, *14*, R130. [PubMed]

35. Toya, T.; Hakuno, D.; Shiraishi, Y.; Kujiraoka, T.; Adachi, T. Arginase inhibition augments nitric oxide production and facilitates left ventricular systolic function in doxorubicin-induced cardiomyopathy in mice. *Physiol. Rep.* **2014**, *2*, e12130. [CrossRef] [PubMed]

36. Kovamees, O.; Shemyakin, A.; Eriksson, M.; Angelin, B.; Pernow, J. Arginase inhibition improves endothelial function in patients with familial hypercholesterolaemia irrespective of their cholesterol levels. *J. Intern. Med.* **2016**, *279*, 477–484. [CrossRef] [PubMed]

37. Grönros, J.; Jung, C.; Lundberg, J.O.; Cerrato, R.; Östenson, C.-G.; Pernow, J. Arginase inhibition restores in vivo coronary microvascular function in type 2 diabetic rats. *Am. J. Physiol. Heart Circ. Physiol.* **2011**, *300*, H1174–H1181. [CrossRef] [PubMed]

38. Morris, C.R.; Poljakovic, M.; Lavrisha, L.; Machado, L.; Kuypers, F.A.; Morris, S.M., Jr. Decreased arginine bioavailability and increased serum arginase activity in asthma. *Am. J. Respir. Crit. Care Med.* **2004**, *170*, 148–153. [CrossRef] [PubMed]

39. El-Bassossy, H.M.; El-Fawal, R.; Fahmy, A.; Watson, M.L. Arginase inhibition alleviates hypertension in the metabolic syndrome. *Br. J. Pharmacol.* **2013**, *169*, 693–703. [CrossRef] [PubMed]

40. Buga, G.M.; Singh, R.; Pervin, S.; Rogers, N.E.; Schmitz, D.A.; Jenkinson, C.P.; Cederbaum, S.D.; Ignarro, L.J. Arginase activity in endothelial cells: Inhibition by NG-hydroxy-L-arginine during high-output NO production. *Am. J. Physiol. Heart Circ. Physiol.* **1996**, *271*, H1988–H1998.

41. Ryoo, S.; Lemmon, C.A.; Soucy, K.G.; Gupta, G.; White, A.R.; Nyhan, D.; Shoukas, A.; Romer, L.H.; Berkowitz, D.E. Oxidized low-density lipoprotein–dependent endothelial arginase II activation contributes to impaired nitric oxide signaling. *Circ. Res.* **2006**, *99*, 951–960. [CrossRef] [PubMed]

42. Zhu, W.; Chandrasekharan, U.M.; Bandyopadhyay, S.; Morris, S.M.; DiCorleto, P.E.; Kashyap, V.S. Thrombin induces endothelial arginase through AP-1 activation. *Am. J. Physiol. Cell Physiol.* **2010**, *298*, C952–C960. [CrossRef] [PubMed]

43. Hu, H.; Moon, J.; Chung, J.H.; Kim, O.Y.; Yu, R.; Shin, M.-J. Arginase inhibition ameliorates adipose tissue inflammation in mice with diet-induced obesity. *Biochem. Biophys. Res. Commun.* **2015**, *464*, 840–847. [CrossRef] [PubMed]

44. Bivalacqua, T.J.; Hellstrom, W.J.; Kadowitz, P.J.; Champion, H.C. Increased expression of arginase II in human diabetic corpus cavernosum: In diabetic-associated erectile dysfunction. *Biochem. Biophys. Res. Commun.* **2001**, *283*, 923–927. [CrossRef] [PubMed]

45. Romero, M.J.; Platt, D.H.; Tawfik, H.E.; Labazi, M.; El-Remessy, A.B.; Bartoli, M.; Caldwell, R.B.; Caldwell, R.W. Diabetes-induced coronary vascular dysfunction involves increased arginase activity. *Circ. Res.* **2008**, *102*, 95–102. [CrossRef] [PubMed]

46. Olivon, V.C.; Fraga-Silva, R.A.; Segers, D.; Demougeot, C.; de Oliveira, A.M.; Savergnini, S.S.; Berthelot, A.; de Crom, R.; Krams, R.; Stergiopulos, N. Arginase inhibition prevents the low shear stress-induced development of vulnerable atherosclerotic plaques in ApoE−/− mice. *Atherosclerosis* **2013**, *227*, 236–243. [CrossRef] [PubMed]

47. Sansbury, B.E.; Hill, B.G. Regulation of obesity and insulin resistance by nitric oxide. *Free Radic. Biol. Med.* **2014**, *73*, 383–399. [CrossRef] [PubMed]

48. Kim, F.; Pham, M.; Maloney, E.; Rizzo, N.O.; Morton, G.J.; Wisse, B.E.; Kirk, E.A.; Chait, A.; Schwartz, M.W. Vascular inflammation, insulin resistance, and reduced nitric oxide production precede the onset of peripheral insulin resistance. *Arterioscler. Thromb. Vasc. Biol.* **2008**, *28*, 1982–1988. [CrossRef] [PubMed]

49. Bender, S.; Herrick, E.; Lott, N.; Klabunde, R. Diet-induced obesity and diabetes reduce coronary responses to nitric oxide due to reduced bioavailability in isolated mouse hearts. *Diabetes Obes. Metab.* **2007**, *9*, 688–696. [CrossRef] [PubMed]

50. Gruber, H.; Mayer, C.; Mangge, H.; Fauler, G.; Grandits, N.; Wilders-Truschnig, M. Obesity reduces the bioavailability of nitric oxide in juveniles. *Int. J. Obes.* **2008**, *32*, 826–831. [CrossRef] [PubMed]

51. Sansbury, B.E.; Cummins, T.D.; Tang, Y.; Hellmann, J.; Holden, C.R.; Harbeson, M.A.; Chen, Y.; Patel, R.P.; Spite, M.; Bhatnagar, A. Overexpression of endothelial nitric oxide synthase prevents diet-induced obesity and regulates adipocyte phenotypenovelty and significance. *Circ. Res.* **2012**, *111*, 1176–1189. [CrossRef] [PubMed]

52. Jobgen, W.S.; Fried, S.K.; Fu, W.J.; Meininger, C.J.; Wu, G. Regulatory role for the arginine-nitric oxide pathway in metabolism of energy substrates. *J. Nutr. Biochem.* **2006**, *17*, 571–588. [CrossRef] [PubMed]

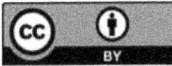

nutrients

MDPI

Article

A Protein Diet Score, Including Plant and Animal Protein, Investigating the Association with HbA1c and eGFR—The PREVIEW Project

Grith Møller [1,*], Diewertje Sluik [2], Christian Ritz [1], Vera Mikkilä [3], Olli T. Raitakari [4,5], Nina Hutri-Kähönen [6], Lars O. Dragsted [1], Thomas M. Larsen [1], Sally D. Poppitt [7], Marta P. Silvestre [7], Edith J.M. Feskens [2], Jennie Brand-Miller [8] and Anne Raben [1]

[1] Department of Nutrition, Exercise and Sports, Faculty of Science, University of Copenhagen, Rolighedsvej 26, 1958 Frederiksberg C, Denmark; ritz@nexs.ku.dk (C.R.); ldra@nexs.ku.dk (L.O.D.); tml@nexs.ku.dk (T.M.L.); ara@nexs.ku.dk (A.R.)
[2] Division of Human Nutrition, Wageningen University, Stippeneng 4, 6708 WE Wageningen, The Netherlands; Diewertje.sluik@wur.nl (D.S.); edith.feskens@wur.nl (E.J.M.F.)
[3] Department of Food and Environmental Sciences, University of Helsinki, 00014 Helsinki, Finland; vera.mikkila@aka.fi
[4] Research Centre of Applied and Preventive Cardiovascular Medicine, Kiinamyllynkatu 10, University of Turku, 20520 Turku, Finland; olli.raitakari@uta.fi
[5] Department of Clinical Physiology and Nuclear Medicine, Turku University Hospital, 20521 Turku, Finland
[6] Department of Pediatrics, Tampere University Hospital and Faculty of Medicine and Life Sciences, University of Tampere, 33014 Tampere, Finland; nina.hutri-kahonen@uta.fi
[7] Human Nutrition Unit, School of Biological Sciences, 18 Carrick Place, Mt Eden, University of Auckland, Auckland 1024, New Zealand; s.poppitt@auckland.ac.nz (S.D.P.); m.silvestre@auckland.ac.nz (M.P.S.)
[8] School of Life and Environmental Sciences & Charles Perkins Centre, University of Sydney, Camperdown, NSW 2006, Australia; jennie.brandmiller@sydney.edu.au
* Correspondence: gmp@nexs.ku.dk; Tel.: +45-35-33-48-18

Received: 7 June 2017; Accepted: 11 July 2017; Published: 17 July 2017

Abstract: Higher-protein diets have been advocated for body-weight regulation for the past few decades. However, the potential health risks of these diets are still uncertain. We aimed to develop a protein score based on the quantity and source of protein, and to examine the association of the score with glycated haemoglobin (HbA1c) and estimated glomerular filtration rate (eGFR). Analyses were based on three population studies included in the PREVIEW project (PREVention of diabetes through lifestyle Intervention and population studies in Europe and around the World): NQplus, Lifelines, and the Young Finns Study. Cross-sectional data from food-frequency questionnaires (n = 76,777 subjects) were used to develop a protein score consisting of two components: 1) percentage of energy from total protein, and 2) plant to animal protein ratio. An inverse association between protein score and HbA1c (slope -0.02 ± 0.01 mmol/mol, $p < 0.001$) was seen in Lifelines. We found a positive association between the protein score and eGFR in Lifelines (slope 0.17 ± 0.02 mL/min/1.73 m^2, $p < 0.0001$). Protein scoring might be a useful tool to assess both the effect of quantity and source of protein on health parameters. Further studies are needed to validate this newly developed protein score.

Keywords: protein diet score; HbA1c; eGFR; healthy subjects; population studies

1. Introduction

A diet rich in protein, ranging from 1.2 to 1.6 g protein/kg/day, may improve body weight regulation [1–3]. Protein-rich diets also appear to supplement other strategies, such as energy restriction and physical activity, to combat the global obesity epidemic [4]. As obesity is an independent risk factor for type 2 diabetes (T2D), higher protein diets for weight regulation and maintenance might also be beneficial for the prevention of T2D [5]. Although the total amount of protein may be important, the source of protein will influence other components of the diet, such as dietary fibre and micronutrients. Therefore, protein source is likely to be an important determinant for health outcomes [6]. Dietary guidelines suggest moving towards a more plant-based diet [7]. Plant-derived diets provide a number of phytochemicals that have been associated with protection against many chronic diseases, but conversely compared to dietary proteins from animal sources, plant proteins lack sufficient amounts of key essential amino acids. In most industrialised countries, animal protein is the main source of dietary protein rather than plant protein, and is therefore often a differentially increased choice when total protein intake is increased. However, the consumption of animal products, especially red and processed meat, has been associated with an increased risk of diseases such as cancer, T2D and cardiovascular diseases [8–10]. The optimal plant to animal protein ratio in the diet has not yet been established.

Firstly, we considered whether a higher protein intake might be associated with lower glycated haemoglobin (HbA1c). HbA1c levels measure average blood glucose concentration over the previous six to eight weeks; high concentrations are a risk factor for T2D. A recent meta-analysis of 32 randomised controlled trials showed a long-term positive effect of higher-protein diets on body weight management, which in turn could lead to lower HbA1c [11]. Several dietary intervention studies have also shown that higher protein diets can lower HbA1c directly, at least among T2D patients [12]. Secondly, we considered whether a higher protein intake may be associated with elevated estimated glomerular filtration rate (eGFR), an adverse indicator of renal function, since carefully controlled dietary studies show that higher protein diets may increase this marker of kidney function [13]. The current concern for adverse renal effects of higher protein diets derives from the detrimental effects of induced glomerular hyperfiltration [14]. Thirdly, with respect to protein quality, there are several lines of epidemiological evidence indicating that an increased consumption of plant protein may be associated with a reduced risk of cardiovascular disease, T2D [5,15] and inflammation [16], which might be ascribed in part to lower levels of HbA1c.

In the past three decades, studies have clearly shown that the relationship between dietary intake and health is very complex, with many interactions [17]. For all these reasons, examining composite indices of food and nutrient intake can be useful. Recently, a low-carbohydrate diet score was developed by Halton et al. [18] to classify women in the Nurses' Health Study according to their relative levels of fat, protein—including animal and vegetable protein—and carbohydrate intake. This score was used to prospectively examine the association with the risk of coronary heart disease in this cohort.

A scoring tool to specifically assess quantity, as well as the source, of protein intake has to our knowledge not previously been developed. Therefore, we aimed to develop a protein diet score based on dietary protein quantity and source—plant or animal—as a tool to investigate the role of protein in T2D-related adverse metabolic health. We hypothesised that a protein score with a higher protein energy percentage ($E\%$) within the acceptable macronutrient distribution range for protein [19], in combination with a higher plant to animal protein ratio, would be associated with a lower HbA1c level and possibly also an increase in eGFR.

2. Materials and Methods

2.1. Study Design and Population

This study included cross-sectional data from two Dutch and one Finnish observational studies, NQplus, Lifelines and The Young Finns Study, all part of the PREVIEW project (PREVention of diabetes through lifestyle Intervention and population studies in Europe and around the World) www.previewstudy.com, The overall aim of PREVIEW is to investigate the impact of a higher-protein, low glycemic index (GI) diet and physical activity regime for the prevention of T2D in overweight and obese adults and children at high risk of developing this disease [20].

The Nutrition Questionnaires plus study (the NQplus study) is a longitudinal observational study in Dutch adults within the surroundings of Wageningen, the Netherlands. Its main aims are to develop a national dietary assessment reference database for the future development and improvement of dietary assessment methods, to validate newly developed food frequency questionnaires (FFQs), and to study dietary factors and intermediate health outcomes. A total of 2048 individuals aged from 20–70 years took part in the study [21,22].

Lifelines is a large observational population-based cohort study of both adults and children conducted in the north of the Netherlands [23]. The overall aim of this study was to gain insight into the etiology of healthy aging in the general population. Lifelines was initiated in 2006 and baseline data have been collected for 167,729 individuals, aged 6 months–93 years. Regular follow-up measurements are planned.

The Young Finns Study is a multi-centre follow-up study in Finland. Its main goals are to determine the contribution made by childhood lifestyle, biological, and psychological measures to the risk of cardiovascular diseases in adulthood. At baseline in 1980, 3596 subjects aged 3–18 years were included, and the same subjects have now been followed for more than 30 years [23]. For the purposes of this cross-sectional investigation, we used measurements from the 2007 follow-up, when subjects were 30–45 years of age.

All subjects at baseline who had missing data on the FFQ, or subjects who had implausibly high (>3500 kcal) or low (<500 kcal) daily energy intake on the FFQ, were excluded [18]. Furthermore, subjects with missing values in either exposure or outcome variables were omitted. Also, subjects with a history of diabetes, hypertension, hypercholesterolemia, cardiovascular disease, cancer or kidney disease were excluded, because these diseases can cause alterations in the habitual diet. After these exclusions, a total of 76,777 subjects from Lifelines ($n = 75,131$), NQplus ($n = 492$), and The Young Finns Study ($n = 1154$) remained in the current analysis.

2.2. Assessment of Diet

NQplus used a validated 180 item semi-quantitative general FFQ to assess usual dietary intake [24,25]. Answer categories for frequency questions ranged between never per month to 6–7 days per week, and portion sizes were estimated using typical portion size estimates (e.g., glass, slice) and commonly used household measures. Average daily nutrient intakes were calculated by multiplying the frequency of consumption by portion size and nutrient content per gram using the Dutch food composition table of 2011 [26]. With respect to the definition of animal and vegetable protein, the Dutch food composition table distinguishes between these sources and was used for both NQplus and Lifelines.

In Lifelines, a newly developed FFQ consisting of 110 items was used to estimate intake of energy, fat, carbohydrate, protein and alcohol. Responses to food frequency questions ranged between never per month to 6–7 days per week, and portion sizes were estimated using typical portion size estimates and commonly used household measures. Average daily nutrient intakes were calculated by multiplying frequency of consumption by portion size and nutrient content per gram using the Dutch food composition table of 2011 [26].

In the Young Finns Study, a validated 131-item quantitative FFQ was used [27]. The food items were presented in 12 subgroups, e.g., dairy products, vegetables, or fruits and berries. After each subgroup, there were empty lines for subjects to add foods not listed in the questionnaire. The portion sizes were fixed and, if possible, specified using typical portion size estimates. The nine frequency categories ranged from never or seldom to six or more times a day. The food consumption and nutrient intakes were calculated by multiplying the frequency of food consumption by fixed portion sizes to obtain the weight of each listed food item consumed as an average per day [28]. The Finnish food composition database of 2008 was used for the nutrient calculations [29]. The database does not distinguish between animal or plant protein as separate nutrients; therefore, all foods were first classified into either "animal" or "plant" foods. Protein intakes were calculated by the source using these classes.

2.3. Calculation of the Protein Score

Following the methodology of Halton et al. [18], a protein score was developed based on relative cut-off points i.e., the population distribution. The scoring was set according to the hypothesis that a higher protein intake, as well as a higher plant to animal protein ratio, would be associated with improved markers of health outcomes, including a lower HbA1c (a measure of average blood glucose concentrations in the previous 6–8 weeks) and higher eGFR (a measure of good kidney function). Each study population was divided into 11 strata according to total protein intake (expressed as *E*%), and 11 strata according to plant to animal protein ratio. Subjects in the highest stratum of protein intake received 10 points, subjects in the next stratum received 9 points, and so on, down to subjects in the lowest stratum, who received 0 points. In terms of calculating plant to animal protein ratio, those with the highest intake of plant to animal protein received 10 points, and those with the lowest plant to animal protein ratio received 0 points. The sum of the points of each of the two components created the overall protein diet score, which ranged from 0 to 20 points. Therefore, a higher score reflects a higher energy percentage of total protein, and a higher plant to animal protein ratio, while a lower score reflects a lower protein and a lower plant to animal protein ratio. Each component of the score was also considered separately.

2.4. Validation of the Protein Score in NQplus Using a Urinary Biomarker

Nitrogen (N) from 24-h urine was determined in NQplus by the Kjeldahl technique (Foss KjeltecTM 2300 analyser, Foss Analytical, Hilleroed, Denmark). This allowed us to evaluate the validity of the protein *E*% component score based on FFQ versus nitrogen excretion in urine, assuming N balance. Adjustments for incomplete urine samples were also done by para-aminobenzoic acid [30].

An attenuation factor, usually between 0 and 1, was defined as the correlation between the self-reported N intakes using the FFQ and the measured N losses (assumed to be "true" intake) using the urinary biomarker [30,31].

2.5. Risk Factor Assessment

In NQplus, fasting venous blood was collected, and immediately centrifuged and stored at −80 °C until further analyses. Serum creatinine was determined using enzymatic methods via a Dimension Vista 1500 automated analyser or Roche Modular P800 chemistry analyser (Roche, Basel Switzerland). HbA1c was determined with a high-performance liquid chromatographic (HPLC) measurement technology using an ADAMSTM A1c HA-8160 analyser (A. Menarini Diagnostics, Florence, Italy). eGFR was estimated using the chronic kidney disease epidemiology collaboration creatinine equation (CKD-EPI) [32].

In Lifelines, fasting blood samples were processed on the day of collection and stored at −80 °C until analysis. Serum creatinine was measured on a Roche Modular P chemistry analyser (Grenzacherstrasse, Switzerland). The HbA1c level was measured using a turbidimetric inhibition immunoassay (COBAS INTEGRA 800 CTS analyser; Roche Diagnostics, Almere, the Netherlands), but standardised against the reference method of the International Federation of Clinical Chemistry and Laboratory Medicine (IFCC). eGFR was estimated using the chronic kidney disease epidemiology collaboration creatinine equation (CKD-EPI) [32].

In the Young Finns Study, fasting blood samples were collected and stored at −70 °C until analysis. Serum creatinine was determined photometrically (Creatinine reagent, Dublin, Ireland) on an AU400 analyser (Olympus, Tokyo, Japan). eGFR was estimated using the Modification of Diet in Renal Disease (MDRD) formula [33]. The HbA1c fraction in blood was measured by an ARCHITECT ci8200 analyser (Abbott Laboratories, Abbott Park, IL, USA). The concentration of HbA1c was measured immunoturbidimetrically with the microparticle agglutination inhibition method (HbA1c reagent; Thermo Fisher Scientific, Waltham, MA, USA).

2.6. Statistical Analyses

All statistical analyses were performed using *R* version 3.2.0 [34], and IBM SPSS Statistics 22. Separate but similar analyses as detailed below were carried out for each of the three studies. Associations between total protein score, HbA1c and eGFR were evaluated by means of analysis of covariance (ANCOVA). Furthermore, associations between the single components of the protein score (plant to animal protein ratio, animal protein (*E*%), plant protein (*E*%), and total protein intake (*E*%)) and HbA1c and eGFR were investigated using ANCOVA. The protein score and its components were adjusted for total energy intake by means of the residual method [35] before entering the analyses. Both unadjusted and adjusted analyses of associations between total protein score, HbA1c and eGFR were performed. The adjustment for possible confounders included: age (years), gender (male/female), education (low, medium and high), alcohol (0 g/day, 0–6 g/day, 6–12 g/day, ≥12 g/day), smoking status (never, former, current <10 cigarettes/day, current ≥10 cigarettes/day) and exercise. Low education meant no education or primary education; medium education meant lower or preparatory vocational education, lower general secondary education, intermediate vocational education or apprenticeship, higher general secondary education, or pre-university secondary education; high education meant higher vocational education or university). Smoking status was included as a confounding factor, because smoking has been associated with increased T2D risk [36] and may be an independent risk factor in the progression of kidney disease [37]. Light intense, moderate intense, and intense physical activity were measured in the metabolic equivalent of the task in minutes per week.

Potential effect modification was assessed through stratified analyses for age, gender, and BMI categories. A *p*-value < 0.05 was considered statistically significant.

3. Results

3.1. Characteristics of the Study Populations

The average protein diet score ranged from 8.0 in the lower quartile to 12.0 in the upper quartile in NQplus, Lifelines and the Young Finns Study (Table 1). In NQplus, Lifelines and the Young Finns Study, 50% of the subjects had a protein score between 8.0–12.0. The mean daily protein intake ranges were 13.1–15.9 *E*% in NQplus, 13.3–16.0 *E*% in Lifelines, and 16.0–19.0 *E*% in the Young Finns Study. The median age of 39.0 years in the Young Finns Study was lower compared to NQplus (53.0 years) and Lifelines (44.0 years). In the Young Finns Study, median physical activity was 792 MET min/week, as compared with NQplus (2376 MET min/week) and Lifelines (2205 MET min/week). Furthermore, the median daily intake of animal protein was larger in the Young Finns Study (12.3 *E*%), as compared with NQplus (7.7 *E*%) and Lifelines (8.4 *E*%). In addition, the median intake of cereals was higher in both NQplus (190 g/day) and Lifelines (181 g/day) than in the Young Finns Study (124 g/day) (Table 1).

In NQplus, we evaluated the validity of the protein score against nitrogen excretion in urine, after adjusting for incomplete urine samples. The attenuation factor for the protein score was 0.48, indicating a 48% average concordance between self-reported protein intake and the urine biomarker of protein intake.

Table 1. Characteristics of the study populations (*n* =76,777).

Study	NQplus (*n* = 492)	Lifelines (*n* = 75,131)	Young Finns Study (*n* = 1154)
Age-years	53.0 (44.0; 60.0)	42.0 (32.0; 49.0)	39.0 (33.0; 42.0)
Age <44 years % (no.)	24.6 (121)	59.9 (44,992)	83.3 (961)
Age >44 years % (no.)	75.4 (371)	40.1 (30,139)	16.7 (193)
Males-% (no.)	61.0 (312)	38.8 (29,145)	59.7 (691)

Table 1. *Cont.*

Study	NQplus (*n* = 492)	Lifelines (*n* = 75,131)	Young Finns Study (*n* = 1154)
Age <44 years (no.) (M/F)	(265/227)	(16,969/28,023)	(574/387)
Age >44 years (no.) (M/F)	(47/74)	(12,176/17,963)	(117/76)
Education-% (no.)			
- Low	0.4 (2)	1.7 (1253)	56.7 (655)
- Medium	42.3 (208)	63.9 (48,038)	22.95 (264)
- High	57.3 (282)	34.2 (25,729)	20.4 (235)
Body mass index-kg/m^2	24.8 (22.7; 26.9)	24.7 (22.6; 27.3)	25.0 (22.4; 27.8)
Physical activity-MET–min/week	2376 (1380; 2950)	2205 (1260; 3582)	792 (180.0; 1899)
Smoking status-% (no.)			
- Never	54.7 (268)	50.3 (37,821)	53.0 (611)
- Former	37.4 (184)	27.8 (20,895)	23.8 (275)
- Current <10 cigarettes/day	3.4 (17)	10.5 (7881)	15.5 (179)
- Current ≥10 cigarettes/day	4.5 (22)	11.4 (8534)	7.7 (89)
HbA1c (mmol/mol)	35.5 (33.3; 37.0)	36 (34.0; 38.0)	36.0 (34.0; 38.0)
eGFR (mL/min/1.73 m^2)	91.1 (81.7; 100.1)	100.0 (89.3; 109.5)	100.5 (90.2; 107.9)
Energy intake-calories/day	2039 (1728; 2456)	1983 (1639; 2386)	2217 (1834; 2653)
Protein diet score	10.0 (8.0; 12.0)	10.0 (8.00; 12.0)	10.0 (9.0; 12.0)
Total protein intake			
- Total protein-(*E*%/day)	14.6 (13.1; 15.9)	14.6 (13.3; 16.0)	17.4 (16.0; 19.0)
- Protein-(g/kg body weight/day)	0.99 (0.79; 1.17)	0.95 (0.78; 1.13)	1.3 (1.1; 1.6)
Animal protein-(*E*%/day)	7.7 (6.3; 9.3)	8.4 (7.1; 9.9)	12.3 (10.8; 14.0)
Plant protein-(*E*%/day)	6.6 (5.9; 7.4)	6.1 (5.5; 6.7)	3.8 (3.2; 4.3)
Plant to animal protein ratio	0.9 (0.7; 1.1)	0.72 (0.58; 0.90)	0.3 (0.2; 0.4)
Red meat-(g/day)	34.8 (19.2; 45.5)	38.6 (23.4; 50.5)	79.4 (55.5; 106.3)
Processed meat-(g/day)	16.9 (6.1; 31.1)	17.6 (8.4; 31.1)	38.1 (23.0; 64.5)
Poultry-(g/day)	9.5 (5.3; 15.0)	9.6 (6.1; 15.0)	26.0 (20.3; 60.8)
Fish-(g/day)	14.5 (8.2; 16.2)	10.5 (4.2; 16.4)	24.0 (16.6; 36.2)
Eggs-(g/day)	8.9 (7.1; 17.9)	7.2 (4.5; 17.9)	19.3 (13.9; 25.9)
Dairy-(g/day)	324.0 (211.8; 456.6)	295.7 (186.0; 426.1)	546.6 (343.4; 779.7)
Cereals-(g/day)	190.4 (140.3; 254.0)	181.2 (137.5; 234.0)	123.9 (91.8; 166.7)
Legumes-(g/day)	35.7 (19.2; 67.3)	4.4 (0.0; 13.3)	8.2 (4.7; 12.5)
Total carbohydrate			
- Total carbohydrate-(*E*%/day)	43.3 (39.7; 47.1)	45.2 (41.8; 48.7)	46.1 (42.4; 49.8)
- Total carbohydrate-(g/day)	220 (178.5; 269.2)	223.3 (182.0; 271.4)	254.7 (206.7; 309.2)
Total fat			
- Total fat-(*E*%/day)	35.6 (31.7; 39.2)	35.4 (32.1; 38.4)	32.6 (29.5; 35.6)
- Total fat-(g/day)	80.8 (62.9; 102.6)	77.6 (61.4; 96.4)	79.6 (64.4; 96.8)
Alcohol consumption-(g/day) % (no)			
- 0 g/day	3.9 (19)	2.5 (1875)	0.8 (9)
- >0–6 g/day	41.7 (205)	54.4 (40,775)	56.2 (646)
- 6–12 g/day	21.1 (104)	23.0 (17,243)	24.6 (283)
- >12 g/day	33.3 (164)	20.3 (15,238)	18.4 (212)
Glycemic index	53.1 (50.7; 55.4)	56.0 (54.1; 57.8)	51.0 (48.3; 53.8)
Glycemic load	117.4 (93.1; 146.7)	125.0 (100.8; 153.2)	129.8 (104.7; 159.9)

Characteristics are shown as median and IQR: interquartile range or as % (no.). eGFR: estimated glomerular filtration rate; *E*%: energy percentage; g: gram; HbA1c: glycated hemoglobin; low education: no education or primary education; medium education: lower or preparatory vocational education, lower general secondary education, intermediate vocational education or apprenticeship, higher general secondary education, or pre-university secondary education; high education: higher vocational education or university; F: females; M: males; MET: metabolic equivalent of task.

3.2. Association between Protein Diet Score and HbA1c

There were no associations between the protein diet score and HbA1c in either NQplus, Lifelines or the Young Finns Study. After adjustments, an inverse association between the protein diet score and HbA1c (slope −0.02 ± 0.01 mmol/mol, *p* < 0.001, Table 2) was seen in Lifelines.

Table 2. Associations of glycated haemoglobin (HbA1c) and estimated glomerular filtration rate (eGFR) (estimate ± SE) across quintiles energy-adjusted protein diet score and quintiles of its energy-adjusted components.

Study	NQplus (n = 492)			Lifelines (n = 75,131) **			Young Finns Study (n = 1154)		
Variable	Slope ± SE	p-Value	R²	Slope ± SE	p-Value	R²	Slope ± SE	p-Value	R²
HbA1c									
Protein diet score									
- Unadjusted	−0.04 ± 0.04	0.368	0.002	−0.0003 ± 0.01	0.95	0	0.01 ± 0.03	0.743	0
- Adjusted	−0.02 ± 0.04	0.722	0.229	−0.02 ± 0.01	<0.001	0.154	−0.02 ± 0.03	0.635	0.088
Total protein (E%)									
- Unadjusted	0.03 ± 0.06	0.671	0.0003	0.07 ± 0.01	<0.001	0.002	0.05 ± 0.04	0.211	0.001
- Adjusted	−0.04 ± 0.06	0.480	0.229	−0.03 ± 0.01	<0.001	0.154	0.0006 ± 0.02	0.988	0.088
Plant to animal protein ratio									
- Unadjusted	−0.49 ± 0.27	0.072	0.006	−0.19 ± 0.039	<0.001	0.001	−0.44 ± 0.66	0.505	0.0003
- Adjusted	−0.06 ± 0.26	0.823	0.229	−0.04 ± 0.03	0.142	0.154	−0.17 ± 0.71	0.810	0.089
eGFR									
Protein diet score									
- Unadjusted	0.53 ± 0.21	0.02	0.013	−0.08 ± 0.02	<0.0001	0.000	−0.16 ± 0.12	0.164	0.002
- Adjusted	0.32 ± 0.18	0.074	0.447	0.17 ± 0.02	<0.0001	0.391	0.08 ± 0.12	0.474	0.152
Total protein (E%)									
- Unadjusted	−0.74 ± 0.31	0.02	0.012	−0.601 ± 0.03	<0.0001	0.007	0.12 ± 0.15	0.445	0.0005
- Adjusted	−0.56 ± 0.25	0.02	0.449	0.08 ± 0.02	<0.0001	0.390	−0.02 ± 0.15	0.904	0.152
Plant to animal protein ratio									
- Unadjusted	6.46 ± 1.29	<0.0001	0.048	1.32 ± 0.09	<0.0001	0.003	−2.28 ± 2.52	0.367	0.0007
- Adjusted	3.96 ± 1.04	<0.001	0.460	1.14 ± 0.10	<0.001	0.391	2.17 ± −2.61	0.405	0.152

Change in HbA1c (mmol/mol) and eGFR (mL/min/1.73 m²) respectively, per 1 unit change in protein score. ** n = 69462 due to missing values of HbA1c model adjusted for age, gender, education (low/middle/high), alcohol (0 g/day, >0–6 g/day, 6–12 g/day, ≥12 g/day), smoking status (never, former, current <10 cigarettes/day, current ≥10 cigarettes/day), light intense, moderate intense, and intense physical activity (MET: minutes/week); total fat (E%), GI and BMI. Abbreviations: eGFR: estimated glomerular filtration rate, E%: energy percentage, HbA1c: glycated hemoglobin.

3.3. Association between Total E% and HbA1c

There was a positive association between total protein (*E%*) and HbA1c in Lifelines (slope 0.07 ± 0.01 mmol/mol, $p < 0.001$, Table 2). After adjustments, we found an inverse association between the total protein intake (*E%*) and HbA1c in Lifelines (slope -0.03 ± 0.01 E%/mmol/mol, $p < 0.001$, Table 2). In NQplus and the Young Finns Study, no associations were found, neither in the basic model nor after adjustments.

3.4. Association of Plant to Animal Protein Ratio and HbA1c

In Lifelines, we found an inverse association (slope -0.19 ± 0.04 mmol/mol, $p < 0.001$, Table 2) between the plant to animal protein ratio and HbA1c in the unadjusted model. After adjustments, this association did not remain.

3.5. Association between Protein Diet Score and eGFR

For eGFR, we found a positive association between the protein diet score and eGFR in NQplus (slope 0.53 ± 0.21 mL/min/1.73 m^2, $p = 0.02$, Table 2), and an inverse association between the protein diet score and eGFR in Lifelines (slope -0.08 ± 0.02 mL/min/1.73 m^2, $p < 0.0001$, Table 2). After adjustments, a positive association was only detected in Lifelines (slope 0.17 ± 0.02 mL/min/1.73 m^2, $p < 0.0001$, Table 2). We found no significant association between the protein diet score and eGFR in the Young Finns Study.

3.6. Association Total Protein E% and eGFR

Before adjustments, we found an inverse association in both NQplus (slope -0.74 ± 0.31 E%/mL/min/1.73 m^2, $p = 0.02$, Table 2) and Lifelines (slope -0.60 ± 0.03 E%/mL/min/1.73 m^2, $p < 0.0001$, Table 2), between the total protein intake (*E%*) and eGFR. For Lifelines, the association changed into a positive association after adjustments (slope 0.08 ± 0.02 E%/mL/min/1.73 m^2, $p < 0.0001$, Table 2). However, in NQplus (slope -0.56 ± 0.25 E%/mL/min/1.73 m^2, $p = 0.02$, Table 2), the inverse association persisted after further adjustments.

3.7. Association between Plant to Animal Protein Ratio and eGFR

Adjusted analyses showed a positive association between the plant to animal protein ratio and eGFR in both NQplus (slope: 3.96 ± 1.04 mL/min/1.73 m^2, $p < 0.001$, Table 2) and Lifelines (slope: 1.14 ± 0.10 mL/min/1.73 m^2, $p < 0.001$, Table 2). Unadjusted analyses also showed positive associations.

For the adjusted analyses, the variability of R-squared ranged from 0.00–0.23 for protein score versus. HbA1c and between 0.00–0.45 for protein score versus eGFR, respectively.

The relationship between the protein diet score and either HbA1c or eGFR was not qualitatively modified by age, gender, or BMI (Table 3).

Table 3. Stratified analyses of the associations of HbA1c and eGFR (estimate $\pm$ SE).

Variable	NQPlus (*n* = 492)	Lifelines (*n* = 75,131)	Young Finns Study (*n* = 1154)
	Slope $\pm$ SE	Slope $\pm$ SE	Slope $\pm$ SE
HbA1c			
Age			
<44 years	-0.073 ± 0.104	0.149 ± 0.022 *	-0.013 ± 0.033
≥44 years	-0.250 ± 0.036 *	0.219 ± 0.024 *	0.016 ± 0.094
Gender			
Men	-0.012 ± 0.058	-0.016 ± 0.008 *	-0.008 ± 0.039
Women	0.0004 ± 0.072	-0.020 ± 0.006 *	0.005 ± 0.056

Table 3. *Cont.*

Variable	NQPlus (*n* = 492)	Lifelines (*n* = 75,131)	Young Finns Study (*n* = 1154)
	Slope ± SE	Slope ± SE	Slope ± SE
BMI			
<25 kg/m^2	−0.009 ± 0.055	−0.012 ± 0.006	−0.039 ± 0.041
25–30 kg/m^2	−0.021 ± 0.076	−0.033 ± 0.008 *	0.005 ± 0.048
≥30 kg/m^2	−0.012 ± 0.044	0.005 ± 0.018	−0.012 ± 0.031
eGFR			
Age			
<44 years	0.040 ± 0.414	−0.019 ± 0.006 *	0.131 ± 0.129
≥44 years	0.424 ± 0.199	−0.012 ± 0.008	−0.053 ± 0.275
Gender			
Men	0.191 ± 0.277	0.189 ± 0.022 *	0.016 ± 0.165
Women	0.124 ± 0.319	0.137 ± 0.022 *	−0.098 ± 0.181
BMI			
<25 kg/m^2	0.227 ± 0.234	0.164 ± 0.022 *	−0.014 ± 0.167
25–30 kg/m^2	0.252 ± 0.299	0.179 ± 0.03 *	−0.024 ± 0.193
≥30 kg/m^2	0.858 ± 0.822	0.117 ± 0.049 *	0.621 ± 0.333

Change in age (years), gender, and BMI (kg/m^2) respectively, per 1 unit change in protein score. Model adjusted for age, gender (except for gender-stratified models), education (low/middle/high), alcohol (0 g/day, >0–6 g/day, 6–12 g/day, ≥12 g/day), smoking status (never, former, current <10 cigarettes/day, current ≥10 cigarettes/day), light intense, moderate intense, and intense physical activity (MET: minutes/week), Fat (en%), GI and BMI (kg/m^2); * $p < 0.05$.

4. Discussion

In the current cross-sectional study, we aimed (1) to develop a protein score capturing both relative quantity and source (plant versus animal) of dietary protein and (2) to examine the association between this score and markers of diabetes and renal function. We developed a protein score with a maximum range from 0 to 20 based on the FFQ data from the study populations investigated. In practice, the scores ranged between 8.0 and 12.0 across all three populations. The significant associations shown in Lifelines were partly reproduced by NQplus and the Young Finns Study, although in these smaller sample size studies, trends were more heterogeneous and affected by adjustment for potential confounders. In particular, the associations between the total protein score and both risk markers HbA1c and eGFR showed consistent patterns across all cohorts when compared to results for the separate components, i.e., animal and plant protein levels (Table S1). A higher total protein diet score was associated with a lower HbA1c and an increase in eGFR after adjustment for the potential confounders in Lifelines, but with no significant relationship in NQplus or the Young Finns Study.

Dietary protein has previously been shown to be beneficial, leading to better glycemic control in T2D [38]; hence, a higher protein diet has been advocated for glycemic control in individuals with T2D [39]. However, when evaluating the association between a higher protein score and HbA1c, it must also be taken into account that dietary protein will always substitute either carbohydrate and/or fat. In a recent study, even a relatively small variation in the proportion of fat and carbohydrates were significantly associated with metabolic risk factors in patients with T2D [40]. Although we adjusted for fat E%, residual confounding by other substances related to meat intake might be present. Previous studies have suggested several plausible mechanisms linking red and processed meat metabolites, including sodium, heme iron, saturated fatty acids, advanced glycation end products, nitrites and nitrates, to an increased risk of T2D [41–43]. In Lifelines, the protein score, protein intake and plant protein were associated with lower HbA1c. The optimal amount and quality of protein for prevention of T2D is still controversial [44]. In a recent study by Virtanen et al., high protein intake was not independently associated with risk of T2D, but the quality of protein was of importance, favouring plant over animal protein in the prevention of T2D [44]. In the study of Malik et al. [10], conducted in three ongoing prospective cohort studies: Nurses' Health Study (NHS), Nurses' Health Study II (NHS II) and Health Professionals Follow-up Study (HPFS)), a higher intake of total protein (*E*%) was positively associated with a higher risk of T2D, but this was shown to be largely due to animal protein intake. In contrast, intake of plant protein was associated with a lower risk of T2D. Results from the European Prospective Investigation into Cancer and Nutrition (EPIC)-NL study [45] also suggested a significantly increased diabetes risk over the quartiles of total protein intake after initial dietary adjustments. However, after further adjustment for waist circumference and BMI, the association was no longer significant. Similar results were observed for animal protein intake (*E*%), whereas vegetable protein intake was not related to T2D [45]. These results are consistent with the current findings observed in our dataset, which show an inverse association between plant protein intake and HbA1c. In the (EPIC)-InterAct case-cohort study [46], diabetes incidence was 17% higher in individuals with the highest protein intake, again largely explained by animal protein intake.

In contrast to these studies, we did not find the same association between total and animal protein and increased HbA1c values. This may be explained by differences in study population and the range of protein intakes. In the present analyses, median protein intake ranged from 0.95 to 1.3 g protein/kg body weight/day across the studies, which is within the daily recommended intake for adults [47]. Furthermore, variation in the protein diet score was low, reflected in the fact that 50% of the population had a range of 8.0 to 12.0. In addition, the difference in the findings may be due to differences in definitions of sources of animal protein or misclassification. The correlation between self-reported protein intake and urinary excretion of total nitrogen measured in the NQplus study was 48%.

Higher protein diet score and total protein intake was related to an increase in eGFR in Lifelines. In NQplus, we found an inverse association between total protein and eGFR. Based on data from the National Health and Nutrition Examination Survey (NHANES), Berryman et al. found no significant associations between total protein intake, or intake of animal or plant protein, and eGFR [48]. Similar results were found in a prospective cohort study by Halbesma et al. [49] and in the Nurses' Health Study [50]. We suspect that differential residual confounding may be partly the cause of these discrepancies. In contrast, in a sub-study of the OmniHeart Trial, in a randomised three-period crossover feeding design, a protein-rich diet (48% plant-based) increased eGFR compared to diets rich in carbohydrates and unsaturated fat [51]. Similar to these findings, Frank et al. [13] showed a significant increase in eGFR with a higher protein diet in a randomised, crossover feeding study. According to Marckmann et al., an increase in eGFR is explained by an acute increase in renal plasma flow and eGFR due to a higher protein intake. The increase is maintained over weeks to months if protein intake is kept high. This condition, glomerular hyperfiltration, may have serious long-term effects on renal health [52]. In contrast, Bankir et al. stated that an increase in eGFR is likely to be a normal adaptation of the kidney to increased protein intake, and hence leads to higher urinary urea concentration [53], rather than being a reflection of poor renal function.

The strengths of the protein diet score developed in our study include easy calculations from FFQ data, as well as simple application and qualitative interpretation e.g., in term of risk prediction. However, a limitation in this protein score is that it is only applicable once population strata are generated. Limitations of FFQ data also apply to the protein score, and include potential confounding and measurement error [54]. Furthermore, it may be comparable across populations because of the use of percentile groups in a relative ranking, and adjustments for protein quality. The present study showed that the protein score was comparable across three study populations within northern Europe with a large number of participants. It can be argued that confounding is also controlled when protein quantity and source are considered simultaneously, in contrast to when the two elements of the score are analysed separately.

By nature, a weakness of the protein score is that it aggregates and condenses information, possibly capturing only some features of the dietary energy composition. Also, the score may not be directly applicable, i.e., quantitatively interpretable, in clinical practice because it is based on the above mentioned relative cut-off points. Our study also has other limitations. As with any cross-sectional investigations, conclusions regarding causality cannot be drawn and long-term intake patterns may not necessarily be captured. In addition, there are large differences in sample size between the trials, which may be responsible for the presence of significant effects in the Lifelines study, but the lack of such effects in the two other studies. However, the overall magnitude of the associations is very small, and thus unlikely to be of any clinical significance.

A weak point in all dietary analysis studies is the validity of self-reported dietary data, which is always debatable. The inherent limitations of over- and underreporting in self-reported dietary data must be acknowledged. In addition, absolute protein is often underreported with FFQ [31]. In the current study, we validated the FFQ used in NQplus with a urinary biomarker. It showed a reasonable agreement, with an attenuation factor of 0.48. This value is quite high when compared with a similar large study from Freedman et al. [31], which pooled five large US validation cohorts of dietary self-report instruments. They found an average attenuation factor for reported protein intake by FFQ of only 0.17.

5. Conclusions

In conclusion, we developed a protein diet score using cross-sectional data from three large European population studies. The protein score was comparable across these diverse study populations. We found some evidence that a higher protein score (higher intake of total protein and plant to animal protein) was associated with lower HbA1c values and with a higher eGFR. This study provides some evidence supporting the notion that both quantity and source of proteins (plant to animal protein ratio) are determining factors on their effect on HbA1c and eGFR. However, further studies are needed to clarify the usefulness of the novel protein score in long-term population and intervention studies, as well as in other health conditions.

Supplementary Materials: The following are available online at www.mdpi.com/2072-6643/9/7/763/s1, Table S1: Associations of HbA1c and eGFR (mean ± SE) across quintiles energy-adjusted protein diet score and quintiles of its energy-adjusted components.

Acknowledgments: The study was funded by EU FP7, (# 312057), the Danish Technological Institute and The Danish Agriculture & Food Council. The NQplus study was core funded by ZonMw (ZonMw, Grant 91110030). The Lifelines Biobank initiative has been made possible by funds from FES (Fonds Economische Structuurversterking), SNN (Samenwerkingsverband Noord Nederland) and REP (Ruimtelijk Economisch Programma). The Young Finns Study has been financially supported by the Academy of Finland: grants 286284 (T.L.), 134309 (Eye), 126925, 121584, 124282, 129378 (Salve), 117787 (Gendi), and 41071 (Skidi); the Social Insurance Institution of Finland; Kuopio, Tampere and Turku University Hospital Medical Funds (grant X51001); Juho Vainio Foundation; Paavo Nurmi Foundation; Finnish Foundation of Cardiovascular Research; Finnish Cultural Foundation; Tampere Tuberculosis Foundation; Emil Aaltonen Foundation; and Yrjö Jahnsson Foundation.

Author Contributions: J.B.M. and A.R. designed the research. E.J.M.F., O.T.R., N.H.K. and V.M. provided essential materials. G.M., C.R. and D.S. performed the statistical analysis, G.M. wrote the paper. L.O.D., T.M.L., S.D.P. and M.P.S. contributed to manuscript draft and revision. A.R. had primary responsibility for the final content. All authors read and approved the final manuscript.

Conflicts of Interest: J.B.M. is president of the Glycemic Index Foundation, a non-profit food endorsement programme, manager of a GI testing service at the University of Sydney and the co-author of books about the GI foods. S.D.P. holds the Fonterra Chair in Human Nutrition at the University of Auckland. None of the other authors declare a conflict of interest.

References

1. Larsen, T.M.; Dalskov, S.-M.; van Baak, M.; Jebb, S.A.; Papadaki, A.; Pfeiffer, A.F.H.; Martinez, J.A.; Handjieva-Darlenska, T.; Kunešová, M.; Pihlsgård, M.; et al. Diets with high or low protein content and glycemic index for weight-loss maintenance. *N. Engl. J. Med.* **2010**, *363*, 2102–2113. [CrossRef] [PubMed]
2. Austin, G.L.; Ogden, L.G.; Hill, J.O. Trends in carbohydrate, fat, and protein intakes and association with energy intake in normal-weight, overweight, and obese individuals: 1971–2006. *Am. J. Clin. Nutr.* **2011**, *93*, 836–843. [CrossRef] [PubMed]

3.   Skov, A.R.; Toubro, S.; Rønn, B.; Holm, L.; Astrup, A. Randomized trial on protein vs carbohydrate in ad libitum fat reduced diet for the treatment of obesity. *Int. J. Obes. Relat. Metab. Disord.* **1999**, *23*, 528–536. [CrossRef] [PubMed]

4.   Leidy, H.J.; Clifton, P.M.; Astrup, A.; Wycherley, T.P.; Westerterp-Plantenga, M.S.; Luscombe-Marsh, N.D.; Woods, S.C.; Mattes, R.D. The role of protein in weight loss and maintenance. *Am. J. Clin. Nutr.* **2015**, *101*, 1320S–1329S. [CrossRef] [PubMed]

5.   Shang, X.; Scott, D.; Hodge, A.M.; English, D.R.; Giles, G.G.; Ebeling, P.R.; Sanders, K.M. Dietary protein intake and risk of type 2 diabetes: Results from the Melbourne Collaborative Cohort Study and a meta-analysis of prospective studies. *Am. J. Clin. Nutr.* **2016**. [CrossRef] [PubMed]

6.   Song, M.; Fung, T.T.; Hu, F.B.; Willett, W.C.; Longo, V.D.; Chan, A.T.; Giovannucci, E.L. Association of Animal and Plant Protein Intake With All-Cause and Cause-Specific Mortality. *JAMA Intern. Med.* **2016**, *176*, 1453–1463. [CrossRef] [PubMed]

7.   Dietary Guidelines for Americans 2015–2020 8th Edition. December 2015. Available online: http://health. gov/dietaryguidelines/2015/guidelines/ (accessed on 10 February 2017).

8.   Abete, I.; Romaguera, D.; Vieira, A.R.; Lopez de Munain, A.; Norat, T. Association between total, processed, red and white meat consumption and all-cause, CVD and IHD mortality: A meta-analysis of cohort studies. *Br. J. Nutr.* **2014**, *112*, 762–775. [CrossRef] [PubMed]

9.   Demeyer, D.; Mertens, B.; De Smet, S.; Ulens, M. Mechanisms Linking Colorectal Cancer to the Consumption of (Processed) Red Meat: A Review. *Crit. Rev. Food Sci. Nutr.* **2015**, *8398*, 2747–2766. [CrossRef] [PubMed]

10. Malik, V.S.; Li, Y.; Tobias, D.K.; Pan, A.; Hu, F.B. Dietary Protein Intake and Risk of Type 2 Diabetes in US Men and Women. *Am. J. Epidemiol.* **2016**, *183*, 715–728. [CrossRef] [PubMed]

11. Clifton, P.M.; Condo, D.; Keogh, J.B. Long term weight maintenance after advice to consume low carbohydrate, higher protein diets—A systematic review and meta analysis. *Nutr. Metab. Cardiovasc. Dis.* **2014**, *24*, 224–235. [CrossRef] [PubMed]

12. Gannon, M.C.; Hoover, H.; Nuttall, F.Q. Further decrease in glycated hemoglobin following ingestion of a LoBAG30 diet for 10 weeks compared to 5 weeks in people with untreated type 2 diabetes. *Nutr. Metab.* **2010**, *7*, 64. [CrossRef] [PubMed]

13. Frank, H.; Graf, J.; Amann-Gassner, U.; Bratke, R.; Daniel, H.; Heemann, U.; Hauner, H. Effect of short-term high-protein compared with normal-protein diets on renal hemodynamics and associated variables in healthy young men. *Am. J. Clin. Nutr.* **2009**, *90*, 1509–1516. [CrossRef] [PubMed]

14. Brenner, B.M.; Meyer, T.W.; Hostetter, T.H. Dietary protein intake and the progressive nature of kidney disease: The role of hemodynamically mediated glomerular injury in the pathogenesis of progressive glomerular sclerosis in aging, renal ablation, and intrinsic renal disease. *N. Engl. J. Med.* **1982**, *307*, 652–659. [PubMed]

15. Nothlings, U.; Schulze, M.B.; Weikert, C.; Boeing, H.; van der Schouw, Y.T.; Bamia, C.; Benetou, V.; Lagiou, P.; Krogh, V.; Beulens, J.W.J.; et al. Intake of Vegetables, Legumes, and Fruit, and Risk for All-Cause, Cardiovascular, and Cancer Mortality in a European Diabetic Population. *J. Nutr.* **2008**, *138*, 775–781. [PubMed]

16. Hermsdorff, H.H.M.; Zulet, M.Á.; Abete, I.; Martínez, J.A. A legume-based hypocaloric diet reduces proinflammatory status and improves metabolic features in overweight/obese subjects. *Eur. J. Nutr.* **2011**, *50*, 61–69. [CrossRef] [PubMed]

17. Kant, A.K. Indexes of overall diet quality: A review. *J. Am. Diet. Assoc.* **1996**, *96*, 785–791. [CrossRef]

18. Halton, T.L.; Willett, W.C.; Liu, S.; Manson, J.E.; Albert, C.M.; Rexrode, K.; Hu, F.B. Low-carbohydrate-diet score and the risk of coronary heart disease in women. *N. Engl. J. Med.* **2006**, *355*, 1991–2002. [CrossRef] [PubMed]

19. Institute of Medicine. Dietary Reference Intakes for Energy, Carbohydrate, Fiber, Fat, Fatty Acids, Cholesterol, Protein, and Amino Acids. (Macronutrients). 2005. Available online: http://www.nap.edu (accessed on 12 February 2017).

20. Raben, A.; Fogelholm, M.; Feskens, E.J.M.; Westerterp-Plantenga, M.; Schlicht, W.; Brand-Miller, J. PREVIEW: PREVention of diabetes through lifestyle Intervention and population studies in Europe and around the World: On behalf of the PREVIEW consortium. *Obes. Facts* **2013**, *6*, 194.

21. Sluik, D.; Brouwer-Brolsma, E.M.; de Vries, J.H.M.; Geelen, A.; Feskens, E.J.M. Associations of alcoholic beverage preference with cardiometabolic and lifestyle factors: The NQplus study. *BMJ Open* **2016**, *6*, e010437. [CrossRef] [PubMed]

22. Van Lee, L.; Feskens, E.J.M.; Meijboom, S.; van Huysduynen, E.J.H.; van't Veer, P.; de Vries, J.H.M.; Geelen, A. Evaluation of a screener to assess diet quality in The Netherlands. *Br. J. Nutr.* **2016**, *115*, 517–526. [CrossRef] [PubMed]

23. Scholtens, S.; Smidt, N.; Swertz, M.A.; Bakker, S.J.L.; Dotinga, A.; Vonk, J.M.; van Dijk, F.; van Zon, S.K.R.; Wijmenga, C.; Wolffenbuttel, B.H. R.; Stolk, R.P. Cohort Profile: LifeLines, a three-generation cohort study and biobank. *Int. J. Epidemiol.* **2015**, *44*, 1172–1180. [CrossRef] [PubMed]

24. Feunekes, G.I.J.; Van Staveren, W.A.; De Vries, J.H.M.; Burema, J.; Hautvast, J.G. Relative and biomarker-based validity of a food-frequency questionnaire estimating intake of fats and cholesterol. *Am. J. Clin. Nutr.* **1993**, *58*, 489–496. [PubMed]

25. Siebelink, E.; Geelen, A.; de Vries, J.H.M. Self-reported energy intake by FFQ compared with actual energy intake to maintain body weight in 516 adults. *Br. J. Nutr.* **2011**, *106*, 274–281. [CrossRef] [PubMed]

26. NEVO-Tabel. *Nederlands Voedingsstoffen-Tabel (NEVO-Tabel) 2011 (Dutch National Food Composition Table 2011) version 3*; RIVM/Dutch Nutrition Centre: Bilthoven, The Netherlands, 2011.

27. Männistö, S.; Virtanen, M.; Mikkonen, T.; Pietinen, P. Reproducibility and Validity of a Food Frequency Questionnaire in a Case-Control Study on Breast Cancer. *J. Clin. Epidemiol.* **1996**, *494*, 401–409. [CrossRef]

28. Paalanen, L.; Männistö, S.; Virtanen, M.J.; Knekt, P.; Räsänen, L.; Montonen, J.; Pietinen, P. Validity of a food frequency questionnaire varied by age and body mass index. *J. Clin. Epidemiol.* **2006**, *59*, 994–1001. [CrossRef] [PubMed]

29. National Public Health Institute of Finland. Fineli. Finnish Food Composition Database. Release 7. Helsinki, Finland, the National Public Health Institute, Nutrition Unit. 2007. Available online: http://www.fineli.fi/ (accessed on 11 July 2016).

30. Sluik, D.; Geelen, A.; de Vries, J.H.M.; Eussen, S.J.P.M.; Brants, H.A.M.; Meijboom, S.; van Dongen, M.C.J.M.; Bueno-de-Mesquita, H.B.; Wijckmans-Duysens, N.E.G.; van't Veer, P.; et al. A national FFQ for The Netherlands (the FFQ-NL 1.0): Validation of a comprehensive FFQ for adults. *Br. J. Nutr.* **2016**, *116*, 913–923. [CrossRef] [PubMed]

31. Freedman, L.S.; Commins, J.M.; Moler, J.E.; Arab, L.; Baer, D.J.; Kipnis, V.; Midthune, D.; Moshfegh, A.J.; Neuhouser, M.L.; Prentice, R.L.; et al. Pooled Results From 5 Validation Studies of Dietary Self-Report Instruments Using Recovery Biomarkers for Energy and Protein Intake. *Am. J. Epidemiol.* **2014**, *180*, 172–188. [CrossRef] [PubMed]

32. Levey, A.S.; Stevens, L.A.; Schmid, C.H.; Zhang, Y.L.; Castro, A.F.; Feldman, H.I.; Kusek, J.W.; Eggers, P.; Van Lente, F.; Greene, T.; et al. A new equation to estimate glomerular filtration rate. *Ann. Intern Med.* **2009**, *150*, 604–612. [CrossRef] [PubMed]

33. Levey, A.S.; Bosch, J.P.; Lewis, J.B.; Greene, T.; Rogers, N.; Roth, D. A More Accurate Method to Estimate Glomerular Filtration Rate from Serum Creatinine: A New Prediction Equation. *Ann. Intern. Med.* **1999**, *130*, 461–470. [CrossRef] [PubMed]

34. R Development Core Team. R: A Language and Environment for Statistical Computing. Available online: http://www.R-project.org/ (accessed on 24 April 2016).

35. Willett, W.C.; Howe, G.R.; Kushi, L.H. Adjustment for total energy intake in epidemiologic studies. *Am. J. Clin. Nutr.* **1997**, *65*, 1220S–1228S. [PubMed]

36. Maddatu, J.; Anderson-Baucum, E.; Evans-Molina, C. Smoking and the risk of type 2 diabetes. *Transl Res.* **2017**, *184*, 101–107. [CrossRef] [PubMed]

37. Hallan, S.; Orth, S. Smoking is a risk factor in the progression to kidney failure. *Kidney Int.* **2011**, *80*, 516–523. [CrossRef] [PubMed]

38. Halton, T.L.; Liu, S.; Manson, J.E.; Hu, F.B. Low-carbohydrate-diet score and risk of type 2 diabetes in women. *Am. J. Clin. Nutr.* **2008**, *87*, 339–346. [PubMed]

39. Feinman, R.D.; Pogozelski, W.K.; Astrup, A.; Bernstein, R.K.; Fine, E.J.; Westman, E.C.; Accurso, A.; Frassetto, L.; Gower, B.A.; McFarlane, S.I.; et al. Dietary carbohydrate restriction as the first approach in diabetes management: Critical review and evidence base. *Nutrition* **2015**, *31*, 1–13. [CrossRef] [PubMed]

40. Vitale, M.; Masulli, M.; Rivellese, A.A.; Babini, A.C.; Boemi, M.; Bonora, E.; Buzzetti, R.; Ciano, O.; Cignarelli, M.; Cigolini, M.; et al. Influence of dietary fat and carbohydrates proportions on plasma lipids, glucose control and low-grade inflammation in patients with type 2 diabetes—The TOSCA.IT Study. *Eur. J. Nutr.* **2016**, *55*, 1645–1651. [CrossRef] [PubMed]

41. Kim, Y.; Keogh, J.; Clifton, P. A review of potential metabolic etiologies of the observed association between red meat consumption and development of type 2 diabetes mellitus. *Metabolism* **2015**, *64*, 768–779. [CrossRef] [PubMed]

42. Aune, D.; Ursin, G.; Veierød, M.B. Meat consumption and the risk of type 2 diabetes: A systematic review and meta-analysis of cohort studies. *Diabetologia* **2009**, *52*, 2277–2287. [CrossRef] [PubMed]

43. Feskens, E.J.M.; Sluik, D.; Van Wondenbergh, G.J. Meat Consumption, Diabetes, and its Complications. *Curr. Diabetes Rep.* **2013**, *13*, 298–306. [CrossRef] [PubMed]

44. Virtanen, H.E.K.; Koskinen, T.T.; Voutilainen, S.; Mursu, J.; Tuomainen, T.P.; Kokko, P.; Virtanen, J.K. Intake of different dietary proteins and risk of type 2 diabetes in men: The Kuopio Ischaemic Heart Disease Risk Factor Study. *Br. J. Nutr.* **2017**, *117*, 882–893. [CrossRef] [PubMed]

45. Sluijs, I.; Beulens, J.W.J.; Spijkerman, A.M.W.; Grobbee, D.E.; Van Der Schouw, Y.T. Dietary intake of total, animal, and vegetable protein and risk of type 2 diabetes in the European Prospective Investigation into Cancer and Nutrition (EPIC)-NL study. *Diabetes Care* **2010**, *33*, 43–48. [CrossRef] [PubMed]

46. Raitakari, O.T.; Juonala, M.; Rönnemaa, T.; Keltikangas-Järvinen, L.; Räsänen, L.; Pietikäinen, M.; Hutri-Kähönen, N.; Taittonen, L.; Jokinen, E.; Marniemi, J.; et al. Cohort profile: The cardiovascular risk in young Finns study. *Int. J. Epidemiol.* **2008**, *37*, 1220–1226. [CrossRef] [PubMed]

47. Nordic Nutrition Recommendations 2012. In *Integrating Nutrition and Physical Activity*, 5th ed.; Nordic Council of Ministers: Copenhagen, Denmark, 2014.

48. Berryman, C.E.; Agarwal, S.; Lieberman, H.R.; Fulgoni, V.L.; Pasiakos, S.M. Diets higher in animal and plant protein are associated with lower adiposity and do not impair kidney function in US adults. *Am. J. Clin. Nutr.* **2016**, *104*, 743–749. [CrossRef] [PubMed]

49. Halbesma, N.; Bakker, S.J.L.; Jansen, D.F.; Stolk, R.P.; De Zeeuw, D.; De Jong, P.E.; Gansevoort, R.T. High Protein Intake Associates with Cardiovascular Events but not with Loss of Renal Function. *J. Am. Soc. Nephrol.* **2009**, *20*, 1797–1804. [CrossRef] [PubMed]

50. Knight, E.L.; Stampfer, M.J.; Hankinson, S.E.; Spiegelman, D.; Curhan, G.C. The impact of protein intake on renal function decline in women with normal renal function or mild renal insufficiency. *Ann. Intern. Med.* **2003**, *138*, 460–467. [CrossRef] [PubMed]

51. Juraschek, S.P.; Appel, L.J.; Anderson, C.A.M.; Miller, E.R. Effect of a High-Protein Diet on Kidney Function in Healthy Adults: Results From the OmniHeart Trial. *Am. J. Kidney Dis.* **2013**, *61*, 547–554. [CrossRef] [PubMed]

52. Marckmann, P.; Osther, P.; Pedersen, A.N.; Jespersen, B. High-Protein Diets and Renal Health. *J. Ren. Nutr.* **2015**, *25*, 1–5. [CrossRef] [PubMed]

53. Bankir, L.; Bouby, N.; Trinh-Trang-Tan, M.-M.; Ahloulay, M.; Promeneur, D. Direct and indirect cost of urea excretion. *Kidney Int.* **1996**, *49*, 1598–1607. [CrossRef] [PubMed]

54. Keogh, R.H.; Carroll, R.J.; Tooze, J.A.; Kirkpatrick, S.I.; Freedman, L.S. Statistical issues related to dietary intake as the response variable in intervention trials. *Stat. Med.* **2016**, *35*, 4493–4508. [CrossRef] [PubMed]

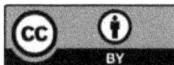

nutrients

MDPI

Review

Precision Nutrition: A Review of Personalized Nutritional Approaches for the Prevention and Management of Metabolic Syndrome

Juan de Toro-Martín [1,2], Benoit J. Arsenault [3,4], Jean-Pierre Després [4,5] and Marie-Claude Vohl [1,2,*]

1   Institute of Nutrition and Functional Foods (INAF), Laval University, Quebec City, QC G1V 0A6, Canada; juan.de-toro-martin.1@ulaval.ca
2   School of Nutrition, Laval University, Quebec City, QC G1V 0A6, Canada
3   Department of Medicine, Faculty of Medicine, Laval University, Quebec City, QC G1V 0A6, Canada; benoit.arsenault@criucpq.ulaval.ca
4   Quebec Heart and Lung Institute, Quebec City, QC G1V 4G5, Canada; jean-pierre.despres@criucpq.ulaval.ca
5   Department of Kinesiology, Faculty of Medicine, Laval University, Quebec City, QC G1V 0A6, Canada
*   Correspondence: marie-claude.vohl@fsaa.ulaval.ca; Tel.: +1-418-656-2131 (ext. 4676)

Received: 6 July 2017; Accepted: 18 August 2017; Published: 22 August 2017

Abstract: The translation of the growing increase of findings emerging from basic nutritional science into meaningful and clinically relevant dietary advices represents nowadays one of the main challenges of clinical nutrition. From nutrigenomics to deep phenotyping, many factors need to be taken into account in designing personalized and unbiased nutritional solutions for individuals or population sub-groups. Likewise, a concerted effort among basic, clinical scientists and health professionals will be needed to establish a comprehensive framework allowing the implementation of these new findings at the population level. In a world characterized by an overwhelming increase in the prevalence of obesity and associated metabolic disturbances, such as type 2 diabetes and cardiovascular diseases, tailored nutrition prescription represents a promising approach for both the prevention and management of metabolic syndrome. This review aims to discuss recent works in the field of precision nutrition analyzing most relevant aspects affecting an individual response to lifestyle/nutritional interventions. Latest advances in the analysis and monitoring of dietary habits, food behaviors, physical activity/exercise and deep phenotyping will be discussed, as well as the relevance of novel applications of nutrigenomics, metabolomics and microbiota profiling. Recent findings in the development of precision nutrition are highlighted. Finally, results from published studies providing examples of new avenues to successfully implement innovative precision nutrition approaches will be reviewed.

Keywords: precision nutrition; nutrigenomics; physical activity; deep phenotyping; metabolomics; gut microbiota

---

1. Precision Nutrition

The Road to Tailored Dietary Advices

One of the ultimate goals of the promising field of precision nutrition is the design of tailored nutritional recommendations to treat or prevent metabolic disorders [1]. More specifically, precision nutrition pursuits to develop more comprehensive and dynamic nutritional recommendations based on shifting, interacting parameters in a person's internal and external environment throughout life. To that end, precision nutrition approaches include, in addition to genetics, other factors such as dietary habits, food behavior, physical activity, the microbiota and the metabolome. Following the completion of the mapping of the Human Genome, a cumulative number of association studies have been performed in order to identify the genetic factors that may explain the inter-individual variability of the metabolic response to specific diets. In this sense, while numerous genes and polymorphisms have been already identified as relevant factors in this heterogeneous response to nutrient intake [2–7], clinical evidence supporting these statistical relationships is currently too weak to establish a comprehensive framework for personalized nutritional interventions in most cases [8]. Thus, although most of findings on this topic are still relatively far from giving their fully expected potential in terms of translation and application of this knowledge to precision nutrition [9], some of them have been successfully developed in both the public and the private sectors. On one hand, the hypolactasia diagnosis [10], the celiac disease ruling out [11] or the phenylketonuria screening [12], have allowed the implementation of tailored nutritional advices based on genetic makeup for years, i.e., avoiding lactose-, gluten- and phenylalanine-containing products to at-risk individuals. On the private sector, many companies are already offering genetic tests to customize diets based on the individual response to specific nutrients. For instance, that is the case of genetic tests based on the specific metabolism of caffeine (slow or fast metabolizers) [13,14], the predisposition to weight gain by saturated fat intake [15,16], or the increased risk of developing hypertension by high salt intake [17,18], among others. Together, these nutritional recommendations solely based on genetic background represents a straightforward approach to the concept of personalized nutrition. Although quite similar to the concept of precision nutrition, and sometimes interchangeable, the latter makes reference to a conceptual framework covering a wider set of individual features allowing an effective and dynamic nutritional approach [1]. Thus, while personalized nutrition based on genes is already being implemented successfully based on numerous research studies, such as the ones above mentioned, precision nutrition may still lack sufficient evidence for full implementation given its complexity, as will be reviewed below.

Regarding obesity and metabolic syndrome, recent published studies focusing on gene-environment interactions have revealed important insights about the impact of macronutrient intake in the association of genetic markers with metabolic health, fat mass accumulation or body composition. This is broadly relevant in precision nutrition, since results from these studies, focused on macronutrient intake, open the door to tailor efficiently diets based on the individual genetic makeup. In this regard, recent work by Goni et al. [19] analyzed the usefulness of a genetic risk score (GRS) on obesity prediction, and more interestingly, the impact of macronutrient intake in the predictive value of this GRS. The GRS was built as an additive summary measure of a set of 16 genetic variants (according to the number of risk alleles for each variant) previously associated with obesity (rs9939609, *FTO*; rs17782313, *MC4R*; rs1801282, *PPARG*; rs1801133, *MTHFR* and rs894160, *PLIN1*) and lipid metabolism disturbances (rs1260326, *GCKR*; rs662799, *APOA5*; rs4939833, *LIPG*; rs1800588l, *LIPC*, rs328, *LPL*; rs12740374, *CELSR2*; rs429358 and rs7412, *APOE*; rs1799983, *NOS3*; rs1800777, *CETP* and rs1800206, *PPARA*). After the validation of the GRS, i.e., high risk group (subjects having more than 7 risk alleles) showing increased body mass index (0.93 kg/m^2 greater BMI), body fat mass (1.69% greater BFM), waist circumference (1.94 cm larger WC) and waist-to-hip ratio (0.01 greater WHR), significant interactions between macronutrient intake and GRS prediction values were observed. For instance, higher intake of animal protein was significantly associated with higher BFM in individuals within the high-risk GRS group ($P_{interaction} = 0.032$), whereas higher vegetable protein consumption showed a protective effect among subjects in the low-risk group ($P_{interaction} = 0.003$), as these individuals were characterized by a lower percentage of BFM [19]. Similar trends were reported by Rukh et al., where total protein intake was found to modulate GRS association with obesity in women ($P_{interaction} = 0.039$) [20]. Other studies on gene-macronutrients interactions, in which a GRS developed on the basis of BMI-associated single nucleotide polymorphisms (SNPs) was used, have revealed that high intake of sugar-sweetened beverages [21–23], fried foods [24] or saturated fatty-acids [25] are also able to modulate the risk to develop obesity. Altogether, these results suggest that the accumulation of common polymorphisms at loci known to influence body weight may influence one's predisposition to gain weight when exposed to certain types of diets.

Over the past recent years, it has become increasingly evident that the assessment of dietary patterns provides a more reliable picture of real food intake compared to the assessment of macronutrients intake considered in isolation. In this regard, a recent work focused on the effect of the obesity-associated *MC4R* gene on metabolic syndrome has revealed a relevant gene-diet interaction with dietary patterns [26]. In this case-control study, participants with metabolic syndrome from the Tehran Lipid and Glucose Study [27] were randomly matched with controls by age and sex, leading a total of 815 pairs. Healthy and western dietary patterns were identified by factor analysis based on 25 food groups extracted from a 168-item semi-quantitative food frequency questionnaire (FFQ). The healthy dietary pattern was characterized by high intake of vegetables, legumes, low fat dairy, whole grains, liquid oils and fruits, while the western dietary pattern consisted of high intake of soft drinks, fast foods, sweets, solid oils, red meats, salty snacks, refined grains, high fat dairy, eggs and poultry. Results from this study revealed that carriers of the rare allele in the *MC4R* gene and having the highest score of the western dietary pattern had increased risk (odds ratio—OR) of developing metabolic syndrome (OR = 1.71 (1.04–2.41); P_{trend} = 0.007), as compared to those having lower scores [26]. Similar gene-dietary pattern interactions were revealed in another study linking GRS with WHR and BMI, and different diet scores, ranging from healthier (whole grains, fish, fruits, vegetables, nuts/seeds) to unhealthier (red/processed meats, sweets, sugar-sweetened beverages and fried potatoes) [28]. Results from this study, where more than 68,000 participants from 18 different cohorts were used, showed nominally significant associations between diet score and WHR-GRS, with stronger genetic effect in subjects with a higher diet score ($\beta_{interaction}$ ($SE_{interaction}$) = 4.77 × 10^{-5} (2.32 × 10^{-5}); $P_{interaction}$ = 0.04), i.e., consuming healthier diets [28].

As above mentioned, the scientific community generally agrees that the future of precision nutrition will not be solely based on nutrigenetics [29]. Clearly, factors beyond genetics also need to be considered when designing personalized or tailored diets. In this regard, the usefulness of tailored dietary advices to adequately anticipate individual responses to nutritional intakes is one of the main goals of precision nutrition. In order to attain this goal, and as illustrated in the precision nutrition plate (Figure 1), determinants not only related to nutritional or genetic factors, e.g., lifestyle including physical activity (PA) habits, metabolomics or gut microbiomics, are also emerging as significant contributors that merit consideration in the field of precision nutrition [30–32].

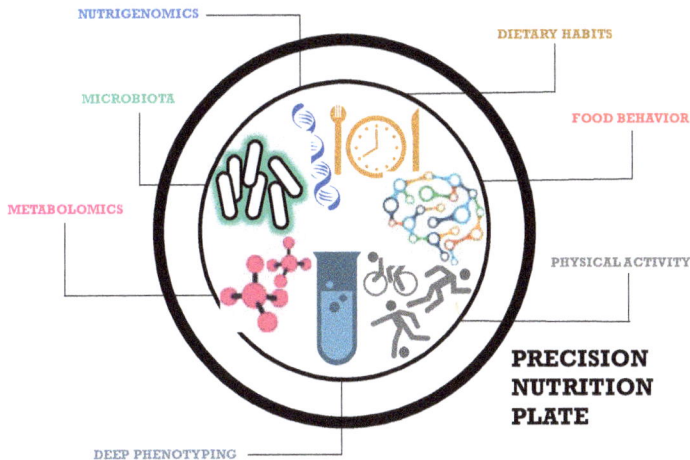

Figure 1. The *precision nutrition plate*. A schematic representation of the main factors worth to consider when approaching precision nutrition.

This is the case of a recent study where the power of a machine-learning algorithm to predict postprandial glucose levels was tested [33]. In this study, the ability of an algorithm to forecast postprandial glycaemia as well as an expert-based prediction was reported. To do that, the high inter-individual variability of postprandial glycemic response was first revealed by using subcutaneous sensors that accurately monitored glucose levels (every 5 min during 7 full days) in a cohort of 800 subjects, resulting in over 1.5 million glucose measurements, corresponding to nearly 47,000 real-life meals and over 5000 standardized meals. A comprehensive profiling including data derived from a FFQ, sleep and PA habits, medical histories, anthropometric measures, blood tests and microbiota profiling was assessed for each participant. These features were then included in the prediction algorithm, which was first tested in the cohort of 800 subjects and further successfully validated in an independent cohort of 100 patients. Further analyses allowed the quantification of the partial contribution of each parameter of the algorithm, from meal nutrient content (carbohydrates, fat, dietary fibers, sodium) to microbiome-based features, in the prediction of postprandial glucose levels. Finally, the predictive performance of the algorithm was examined in a two-arm blinded randomized controlled trial with 26 new participants. In the first arm, after the 1-week profiling, 12 participants were sequentially assigned to an unhealthy or a healthy diet according to the postprandial glycemic responses predicted by the algorithm for each participant. In the second arm, 14 participants followed the same unhealthy and healthy diets, but dietary advices were given by a registered dietitian and a scientist experienced in analyzing continuous glucose monitoring data. The tailored dietary advice in both the predictor and the expert arms resulted in a significant decrease of postprandial glucose levels when participants were assigned to the healthy diet. More specifically, the correlation between postprandial glucose levels measured during the profiling and the intervention weeks was 0.7 in the expert arm, and it reached 0.8 with the algorithm-predicted values. These results, in spite of providing support for the potential of this personalized nutrition approach, should be taken with caution until further studies are completed, since some observations mainly concerning the inter-individual variability in glycemic responses have been recently pointed out [34]. In any case, such an innovative prediction algorithm, which utilizes clinical, nutritional and lifestyle variables, as well as microbiome profiles as input parameters, exemplifies the great possibilities offered by these sophisticated methods for the further implementation of precision nutrition.

According to the International Society of Nutrigenetics/Nutrigenomics (ISNN), the future of precision nutrition should be discussed at three levels: stratification of conventional nutritional guidelines into population subgroups by age, gender and other social determinants, individual approaches issued from a deep and refined phenotyping, and a genetic-directed nutrition based on rare genetic variants having high penetrance and impact on individuals' response to particular foods [29] (Figure 2). This categorization of precision nutrition pillars includes a more in-depth exploration of the challenges that nutrition science must face in next years to evolve in the context of an increasing prevalence of obesity and associated metabolic disorders, resulting largely from the wide-scale adoption of unhealthy feeding behaviors in an *obesogenic* food environment in which it has become increasingly difficult to adhere to healthy dietary patterns.

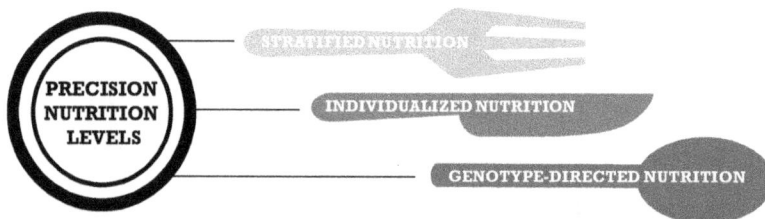

Figure 2. The three levels of precision nutrition according to the International Society of Nutrigenetics/Nutrigenomics (ISNN) [29].

In this regard, a better understanding of the inter-individual variability in the response to diet has been recently identified by the American Society of Nutrition (ASN) as one of the six top research priorities to be addressed in nutrition science to face the forthcoming challenges in population health management [35]. Moreover, the ASN has identified the required tools to attain these research needs for enabling an accurate nutritional impact prediction on health (omics technologies), an enhanced patient information survey (bioinformatics and database management), and a suitable assessment of disease progression and patient response to a nutritional treatment (biomarkers, metabolomics, etc.).

This paper will review the recent advances in the field of precision nutrition, with special emphasis on the novel approaches of dietary habits assessment, food behavior evaluation, PA monitoring, as well as on the novel techniques applied to deep phenotyping, metabotyping and microbiota profiling.

2. Dietary Habits

Fine-Tuning Adherence

The main goal sought with nutritional interventions is to assess potential associations between feeding behaviors and metabolic outcomes such as body composition, insulin sensitivity and markers of the lipoprotein-lipid profile. These potentially causal relationships should then enable to draw conclusions on the clinical relevance of specific nutritional recommendations for population subgroups. Unfortunately, one of the most common obstacles that nutritional science needs to tackle when exploring such associations is that conventional nutritional intervention studies often lack the power to detect subtle effects of diet on metabolic parameters, either because of the short duration of such studies or by the small number of participants involved [36]. The problem resulting from lack of statistical power may be amplified by several additional issues among which inter-individual variability and limited adherence evaluation stand out as potential determinants of modest study outcomes and underestimation of diet effects [37]. Regarding the impact of nutrition on genetic makeup and vice versa, the capacity to accurately monitor food and energy intake remains a major challenge in precision nutrition research.

A better characterization of dietary habits throughout an intervention study will ultimately increase one's chance of generating clear findings. This implies, however, thorough data acquisition in terms of individual food consumption and other factors that could affect adherence evaluation of a particular intervention [38]. The limitations of subjective and memory-based dietary assessment methods (M-BM), such as FFQ, 24-h dietary recall (24H), dietary record (DR) and dietary history (DH) have been known for a long time [39] and continue to be questioned today [40], with under- or over-reporting not being accounted for in many studies, which may lead to biased results in nutritional intervention studies. Other than recall bias inherent in self-reported data, limitations shown by subjective dietary assessment methods comprise the high cost and time-consuming of DH and of multiple 24H and DR, which could also drive to unintentionally changes in participants' diet due to repeated measurements [41]. Since a reliable dietary assessment is key for interpreting diet-induced metabolic outcomes, many approaches aimed at overcoming these issues from different perspectives have been proposed.

Two examples of novel dietary adherence methods are the Mediterranean Diet Adherence Screener (MEDAS) [42,43] and the Mediterranean Lifestyle index (MEDLIFE) [44]. The MEDAS consists of a simple 14-point-instrument to overcome the classical time-consuming FFQ. This time saver questionnaire allows a more robust estimation of Mediterranean diet adherence that can be used in clinical practice. The final MEDAS score ranges from 0 (worst adherence) to 14 (best adherence), according to 9 items from a previously validated index [45], plus three questions on Mediterranean food consumption frequency (nuts per week, sugar-sweetened beverages per day, and tomato sauce with garlic, onion and olive oil per week), and two more questions about Spanish Mediterranean food intake habits (olive oil as the principal source of fat for cooking and preference of white meats—chicken, rabbit, turkey—over red meats—beef, pork, etc.). The MEDAS has been validated within the Prevención with Dieta Mediterránea (PREDIMED) study [46], a primary prevention nutrition-intervention trial that will be presented below. Using a holistic approach, the MEDLIFE index is the first to include PA and social interaction to the classical assessment of food consumption [44]. The MEDLIFE index has been validated with previous diet quality indices, the Alternate Healthy Eating Index (AHEI) [47], the alternate Mediterranean Diet Index (aMED) [48] and the MEDAS [42], and it consists of 28 items divided into three blocks. The first two blocks are dedicated to estimate food consumption frequency and Mediterranean dietary habits, such as the previous MEDAS index [43]. The third block consists of six items that include information about PA (more than 150 min/week or 30 min/day jogging, walking quickly, dancing or doing aerobics) and social habits (time spent sitting, watching television or in front of a computer, sleeping or socializing with friends). The MEDLIFE index is the first to measure other variables beyond food consumption that are part of the Mediterranean lifestyle and it is expected to help in the refinement of association testing between metabolic diseases and diet/lifestyle, as well as in the improvement of measuring adherence to a Mediterranean lifestyle.

Some authors have proposed that more complex and sophisticated statistical methods may help monitoring the adherence of patients to a nutritional intervention, which would lead to a more accurate detection of the potential associations between dietary interventions and metabolic improvements. In this regard, Sevilla-Villanueva et al. [49] have recently reported that adherence evaluation through trajectory analysis allows researchers to observe how study participants evolve during a nutritional intervention depending upon their assigned nutritional group. This artificial intelligence-based approach considers an initial classification of individuals according to the Integrative Multiview Clustering [50], which uses 65 parameters divided in two blocks to group individuals. These two blocks are the baseline block, describing the health condition (biometric measures, tobacco and drug consumption, socio-demographic characteristics, diseases and biomarkers) and the habits block, which describes food habits and PA. This clustering process is performed at the beginning and at the end of the study, creating a trajectory map showing how the individuals belong to one or other final class by observing changes in diet indicators and depending on the initial state and the assigned intervention. Adherence to the intervention was tested in a randomized, parallel, controlled clinical trial with three dietary interventions (Mediterranean diet plus virgin or washed olive oil, and a control group with habitual diet) [51] where the previously mentioned MEDAS was used to assess individual diet scores [42]. By using this approach, researchers are able to unmask dietary changes within a given intervention group and to discriminate participants according to their particular diet trajectories during the study, and not only by their assigned intervention groups. This type of study allows a more specific evaluation of adherence and a more accurate characterization of the impact of the intervention. In any case, the application of these algorithms will likely continue to be influenced by inadequate self-reported-based estimates of energy intake that are, after all, the input parameters of such sophisticated algorithms [52]. In this sense, a recent study has revealed that energy intake under-reporting keeps being a major concern in nutrition research, regardless of self-reporting method [53]. In this study, a total of 200 men and women from the SCAPIS study (Swedish CArdioPulmonary bioImage Study) [54], and aged 50–64 years were recruited and invited to complete a rapid FFQ (the MiniMeal-Q) and a 4-day web-based food record tool (the Riksmaten method). Reported energy intake by the MiniMeal-Q and the Riksmaten method were tested against total energy expenditure measured with the double-labelled water technique in 40 participants. Both methods are widely used in national dietary surveys in Sweden and in large-scale epidemiological studies, and have been partially validated. Results of this study showed that both methods displayed a similar degree of energy intake under-reporting, with a reporting accuracy of 80% and 82% for the for MiniMeal-Q and the Risksmaten methods, respectively [53].

Aiming at a better standardization of adherence monitoring in restricted and free-living individuals, self-reported assessment methods should then be used with caution, and priority should be given to the development of alternative techniques to assess food and energy intake. In this regard, new methods to measure food consumption in a more accurate way are emerging and being validated. A food image-based method, called the Remote Food Photography Method (RFPM) [55], has been recently validated for measuring energy and nutrient intake [56] and has been proposed as a cheap, easy, and reliable method for detecting individual adherence better than classical FFQ. This method involves participants capturing images of their meals and plates waste with a phone camera. These images are further sent to a server where energy and nutrient intake are estimated by validated methods [55]. Another method based on wrist motion tracking aims to give consistent energy intake measurements from daily living by monitoring food bites thanks to a wearable (watch-like) device coupled with a micro-electro-mechanical gyroscope [57]. Although these methods still need to be fine-tuned, they appear to be promising for the optimization of dietary monitoring focused on estimated energy intake and to assess adherence to a nutritional intervention.

Innovative and sophisticated tools to estimate food and energy intake are expected to be further improved and validated, while more precise devices and techniques such as the above mentioned must be developed. Further research is also needed to test whether these *high-tech* methods can be widely used in free-living subjects [58].

3. Food Behavior

Foodstyle Monitoring

In addition to the measurement of total food intake, additional key aspects concerning precision nutrition that must be considered are, for instance, the frequency at which we consume foods throughout the day, the time we have lunch or dinner, and our snacking habits. Again, relying on methods able to collect accurate and valid clinical observations are key priorities as we strive to obtain reliable research results that will ultimately lead to unbiased interpretations.

Innovative technologies in this area are being developed, such as the Universal Eating Monitor (UEM), a table-embedded scale able to precisely quantify the amount of food consumed by a given person over time [59]. Initially conceived to monitor unrestricted eating, currently existing algorithms can be used only under restricted laboratory conditions. Nevertheless, the ability of the UEM to monitor different eating behavior parameters such as eating rate, bite size or food-to-drink ratio makes this tool a potentially useful device in precision nutrition. Accordingly, the Automatic Ingestion Monitor (AIM) is a wearable device designed to monitor the food intake behavior, such as snacking, night eating or weekend overeating, and analyze eating behavior in free living conditions [60]. In this regard, the AIM uses three different sensors (jaw motion, hand gesture and accelerometer) that allow obtaining reliable eating behavior measurements. These systems are two examples of how technology can be implemented to account for inter-individual differences in feeding behavior.

One important aspect of food behavior lies in its interaction with the circadian system, a physiological internal clock working autonomously with rhythms and oscillators synchronized by external time cues, and regulating a variety of physiological functions [61]. Several authors have already shown the relevance of the circadian system in human nutrition. Results from the ONTIME study, a clinical trial focused on the interaction between meal timing, genetics and weight loss showed that carriers of variants at the *PLIN1* locus exhibited lower weight loss within individuals assigned to the group of late lunch eaters (after 15:00), as compared to early lunch eaters (before 15:00) (7.21 ± 0.67 kg vs. 10.63 ± 0.56 kg; $p = 0.001$) [62]. Other food behaviors, such as frequent snacking have also been pinned down to genetics. Garaulet et al. reported that carriers of *PER2* variants displayed extreme snacking, suffered from diet-induced stress and bored-eating, among other behavior atypical patterns [63]. Results of two other recent studies have underscored the relevance of genes linked to the circadian clock in scheduled food behavior. For instance, significant interactions between specific gene variants within the *CLOCK* [64] and the *CRY1* [65] circadian genes, with low-fat diet and carbohydrate intake, respectively, have been identified.

In the first study, the interaction between SNPs at the *CLOCK* locus (rs1801260, rs3749474, rs4580704) with a Mediterranean diet and a low-fat diet was tested in 897 patients with coronary heart disease from the Coronary Diet Intervention with Olive Oil and Cardiovascular Prevention (CORDIOPREV) clinical trial (ClinicalTrials.gov: NCT00924937). After 12 months of intervention, a significant interaction was found between rs4580704 and low-fat dietary pattern for high sensitivity C-reactive protein (hsCRP) levels and the ratio high-density lipoprotein cholesterol/apolipoprotein A1 (HDL/ApoA1). Specifically, after the low-fat diet intervention, rs4580704 major allele carriers (CC) displayed a significant decrease of CRP levels, as compared to minor allele carriers (GG + CG) (~42% vs. ~12.5%; $p < 0.001$) and increased HDL/ApoA1 ratio (~4% vs. ~1.2%; $p < 0.029$), whereas no changes were observed between genotypes after the Mediterranean diet intervention, thereby suggesting that some metabolic disturbances, such as inflammation or dyslipemia, may be improved with personalized nutritional advices based on the genetic background of circadian rhythm [64].

On the other hand, a SNP (rs2287161) at the *CRY1* locus was tested for interaction with carbohydrate intake in predicting insulin resistance [65]. Results showed that increased carbohydrate intake led to a significant increase of fasting insulin ($\beta_{interaction}$ ($SE_{interaction}$) = 0.0040 (0.0015); $P_{interaction}$ = 0.007) and the homeostatic model assessment of insulin resistance (HOMA-IR) ($\beta_{interaction}$ ($SE_{interaction}$) = 0.0040 (0.0016); $P_{interaction}$ = 0.011) only among individuals homozygous for the rs2287161 rare allele. The initial results found in the Mediterranean population of 728 subjects following a Mediterranean diet were further replicated in a North American population of 820 subjects participating in the Genetics of Lipid Lowering Drugs and Diet Network (GOLDN) study.

These and other findings reviewed by Asher & Sassone-Corsi and Oike et al. [66,67] highlight the relevance of chrono-nutrition, i.e., the study of how food components interact with circadian clocks and how meal times affect metabolic processes [67], in the application of precision nutrition. Concretely, these findings point to circadian genetic variability as a relevant factor to be considered when developing scheduled and personalized nutrition programs aimed to face metabolic disorders associated with obesity.

4. Precision Physical Activity

Physical Activity: A Key Factor to Proper Precision Nutrition

There is a wide consensus in the literature that a sedentary lifestyle is one of the main factors contributing to the epidemic of cardiometabolic diseases [68]. Monitoring of PA should be then considered as a central factor when approaching precision nutrition. In words of Betts and González: *An optimal diet can therefore be personalized not only to what an individual is currently doing but to what they should be doing* [1]. In this context, Bouchard et al. have shown that besides the inter-individual variability in the beneficial response to a PA intervention regarding cardiovascular disease (CVD) and type 2 diabetes (T2D) risk factors, some individuals may even experience negative responses, such as a decrease in plasma HDL-C or an increase in systolic blood pressure, fasting plasma insulin and plasma triglyceride (TG) levels [69]. Thus, tailored dietary recommendations should take into account the PA profile of individuals, which will open the door to more integrative interventions, including personalized PA prescriptions. Moreover, not only the inter-individual variability in PA rates is relevant when tailoring nutritional advices, but even greater is the within-individual PA variability with time. In this regard, a recent study has shown the relevance of accounting for day-to-day individual variability of insulin and glucose levels in response to a standardized PA intervention. In this study, 171 sedentary, middle-aged abdominally obese adults were randomly assigned to four exercise groups (non-exercise, a low-amount/low-intensity, high-amount/low-intensity and high-amount/ high-intensity). The intervention consisted of walking on a treadmill five times per week at the required intensity (relative to the cardiorespiratory fitness) for 24 weeks. The day-to-day variability was calculated as the square root of the sum of squared differences of repeat measures (glucose and insulin baseline and 24-week levels in the control group), divided by the total number of paired samples and multiplied by two. Taking into account this individual variability, approximately 80% of the participants did not improve glucose and insulin levels, independently of the PA intensity, underscoring the need for a more comprehensive assessment of the PA-derived metabolic outcomes [70]. This study stressed that within-subject variation must be accurately assessed when evaluating the inter-individual differences in precision nutrition approaches. In this regard, Atkinson & Betherman [71] have proposed a logical framework to identify true inter-individual differences after an intervention, as well as to evaluate their clinical relevance. Such approach includes a comparator arm where standard deviation from the intervention arm should be compared to for the identification of reliable differences among participants.

Recent approaches have started to scrutinize the potential role of PA in previously detected genetic associations with obesity and related metabolic disturbances. For example, it has been reported that a sedentary behavior, estimated as prolonged television watching, accentuates genetic predisposition (measured as GRS) to increased BMI in two prospective cohorts, the Nurses' Health Study and the Health Professionals Follow-up Study [72]. Specifically, an increment of ten points in the GRS was associated with 0.8–3.4 kg/m^2 higher BMI across the different categories of television watching (1–40 h/week; $P_{interaction}$ = 0.001). Recent findings have also reported that the impact of gene variants within *FTO* gene, the first and most strongly obesity-associated gene [73,74], on obesity development is in fact attenuated by PA, i.e., the increase in BMI is 76% more pronounced in inactive individuals carrying the risk allele ($P_{interaction}$ = 0.004) [75]. Additional studies have also reported a protective effect of PA (assessed using self-administered questionnaires) on the impact of obesity-associated genetic variants in the form of aggregated GRS [76,77]. Results from Li et al. [76] revealed that the genetic predisposition to obesity in individuals with high-risk GRS could mitigated by higher levels of PA, as illustrated by BMI differences in physically active vs. sedentary participants. More specifically, the BMI difference between high- and low-risk GRS individuals in the sedentary group amounted to 0.74 kg/m^2, whereas this difference was 0.41 kg/m^2 in the physically active group. These results were also replicated in a meta-analysis of 11 cohorts [77], where a significant but weak association was reported (0.65 kg/m^2 vs. 0.53 kg/m^2). Despite the adequate power to detect small effects and the large number of participants in above-mentioned studies, over 20,000 and 100,000 individuals, respectively, gene × PA interactions are not strong enough to establish causal relationships between increased PA and decreased risk of genetic predisposition to develop obesity, or to use them in clinical practice, as reported by Ahmad et al. [77]. Likewise, a more recent GWAS meta-analysis of 200,452 subjects from 60 previous studies analyzing gene-PA interactions revealed 11 novel loci associated with adiposity, suggesting that accounting for PA could facilitate the uncovering of novel biological determinants of obesity [78]. Nevertheless, the search for PA interactions with obesity-associated loci only provided significant results with the *FTO* gene, showing a decrease of 30% of *FTO* effect in active as compared to sedentary subjects [78]. Although it has been hypothesized that highly penetrant genetic variants may be less influenced by environmental factors [79], it is important to point out that PA is most often estimated by self-reported questionnaires in population studies. In this regard, it is worth highlighting that the majority of studies included in this meta-analysis used self-reported PA data (self-administered or interviewer-administered questionnaires) instead of objective measures (only two studies measured PA by accelerometry), and PA was finally treated as a dichotomous variable (active and inactive individuals) to harmonize this parameter, with the resultant loss of power to detect associations.

It then becomes crucial to replicate these findings with direct and objective measures of PA. In this sense, the recent use of accelerometers to objectively measure PA levels has consistently revealed that both BMI-associated GRS [80] and *FTO* impact on obesity susceptibility [81] are attenuated by higher levels of objectively measured PA. With direct PA measurements, results from the *FTO*-related work [81] are similar to previous findings [75,82], but the attenuation of *FTO* impact on obesity-associated features, such as BMI and WC, is quantitatively more important. These findings could be explained, according to the authors, by the higher precision of PA measurements and its ability to accurately categorize PA intensity into light, moderate or vigorous.

These findings underscore the importance of a reliable assessment of PA for a more accurate interpretation of its potential modulating effect on the association between diet and health outcomes.

Up to now, motion sensors such as accelerometers could be considered as the gold standard to obtain accurate PA measurements [83], and their use in biomedical research in increasing [84,85]. A recent systematic review of the use of accelerometers for measuring PA under free-living conditions revealed that triaxial accelerometers were the most commonly used, followed by biaxial and uniaxial [86]. Among triaxial accelerometers, the most used models in longitudinal assessment of PA in studies related to health and disease [87] were ActiGraph GT3X (ActiGraph LLC, Pensacola, FL, USA) [70,88] and TracmorD (DirectLife, Philips Consumer Lifestyle, Amsterdam, The Netherlands) [81,89]. Nevertheless, these methods have some limitations for large prospective epidemiological studies, e.g., intrusiveness, elevated cost or specialized training for an efficient use [90], limitations that researchers should try to overcome in order to develop precision nutrition approaches that integrate the important notions of energy expenditure and energy balance. In this regard, together with an accurate knowledge of dietary habits, food behaviors, genetics and gut microbiota factors, as well as a precise metabolic phenotyping, precision energy expenditure measurements, including resting energy expenditure (REE), thermic effect of food and activity-related PA should be considered when implementing precision nutrition approaches, as depicted in Figure 3. Regarding activity-related PA, a multidimensional representation of PA (including factors such as occupational PA, sedentary time and leisure activities) has been recently proposed as a way to provide a more comprehensive picture of PA, reducing the bias associated to a unidimensional approach solely based on PA *per se* [91].

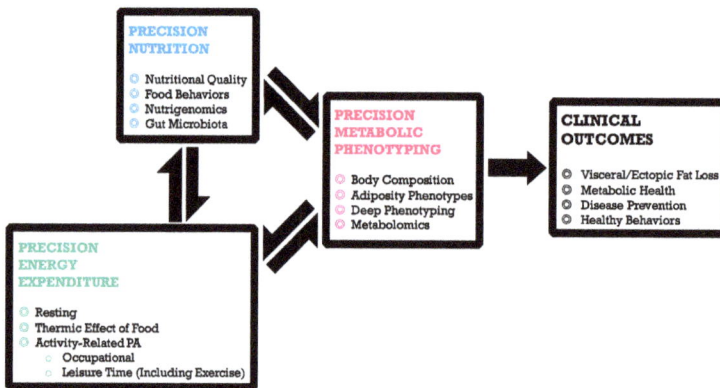

Figure 3. Precision nutrition features and their relationships. PA: physical activity.

5. Deep Phenotyping

High-Quality Phenotypes to Stratify Obesity

The need for precise measures to refine phenotypes emerges as a key pillar to understand inter-individual variability observed for certain pathologies, as well as over time variability for an individual [92]. This is of special relevance when the impact of a given diet or lifestyle advice on specific phenotype features is the pursued goal. Accurate and well-defined disease stratification, taking into account phenotypic heterogeneity, is then required in order to obtain reliable associations in nutritional interventions (Figure 3).

Complex diseases mean complex phenotypes. This is the case of most metabolic disorders, such as obesity, CVD or T2D. The development of new tools or methods with the ability to stratify and distinguish different phenotypes in terms of etiology, severity or underlying mechanisms thus represents a challenge in the field of precision nutrition. In this regard, although obesity is a condition associated with increased risk of T2D, CVD and other metabolic complications, a significant proportion of individuals with excess body weight are characterized by a much healthier metabolic risk profile than what could be expected form their excess adiposity [93], thereby suggesting that BMI does not reflect the actual health status of an individual. On the other hand, individual with a normal BMI may still be characterized by metabolic dysfunction if they carry excess visceral or hepatic fat. Since excess visceral adipose tissue (VAT) accumulation and adipose tissue dysfunction are tightly related to the development of obesity-related metabolic complications [94], it has been proposed that the combined measure of WC and plasma TG levels may represent an inexpensive and useful biomarker of both VAT accumulation and dysfunction, as well as a potential predictor of T2D and CVD risk [95,96]. Results from a study including 21,787 apparently healthy individuals, followed for approximately 10 years as part of the EPIC-Norfolk prospective population study, have shown that the hypertriglyceridemic-waist phenotype (the combination of elevated WC and plasma TG levels) was associated with increased risk (unadjusted hazard ratio—UHR) for coronary artery disease in both men (UHR = 2.40 (2.02–2.87)) and women (UHR = 3.84 (3.20–4.62)) [97].

Several imaging studies have now shown that VAT accumulation has a more deleterious effect than subcutaneous adipose tissue (SAT) on metabolic health [94,98]. Assessment of VAT accumulation represents a challenge when stratifying subjects with abdominal obesity. In this regard, a recent study has shown that epigenetic factors, such as DNA methylation marks, could discriminate VAT from SAT after weight loss surgery [99]. Given that VAT biopsies represents an invasive technique, there is a need to find surrogate biomarkers in more accessible tissues such as blood, allowing a better characterization of obesity in addition to the traditional clinical outcomes, such as BMI or WC. Recent studies have also suggested that whole genome differential methylation patterns derived from blood leukocytes (BL) may be used as surrogates of those derived from VAT. More specifically, a set of differentially methylated cytosine-phosphate-guanine (CpG) sites, common in VAT and BL, were shown to successfully discriminate men with or without metabolic syndrome [100]. These and other results suggest that BL methylation levels could be a good marker of VAT DNA methylation [101], and could then be used to determine the effect of a nutritional intervention on the epigenetic profile, and therefore on metabolic health related to VAT accumulation. Thus, knowledge of epigenetic variations predictive of metabolic complications among individuals with obesity could be of considerable relevance to the field of precision nutrition. For instance, recent studies focusing on DNA methylation differences between responders and non-responders to a weight loss intervention (energy restriction or bariatric surgery) [102–105] suggest that these epigenetic marks may be used as biomarkers to identify high-risk individuals who may be targeted in personalized nutritional programs focused on prevention, management and treatment of obesity.

Robinson has defined deep phenotyping as the precise and comprehensive analysis of phenotypic abnormalities in which the individual components of the phenotype are observed and described [106]. Traditional risk factors for T2D and CVD, such as blood pressure, lipid profile or BMI, are not always representative enough of a given health condition. Rather, in some instances, a thorough, individualized and precise evaluation of a number of metabolic parameters, e.g., continuous glucose monitoring in T2D, could be required [106,107]. This means that a much more detailed phenotyping is required in order to capture the diverse, interindividual and time-dependent, variability of disease manifestations for a better disease stratification.

An example of this extensive phenotyping is the Maastricht Study, where a cohort of 10,000 individuals with an overrepresentation of patients with T2D are being surveyed in a regular basis for T2D traditional risk factors, etiology and associated metabolic disturbances [108]. In this study, traditional (hypertension, dyslipidemia, obesity or inflammation status) and advanced phenotyping techniques (body composition by dual energy X-ray absorptiometry, electrophysiology of the heart, ocular pressure, corneal confocal microscopy or lung function evaluation by spirometry) are being used to elucidate the underlying pathophysiology of T2D and associated metabolic disturbances. This large epidemiological study will likely provide important clues on how detailed phenotyping can be extracted and eventually applied in precision nutrition. In-depth phenotyping methods utilized in this study can be divided into four different approaches: exhaustive biobanking for an efficient risk stratification (whole blood for DNA and RNA extraction, 24 h and morning urine, fasting and post-oral glucose tolerance test serum samples), advanced cardiovascular imaging for better knowledge of T2D-associated CVD risk (microvascular assessment by nail fold microscopy, vascular and cardiac ultrasound), use of accelerometry to objectively measure PA and sedentary time, and the study of psychosocial factors through personality questionnaires. The use of advanced and objective measurements (abdominal fat ultrasound, triaxial accelerometry), combined with traditional and self-reported data (FFQ, PA) represents a strength of this study [108] and a step forward in precision nutrition.

As previously outlined in the *Precision nutrition* section, a similar strategy was carried out by Zeevi et al. in their work about prediction of glycemic responses and personalized nutrition [33]. This work represents a proof-of-concept for the feasibility of individualized prediction of the response to a meal by combining traditional and in-depth measurements, such as FFQ, food diaries, blood tests and microbiome profiling, being able to assign specific diets allowing to successfully lower post-meal blood glucose.

The strengths of deep phenotyping span from providing a much more detailed picture of a given pathology, which allows a better clinical decision-making, to deepening the knowledge of mechanisms governing the progression of the pathology, which improves the evaluation of intervention outcomes. Thus, despite its limitations, such as the high cost, the need for intensive clinical measurements, or the necessity of accurate evaluation by trained professionals, deep phenotyping represents an essential tool for the optimal stratification of diseases to easily and efficiently manage each subtype according to its particular characteristics [107,109]. Translational and precision nutrition approaches shall then profit from this specific and *fine-grained* phenotype information to adequately apply novel and personalized dietary advices.

6. Metabolomics

Towards a Better Characterization of Eating

The accurate understanding of how nutrients are metabolized, and how these metabolites are able to illustrate the body's response to a diet has been previously addressed in many studies [110]. Regarding precision nutrition, metabolomics stands as a cornerstone in the knowledge of the real impact of foods on an individual's health. By identifying food-derived biomarkers, scientists can now determine how different individuals metabolize the same foods distinctly, and how such food products or metabolites may further influence health outcomes in different healthy or unhealthy situations, as well as in atypical conditions, such as intolerances or allergies. In this regard, the standardization of reference values for metabolites is necessary for the further use of them as food-derived biomarkers in the setting of precision nutrition. A recent study carried out in 800 French healthy volunteers where 185 plasma metabolites were analyzed has established a reference dataset for the majority of them [111]. Moreover, this study allowed to differentiate *normal* metabolomes between men and women, elderly and young subjects, and to determine the main sources of variation between population subgroups. As an example, results of this study revealed that individuals with high total cholesterol levels were also characterized by higher plasma sphingomyelins and phosphatidylcholine concentrations [111].

As previously mentioned in the *Dietary habits* section, objective measurement of the adherence to a dietary pattern remains a major challenge of precision nutrition. Recent advances in metabolomics offer a glimpse into promising avenues for better eating characterization. For instance, it could be possible to identify individual foods or nutrients, such as polyphenols, wheat, sugar-sweetened beverages or walnut consumption [112–115]. A further step in metabolomics usefulness is to test its ability to determine the overall picture of an individual food consumption [116]. In this sense, spectroscopic profiling of urine with the use of proton nuclear magnetic resonance (^{1}H-NMR) has recently been validated for the objective measurement of an overall dietary pattern [117]. The 19 participants of this randomized, controlled, crossover trial were assigned to four dietary interventions with a stepwise variance in concordance with the World Health Organization (WHO) healthy eating guidelines. Adherence to the intervention was strictly monitored by food and plate waste weighing, and urine samples were collected daily over three time periods. A global metabolomic profiling with a combination of 16,000 spectral variables was used to generate representative metabolite patterns relevant to each diet. Systematic differences were found in metabolomic profiles between diets 1 and 4 (the most and the least concordant diets to the WHO guidelines). Among individual metabolites, significantly higher concentrations of hippurate (fruit and vegetables), tartrate (grapes) or dimethylamine (fish) were found in the urine of participants assigned to diet 1, as compared to participants assigned to diet 4, while others were significantly lower, such as carnitine (red meat). The ability of this technique to discriminate metabolomic profiles of participants and classify them according to their assigned healthy or unhealthy diet during a nutritional intervention was further successfully validated in free-living populations [117]. However, the low specificity and sensitivity of this method in the discrimination of dietary patterns must be addressed, and some other challenges such as its potential to capture diet dynamics thorough long-term studies have to be considered [118]. The same ^{1}H-NMR technique has also been used to characterize the metabolomic profiles of a whole meal [119]. In this study, a cereal breakfast and an egg and ham breakfast were distinguished by identifying acute metabolomic fingerprints and key discriminatory metabolites in postprandial urine samples. Concretely, phosphocreatine/creatine, citrate and lysine were at higher concentrations after an egg and ham breakfast, whereas erythrose showed a higher concentration after a cereal breakfast [119].

Metabolomics has also been successfully applied in the development of novel population classification methods according to the metabotype, which stands for a group of individuals with similar metabolic profiles, and therefore represents a pillar of *deep phenotyping* [120]. One of the advantages of stratifying population according to the metabolic profile (metabotyping) is the possibility to scale precision nutrition advices to relatively uniform groups of individuals. As an example, since low-grade inflammation is known to be an important factor in insulin resistance development, the search for nutritional strategies focused on alleviating the inflammatory state becomes an attractive approach for precision nutrition [121–123]. In this regard, recent studies based on baseline metabolic profiles, e.g., plasma lipoprotein and fatty acid profiles, cardiometabolic biomarkers or insulin and glucose fasting and postprandial levels, have revealed the ability to *a priori* discriminate between responders and non-responders to a specific treatment or nutritional intervention, as recently reviewed by Riedl et al. [124]. Moreover, preliminary results from a dietary intervention in overweight and obese adolescents (ClinicalTrials.gov: NCT01665742) suggest that the beneficial effects of anti-inflammatory supplements (omega-3 polyunsaturated fatty acids—*n*-3 PUFA—vitamin C, vitamin E, and polyphenols) on insulin sensitivity are limited to the patients with the least favorable metabotype, whose different components (high HOMA-IR and cholesterol levels) also serve as independent predictors of nutritional supplementation outcomes [125].

Emerging evidence suggests that both pre- and post-metabolic profiles in patients undergoing a nutritional intervention can provide valuable information about capabilities of metabotypes to predict a given response to nutrients, and to determine the influence of individual foods, whole meals and dietary patterns on plasma metabolite levels. Thus, the potential of metabolomics has to be further explored in precision nutrition approaches.

7. Microbiota Phenotyping

Diet-Gut Microbiome Interplay

Gut microbiota profiling is becoming a top priority in nutritional interventions, and the impact of specific dietary factors on the ecological diversity of the gut is currently the subject of many ongoing investigations. The development of nutritional interventions based on individual profiles are focused on optimizing gut microbial composition, both richness and diversity, and emerging evidence suggests that gut microbiota profiling should be included as a key feature of precision nutrition [126]. In fact, both composition and diversity of gut microbiota have been identified as potential risk factors for the development of several metabolic disorders including the metabolic syndrome, T2D and CVD [127]. In this regard, the previously discussed study of Zeevi et al. [33] is an example of how gut microbiome profiling could represent a tool allowing accurate glucose response prediction after a meal. In this study, gut microbiota profiling was performed in stool samples of the entire cohort of 800 participants by 16S rRNA and metagenomics sequencing. Numerous microbiome features of composition and function were then integrated into the postprandial glucose response prediction algorithm. The analysis of the contribution of each factor to algorithm predictions revealed 21 beneficial and 28 non-beneficial (decreased or increased predicted postprandial glucose response, respectively) microbiome-based features. For instance, *Eubacterium rectale* abundance was mostly beneficial, whereas *Parabacteroides distasonis* was found to be non-beneficial by the prediction algorithm. Other studies have also highlighted the potential relevance of gut microbiota in tailoring diets. For instance, the FRUVEDomics Study, a behavioral interventional trial (ClinicalTrials.gov ID: NCT03115866), aims at identifying metabolomic and microbiome risk factors that may be subjected to modification through a nutritional intervention, mainly based on increasing fruit and vegetable consumption in young adults at risk for the metabolic syndrome. For that purpose, 36 participants were randomized into three intervention groups. The first one was based on a dietary intake of 50% fruit and vegetables, and the other two groups were based on the same 50% fruit and vegetables plus low refined carbohydrate or low fat. Although it is expected that this trial will be completed in 2019, preliminary results have suggested that individuals with a higher risk of developing metabolic syndrome also exhibited a higher *Firmicutes* to *Bacteroidetes* ratio before the intervention [128–130]. Other than being able to identify different combinations of diets to improve metabolic health, this type of trial is an example of group-based nutritional interventions (at-risk metabolic syndrome young adults). Studies like this have the potential of revealing novel biomarkers, both metabolomic and issued from microbiome profiling, allowing a phenotype refinement that could eventually be used in further individually tailored studies.

A relevant aspect of the gut microbiome is the fact that its composition and diversity can be modulated by host genetic makeup [127]. But even more relevant for the precision nutrition field is the fact that the interaction between diet and host genetic background is also able to modulate the composition of the gut microbiota. A recent study aiming at documenting the impact of host genetics on the gut microbiome found that, in addition to 9 novel loci associated with gut microbial taxonomies and other chromosomal regions related to food preferences, gene-diet interactions regulate *Bifidobacterium* abundance [131]. This study was carried out in three independent Dutch population cohorts: a discovery cohort of 1539 individuals, and two replication cohorts of 534 and 105 individuals, respectively. Interestingly, a functional variant at the lactase (*LCT*) locus, tightly associated with lactase persistence in Europeans [132], was associated with higher abundance of *Bifidobacterium*. Dairy product consumption was not altered significantly by this haplotype, nor by increased *Bifidobacterium* abundance. Nevertheless, the interaction between this haplotype and the intake of dairy products was associated to *Bifidobacterium* abundance [131]. These results pointed out the potential modulation of the microbiome through the interaction between diet and genetic makeup as a target to be considered in further precision nutrition studies [133].

Other examples highlighting the relevance of gut microbiota in precision nutrition have reported its role in the relationship between red meat consumption and the development of atherosclerosis and CVD [134,135]. In these studies, increased fasting plasma levels of trimethylamine (TMA), produced by gut microbiota metabolism, and its proatherogenic metabolite trimethylamine-N-oxide (TMAO) were observed in mice and humans, concomitant with increased risk of atherosclerosis, after oral intake of L-carnitine [134] and phosphatidylcholine [135], both having red meats as a major source. Interestingly, as suggested by Zmora et al. [136], these pieces of work suggest that the general recommendation of reducing the intake of red meat [137] may be better focused on subjects with gut microbial configurations more prone to metabolize such nutrients into proatherogenic species. This study also revealed that the association between red meat intake and mortality could be due to a certain extent to gut microbiota-derived metabolites. Other general recommendations, such as the substitution of sugar consumption by artificial sweeteners, have also revealed that such an approach may not potentially be beneficial for a population subgroup, as reported by Suez et al. [138]. In this study, an increase in the intake of sweeteners led to the development of glucose intolerance in the subgroup of individuals having a sensitive gut microbiota [138]. However, given the high dose of sweetener used (5 mg saccharin/kg body weight—FDA's maximum acceptable daily intake) and the limited number of participants ($n = 7$), the results issued form the study of Suez et al. [138] are still controversial and have generated a broad discussion in the field [139,140]. Although there is mounting evidence supporting the impact of sweeteners on microbiota in rodents [141], larger studies in humans are still needed. In this regard, a recent study has shown that gut bacterial diversity could be affected by recent (four-day food record) sweetener consumption (aspartame and acesulfame potassium) [142].

In summary, recent findings summarized herein suggest a link between microbiome biomarkers and nutritional intervention outcomes [33], the ability of gene-diet interactions to modify gut microbiota composition [131], and the existing link between food consumption, disease development and gut bacteria diversity [134,135]. Altogether, these findings suggest that gut microbiota should be considered when designing individualized nutrition advices.

8. Recent Advances in Precision Nutrition

8.1. From Nutrigenomics to Tailored Nutrition

Genetics have been frequently considered in association studies as an independent factor predisposing to obesity, increased adiposity, T2D and CVD [143–146]. Both GWAS and candidate gene studies have mostly focused on the impact of genetics on metabolic health [147–150]. Although this strategy has identified strong statistical associations, knowledge about the underlying molecular mechanisms affected by these genetic variants, and allowing to interpret their clinical relevance in the development of such pathologies is still scarce [151]. As already mentioned in this review, the physiological consequences of genetic variants and of their interactions with nutrient intake and other lifestyle factors, such as PA [76–78] or dietary habits [19,20,28] have been carried out in the field of precision nutrition.

Besides the fact that interesting findings have emerged from these studies, more ambitious, comprehensive and overarching strategies are currently broadening the knowledge about factors involved in the different response to a given nutritional intervention. This is the case of two large randomized control trials, PREDIMED and Food4me.

8.2. PREDIMED

Given that previous studies have reported that increasing adherence to the Mediterranean diet has beneficial effects on cardiovascular health [152,153], the PREDIMED study was designed as a multicenter, randomized, controlled trial to determine the impact of this diet on cardiovascular outcomes in participants at high cardiovascular risk [46]. The general guidelines to follow the Mediterranean diet were provided to participants as a personalized dietary advice according to their prior adherence to this type of diet, evaluated by the previously mentioned 14-item MEDAS questionnaire [42]. These guidelines consisted in abundant use of olive oil for cooking, generous consumption of vegetables and fresh fruits, legumes, fish or seafood, nuts and seeds, selection of white meats instead of red and processed meats, and cook regularly with tomato, garlic and onion. Further recommendations were focused on reducing the consumption of certain foods, such as butter, sugar-sweetened beverages, pastries or French fries. The unique aspect of this study was the intensive utilization of a constellation of omics techniques (transcriptomics, genomics, epigenomics or metabolomics), the analysis of intermediate phenotypes (plasma lipid concentrations, inflammation markers or blood pressure) and end points (myocardial infarction, stroke, and death from CVD causes), and a robust dietary adherence assessment with a validated 14-item questionnaire [42,154], all of them key pillars in in the field of precision nutrition [155]. The plethora of biomarkers analyzed in the PREDIMED study ranged from genetic, epigenetic and transcriptomic, to proteomic, lipidomic and metabolomic determinants, allowing an in-depth evaluation of the effect of Mediterranean diet on the basis of an integrated framework. For instance, the use of this integrative approach allowed further analysis focused on the genetic makeup, such as the TG-lowering effect of a genetic variant (rs3812316) at the *MLXIPL* locus. Such TG-lowering effect was strengthened in subjects having a high adherence to the Mediterranean diet ($OR = 0.63$ (0.51–0.77); $p = 8.6 \times 10^{-6}$), as compared to those having a low adherence ($OR = 0.88$ (0.70–1.09); $p = 0.219$), which also enhanced the protective effect against myocardial infarction among carriers vs. non-carriers of this SNP ($HR = 0.34$ (0.12–0.93); $p = 0.036$) vs. ($HR = 0.90$ (0.35–2.33); $p = 0.830$), respectively). [156]. Previous nutritional interventions focused on gene-diet interactions have also revealed that TG levels can be modulated by diet depending upon the genetic background [157]. In that study, 210 participants received a daily supplementation of *n*-3 PUFA (5 g of fish oil) during 6 weeks to investigate the interindividual variability in plasma TG response to such supplementation. The GRS built with 10 SNPs showing significant frequency differences between extreme responders (the most significant reduction in plasma TG levels) and non-responders (no change in plasma TG levels) explained 21.5% of the variation in TG response. Another example of the distinctive effect of the Mediterranean diet depending on genetic background was found in a recent case-control study with more than 7000 participants, with or without T2D, issued from the PREDIMED study [158]. A significant interaction was observed between the adherence score to the MEDAS 14-item questionnaire and a GRS formed by two SNPs at the *FTO* and *MC4R* loci in determining T2D risk ($P_{interaction} = 0.006$). Specifically, carriers of the rare alleles of these two loci had higher T2D risk when adherence to the Mediterranean diet was low, but this association disappeared as adherence increased [158].

Metabolomic tools such as liquid chromatography and mass spectrometry are also being used in the PREDIMED study to characterize walnut or cocoa consumption under free-living conditions [115,159], providing a better assessment of dietary exposure to specific nutrients, which might be successfully applied in precision nutrition for the assessment of complex dietary patterns. More examples of gene-diet interactions, metabotyping and the Mediterranean diet impact on gene expression, epigenetic or lipidomic biomarkers emerged from the PREDIMED study are extensively reviewed by Fitó et al. [155].

8.3. Food4Me

Advanced tools and innovative approaches in nutrition assessment are being developed within the Food4Me project (food4me.org). This project, which started in 2011, is carried out by an international consortium focused on the translation of current nutrition knowledge into tailored diets and nutritional advices by meeting three fundamental elements: reliable dietary intake assessment, deep phenotyping (metabotyping), and universal genotyping [160]. The Food4Me project represents a step forward in the potential application of precision nutrition, since in collaboration with stakeholders from different areas (consumers, industry, regulators, etc.) it also seeks to report the attitudes and beliefs of study participants [161], as well as the legal and ethical aspects of this type of nutritional interventions.

Regarding dietary assessment, an innovative web-based tool was tested in a large randomized, controlled trial where participants were randomly assigned to intervention groups for a 6-month period [162]. Nutritional interventions were divided into conventional dietary advice, personalized nutritional advice based on baseline diet and phenotype and, finally, a third group where personalized nutritional advice where based on diet, phenotype and genotype. Baseline diet was evaluated by means of the validated Food4Me online-FFQ [163,164] and phenotypes were assessed by using self-reported anthropometric measurements (body weight, height and upper thigh, waist and hip circumferences) and metabolic parameters (glucose, total cholesterol, carotenoids, *n*-3 fatty acid index and 32 other fatty acids, and vitamin D). Genetic information used for deriving genotype-based personalized nutrition advice was based on loci associated with BMI, weight and WC (*FTO*; rs9939609), *n*-3 PUFA (*FADS1*; rs174546), fat intake (*TCF7L2*; rs7903146), saturated fat (*ApoE(e4)*; rs429358/rs7412) and folate (*MTHFR*; rs1801133). This type of study design was applied to test the efficacy of personalized nutritional advices for improving consumption of a Mediterranean diet [89], that was estimated on the basis of the PREDIMED 14-item questionnaire [42,154]. In this last study, personalized nutritional interventions were divided as previously mentioned (based on baseline diet, phenotype and genotype), plus on the basis of PA, that was evaluated by using the Baecke questionnaire [165] and accelerometer data. Results from this study revealed that adherence scores to a Mediterranean diet were greater among individuals assigned to personalized intervention groups, as compared to the control group (non-personalized general dietary advice) (5.48 ± 0.07 vs. 5.20 ± 0.05, respectively; *p* = 0.002), with the largest differences found when genotype data was included in the analysis of the intervention group (5.63 ± 0.10 vs. 5.38 ± 0.10, respectively; *p* = 0.029). Similarly, a recent randomized controlled trial illustrated how disclosing genetic information can lead to greater behavioral changes in dietary habits than population-based or general nutritional recommendations [166]. Specifically, sodium intake after a 12-month intervention in participants informed that they possessed a risk allele of the *ACE* gene (associated with increased sodium sensitivity) [17,18], and given a targeted recommendation, was significantly reduced as compared to participants in the control group, who received a general recommendation for sodium intake (mean change in mg: −287.3 ± 114.1 vs. 129.8 ± 118.2, *p* = 0.008). On the other hand, the intervention group composed of non-risk *ACE* participants and receiving a general recommendation for sodium intake did not show significant differences as compared to the control group (mean change in mg: −244.2 ± 150.2 vs. 129.8 ± 118.2, *p* = 0.11), suggesting that a targeted nutritional advice based on genotype information impact the intake of specific nutrients in a greater extent than a general recommendation.

It is worth highlighting that the optimal assessment of nutrient intake remains the foundation for personalized nutritional advice in the Food4Me study [160]. In this regard, dietary data was collected by a validated online FFQ [163,164] and participants received regular feedback with practical advice to improve, increase or decrease, the intake of specific nutrients. Likewise, besides traditional parameters (self-reported BMI and WC), deep phenotyping was performed by means of metabolomic measurements (glucose, cholesterol, carotenoids and lipid profile) collected using a dried blood spot technique [162]. Finally, dietary advice was also controlled regarding individual genotype information, that was referred to five diet-responsive SNPs located within genes linked to different anthropometric (body weight) and metabolic functions (total fat, saturated fatty acids, *n*-3 PUFA and folate) [162].

Recent findings from the Food4Me project have revealed promising advances around the three levels stated: dietary intake, deep phenotyping and genotyping. First, it has been reported that a personalized nutritional advice only based on individual baseline diet information (first level) could lead to greater positive changes in nutritional behavior than a conventional dietary advice after a 6-month intervention, i.e., decreased consumption of red meat (8.5%), saturated fat (7.8%) and salt (8.9%), and increased consumption of folate (11.5%), leading to significantly higher Healthy Eating Index (HEI) scores [167,168]. Second, it was also reported that deep phenotyping information could serve as predictor of the response to a nutritional intervention. For instance, baseline fatty acid profiles were able to predict the cholesterol response to a personalized dietary intervention [169]. Finally, regarding genotyping data, although disclosure of information about *FTO* genotype risk had a greater effect on body weight and WC reduction in risk carriers, as compared to the non-personalized control group, these changes were similar to the previously mentioned levels of personalized dietary advice [170]. In line with these results, a previous meta-analysis carried out with data from eight randomized controlled trials revealed that carriage of the *FTO* minor allele was not associated with significant differences in BMI, body weight or WC change in response to a weight loss intervention (dietary, PA or drug-based) [171].

9. Conclusions

Altogether, the studies reviewed herein illustrate the most recent approaches to precision nutrition from different perspectives, highlighting the need for an integrative framework that takes into account the richness of innovative tools and methods in this field. This review was an attempt to stress the most important challenges and issues that nutritional science has to overcome in order to successfully translate basic and clinical knowledge into an effective precision nutrition care.

Up to date, the PREDIMED study and the Food4Me project could be considered as state-of-the-art trials in the field of precision nutrition, and two of the most stimulating wide-scale approaches in this field, that will hopefully provide guidance about how precision nutrition could be used to successfully prevent and manage cardiometabolic disorders. As already mentioned, such integrated approaches have the potential to improve dietary behaviors in an individualized or in a group-based manner, and to generate new and innovative tools, methods and procedures.

It is worth mentioning that although precision nutrition remains in its infancy, it does not take away from the fact that great approaches have been translated into general practice, mainly in the field of nutrigenetics. As extensively reviewed in [172], the large body of evidence supporting this genetic-based approach warrant further progress in this field. At this point, it is important to underscore some limitations encountered by genetic-based nutrition in its translation into general practice, such as the skeptical views of registered dietitians toward genetic testing and the scarcity of such personalized approach in higher education curricula of health professionals [173,174]. In this regard, the feasibility of the whole precision nutrition framework will depend on joint efforts of all actors involved. On one hand, while nutrition professionals are expected to start adopting new diagnosis and follow-up techniques, policy makers should elaborate appropriate policies assuring, among others, an adequate protection of personal information issued from intensive data collection. On the other hand, a substantial part of the task of translating precision nutrition into a widely applicable procedure in nutritional practice remains on private industries, by pursuing the development of precision nutrition tools affordable and accessible to the general population. Thus, as highlighted in the position statement of the International Society of Nutrigenetics/Nutrigenomics [175], ethical and legal aspects around precision nutrition, as well as the built environment and social contexts that influence food consumption have to be considered for a wide and fruitful implementation of this promising concept of *modern nutrition* into the general population.

Acknowledgments: J.T.M. is funded by a postdoctoral fellowship from the Fonds de Recherche du Québec—Santé (FRQS). B.J.A. holds a junior scholarship award from the FRQS. J.-P.D. is Scientific Director of the International Chair on Cardiometabolic Risk at Université Laval. No M.-C.V. holds a Tier 1 Canada Research Chair in Genomics Applied to Nutrition and Metabolic Health.

Author Contributions: J.T.M. wrote the manuscript. B.L., J.-P.D. and M.-C.V. critically reviewed the manuscript. All authors approved the final version of the manuscript.

Conflicts of Interest: The authors declare no conflict of interest.

References

1. Betts, J.A.; Gonzalez, J.T. Personalised nutrition: What makes you so special? *Nutr. Bull.* **2016**, *41*, 353–359. [CrossRef]

2. McMahon, G.; Taylor, A.E.; Davey Smith, G.; Munafò, M.R. Phenotype refinement strengthens the association of AHR and CYP1A1 genotype with caffeine consumption. *PLoS ONE* **2014**, *9*, e103448. [CrossRef] [PubMed]

3. Valleé Marcotte, B.; Cormier, H.; Guénard, F.; Rudkowska, I.; Lemieux, S.; Couture, P.; Vohl, M.C. Novel Genetic Loci Associated with the Plasma Triglyceride Response to an Omega-3 Fatty Acid Supplementation. *J. Nutrigenet. Nutrigenomics* **2016**, *9*, 1–11. [CrossRef] [PubMed]

4. Ouellette, C.; Rudkowska, I.; Lemieux, S.; Lamarche, B.; Couture, P.; Vohl, M.-C. Gene-diet interactions with polymorphisms of the MGLL gene on plasma low-density lipoprotein cholesterol and size following an omega-3 polyunsaturated fatty acid supplementation: A clinical trial. *Lipids Health Dis.* **2014**, *13*, 86. [CrossRef] [PubMed]

5. Rudkowska, I.; Pérusse, L.; Bellis, C.; Blangero, J.; Després, J.-P.; Bouchard, C.; Vohl, M.-C. Interaction between Common Genetic Variants and Total Fat Intake on Low-Density Lipoprotein Peak Particle Diameter: A Genome-Wide Association Study. *J. Nutrigenet. Nutrigenomics* **2015**, *8*, 44–53. [CrossRef] [PubMed]

6. Tremblay, B.L.; Cormier, H.; Rudkowska, I.; Lemieux, S.; Couture, P.; Vohl, M.-C. Association between polymorphisms in phospholipase A2 genes and the plasma triglyceride response to an *n*-3 PUFA supplementation: A clinical trial. *Lipids Health Dis.* **2015**, *14*, 12. [CrossRef] [PubMed]

7. Palatini, P.; Ceolotto, G.; Ragazzo, F.; Dorigatti, F.; Saladini, F.; Papparella, I.; Mos, L.; Zanata, G.; Santonastaso, M. CYP1A2 genotype modifies the association between coffee intake and the risk of hypertension. *J. Hypertens.* **2009**, *27*, 1594–1601. [CrossRef] [PubMed]

8. Ahmadi, K.R.; Andrew, T. Opportunism: A panacea for implementation of whole-genome sequencing studies in nutrigenomics research? *Genes Nutr.* **2014**, *9*, 387. [CrossRef] [PubMed]

9. Özdemir, V.; Kolker, E. Precision Nutrition 4.0: A Big Data and Ethics Foresight Analysis—Convergence of Agrigenomics, Nutrigenomics, Nutriproteomics, and Nutrimetabolomics. *OMIS J. Integr. Biol.* **2016**, *20*, 69–75. [CrossRef] [PubMed]

10. Rasinpera, H.; Savilahti, E.; Enattah, N.S.; Kuokkanen, M.; Tötterman, N.; Lindahl, H.; Järvelä, I.; Kolho, K.-L. A genetic test which can be used to diagnose adult-type hypolactasia in children. *Gut* **2004**, *53*, 1571–1576. [CrossRef] [PubMed]

11. Ludvigsson, J.F.; Bai, J.C.; Biagi, F.; Card, T.R.; Ciacci, C.; Ciclitira, P.J.; Green, P.H.R.; Hadjivassiliou, M.; Holdoway, A.; van Heel, D.A.; et al. Diagnosis and management of adult coeliac disease: Guidelines from the British Society of Gastroenterology. *Gut* **2014**, *63*, 1210–1228. [CrossRef] [PubMed]

12. DiLella, A.G.; Huang, W.M.; Woo, S.L. Screening for phenylketonuria mutations by DNA amplification with the polymerase chain reaction. *Lancet* **1988**, *1*, 497–499. [CrossRef]

13. Cornelis, M.C.; El-Sohemy, A.; Campos, H. Genetic polymorphism of the adenosine A2A receptor is associated with habitual caffeine consumption. *Am. J. Clin. Nutr.* **2007**, *86*, 240–244. [PubMed]

14. Cornelis, M.C.; El-Sohemy, A.; Kabagambe, E.K.; Campos, H. Coffee, CYP1A2 Genotype, and Risk of Myocardial Infarction. *JAMA* **2006**, *295*, 1135. [CrossRef] [PubMed]

15. Corella, D.; Peloso, G.; Arnett, D.K.; Demissie, S.; Cupples, L.A.; Tucker, K.; Lai, C.-Q.; Parnell, L.D.; Coltell, O.; Lee, Y.-C.; et al. APOA2, Dietary Fat, and Body Mass Index. *Arch. Intern. Med.* **2009**, *169*, 1897. [CrossRef] [PubMed]

16. Corella, D.; Tai, E.S.; Sorlí, J.V.; Chew, S.K.; Coltell, O.; Sotos-Prieto, M.; García-Rios, A.; Estruch, R.; Ordovas, J.M. Association between the APOA2 promoter polymorphism and body weight in Mediterranean and Asian populations: Replication of a gene-saturated fat interaction. *Int. J. Obes. (Lond.)* **2011**, *35*, 666–675. [CrossRef] [PubMed]

17. Giner, V.; Poch, E.; Bragulat, E.; Oriola, J.; González, D.; Coca, A.; De La Sierra, A. Renin-angiotensin system genetic polymorphisms and salt sensitivity in essential hypertension. *Hypertension* **2000**, *35*, 512–517. [CrossRef] [PubMed]

18. Poch, E.; González, D.; Giner, V.; Bragulat, E.; Coca, A.; de La Sierra, A. Molecular basis of salt sensitivity in human hypertension. Evaluation of renin-angiotensin-aldosterone system gene polymorphisms. *Hypertension* **2001**, *38*, 1204–1209. [CrossRef] [PubMed]

19. Goni, L.; Cuervo, M.; Milagro, F.I.; Martínez, J.A. A genetic risk tool for obesity predisposition assessment and personalized nutrition implementation based on macronutrient intake. *Genes Nutr.* **2015**, *10*, 1–10. [CrossRef] [PubMed]

20. Rukh, G.; Sonestedt, E.; Melander, O.; Hedblad, B.; Wirfält, E.; Ericson, U.; Orho-Melander, M. Genetic susceptibility to obesity and diet intakes: Association and interaction analyses in the Malmö Diet and Cancer Study. *Genes Nutr.* **2013**, *8*, 535–547. [CrossRef] [PubMed]

21. Olsen, N.J.; Ängquist, L.; Larsen, S.C.; Linneberg, A.; Skaaby, T.; Husemoen, L.L.N.; Toft, U.; Tjønneland, A.; Halkjær, J.; Hansen, T.; et al. Interactions between genetic variants associated with adiposity traits and soft drinks in relation to longitudinal changes in body weight and waist circumference. *Am. J. Clin. Nutr.* **2016**, *104*, 816–826. [CrossRef] [PubMed]

22. Qi, Q.; Chu, A.Y.; Kang, J.H.; Jensen, M.K.; Curhan, G.C.; Pasquale, L.R.; Ridker, P.M.; Hunter, D.J.; Willett, W.C.; Rimm, E.B.; et al. Sugar-Sweetened Beverages and Genetic Risk of Obesity. *N. Engl. J. Med.* **2012**, *367*, 1387–1396. [CrossRef] [PubMed]

23. Brunkwall, L.; Chen, Y.; Hindy, G.; Rukh, G.; Ericson, U.; Barroso, I.; Johansson, I.; Franks, P.W.; Orho-Melander, M.; Renstrom, F. Sugar-sweetened beverage consumption and genetic predisposition to obesity in 2 Swedish cohorts. *Am. J. Clin. Nutr.* **2016**, *104*, 809–815. [CrossRef] [PubMed]

24. Qi, Q.; Chu, A.Y.; Kang, J.H.; Huang, J.; Rose, L.M.; Jensen, M.K.; Liang, L.; Curhan, G.C.; Pasquale, L.R.; Wiggs, J.L.; et al. Fried food consumption, genetic risk, and body mass index: Gene-diet interaction analysis in three US cohort studies. *BMJ* **2014**, *348*, g1610. [CrossRef] [PubMed]

25. Casas-Agustench, P.; Arnett, D.K.; Smith, C.E.; Lai, C.-Q.; Parnell, L.D.; Borecki, I.B.; Frazier-Wood, A.C.; Allison, M.; Chen, Y.-D.I.; Taylor, K.D.; et al. Saturated Fat Intake Modulates the Association between an Obesity Genetic Risk Score and Body Mass Index in Two US Populations. *J. Acad. Nutr. Diet.* **2014**, *114*, 1954–1966. [CrossRef] [PubMed]

26. Koochakpoor, G.; Daneshpour, M.S.; Mirmiran, P.; Hosseini, S.A.; Hosseini-Esfahani, F.; Sedaghatikhayat, B.; Azizi, F. The effect of interaction between Melanocortin-4 receptor polymorphism and dietary factors on the risk of metabolic syndrome. *Nutr. Metab. (Lond.)* **2016**, *13*, 35. [CrossRef] [PubMed]

27. Azizi, F.; Ghanbarian, A.; Momenan, A.A.; Hadaegh, F.; Mirmiran, P.; Hedayati, M.; Mehrabi, Y.; Zahedi-Asl, S. Tehran Lipid and Glucose Study Group. Prevention of non-communicable disease in a population in nutrition transition: Tehran Lipid and Glucose Study phase II. *Trials* **2009**, *10*, 5. [CrossRef] [PubMed]

28. Nettleton, J.A.; Follis, J.L.; Ngwa, J.S.; Smith, C.E.; Ahmad, S.; Tanaka, T.; Wojczynski, M.K.; Voortman, T.; Lemaitre, R.N.; Kristiansson, K.; et al. Gene x dietary pattern interactions in obesity: Analysis of up to 68 317 adults of European ancestry. *Hum. Mol. Genet.* **2015**, *24*, 4728–4738. [CrossRef] [PubMed]

29. Ferguson, L.R.; De Caterina, R.; Görman, U.; Allayee, H.; Kohlmeier, M.; Prasad, C.; Choi, M.S.; Curi, R.; de Luis, D.A.; Gil, Á.; et al. Guide and Position of the International Society of Nutrigenetics/Nutrigenomics on Personalised Nutrition: Part 1 - Fields of Precision Nutrition. *J. Nutrigenet. Nutrigenomics* **2016**, *9*, 12–27. [CrossRef] [PubMed]

30. Allison, D.B.; Bassaganya-Riera, J.; Burlingame, B.; Brown, A.W.; le Coutre, J.; Dickson, S.L.; van Eden, W.; Garssen, J.; Hontecillas, R.; Khoo, C.S.H.; et al. Goals in Nutrition Science 2015–2020. *Front. Nutr.* **2015**, *2*, 1–13. [CrossRef] [PubMed]

31. Corella, D.; Coltell, O.; Mattingley, G.; Sorlí, J.V.; Ordovas, J.M. Utilizing nutritional genomics to tailor diets for the prevention of cardiovascular disease: A guide for upcoming studies and implementations. *Expert Rev. Mol. Diagn.* **2017**, *17*, 495–513. [CrossRef] [PubMed]

32. Srinivasan, B.; Lee, S.; Erickson, D. Precision nutrition—Review of methods for point-of-care assessment of nutritional status. *Curr. Opin. Biotechnol.* **2017**, *44*, 103–108. [CrossRef] [PubMed]

33. Zeevi, D.; Korem, T.; Zmora, N.; Israeli, D.; Rothschild, D.; Weinberger, A.; Ben-Yacov, O.; Lador, D.; Avnit-Sagi, T.; Lotan-Pompan, M.; et al. Personalized Nutrition by Prediction of Glycemic Responses. *Cell* **2015**, *163*, 1079–1095. [CrossRef] [PubMed]

34. Wolever, T.M.S. Personalized nutrition by prediction of glycaemic responses: Fact or fantasy? *Eur. J. Clin. Nutr.* **2016**, *70*, 411–413. [CrossRef] [PubMed]

35. Ohlhorst, S.D.; Russell, R.; Bier, D.; Klurfeld, D.M.; Li, Z.; Mein, J.R.; Milner, J.; Ross, A.C.; Stover, P.; Konopka, E. Nutrition research to affect food and a healthy lifespan. *Adv. Nutr. Int. Rev. J.* **2013**, *4*, 579–584. [CrossRef] [PubMed]

36. Loos, R.J.F.; Janssens, A.C.J.W. Predicting Polygenic Obesity Using Genetic Information. *Cell Metab.* **2017**, *25*, 535–543. [CrossRef] [PubMed]

37. Hebert, J.R.; Frongillo, E.A.; Adams, S.A.; Turner-McGrievy, G.M.; Hurley, T.G.; Miller, D.R.; Ockene, I.S. Perspective: Randomized Controlled Trials Are Not a Panacea for Diet-Related Research. *Adv. Nutr. An Int. Rev. J.* **2016**, *7*, 423–432. [CrossRef] [PubMed]

38. Siebelink, E.; Geelen, A.; de Vries, J.H.M. Self-reported energy intake by FFQ compared with actual energy intake to maintain body weight in 516 adults. *Br. J. Nutr.* **2011**, *106*, 274–281. [CrossRef] [PubMed]

39. Schaefer, E.J.; Augustin, J.L.; Schaefer, M.M.; Rasmussen, H.; Ordovas, J.M.; Dallal, G.E.; Dwyer, J.T. Lack of efficacy of a food-frequency questionnaire in assessing dietary macronutrient intakes in subjects consuming diets of known composition. *Am. J. Clin. Nutr.* **2000**, *71*, 746–751. [PubMed]

40. Archer, E.; Pavela, G.; Lavie, C.J. The Inadmissibility of What We Eat in America and NHANES Dietary Data in Nutrition and Obesity Research and the Scientific Formulation of National Dietary Guidelines. *Mayo Clin. Proc.* **2015**, *90*, 911–926. [CrossRef] [PubMed]

41. Shim, J.-S.; Oh, K.; Kim, H.C. Dietary assessment methods in epidemiologic studies. *Epidemiol. Health* **2014**, *36*, e2014009. [CrossRef] [PubMed]

42. Schroder, H.; Fito, M.; Estruch, R.; Martinez-Gonzalez, M.A.; Corella, D.; Salas-Salvado, J.; Lamuela-Raventos, R.; Ros, E.; Salaverria, I.; Fiol, M.; et al. A Short Screener Is Valid for Assessing Mediterranean Diet Adherence among Older Spanish Men and Women. *J. Nutr.* **2011**, *141*, 1140–1145. [CrossRef] [PubMed]

43. Martínez-González, M.A.; García-Arellano, A.; Toledo, E.; Salas-Salvadó, J.; Buil-Cosiales, P.; Corella, D.; Covas, M.I.; Schröder, H.; Arós, F.; Gómez-Gracia, E.; et al. A 14-item Mediterranean diet assessment tool and obesity indexes among high-risk subjects: The PREDIMED trial. *PLoS ONE* **2012**, *7*, e43134. [CrossRef] [PubMed]

44. Sotos-Prieto, M.; Moreno-Franco, B.; Ordovás, J.; León, M.; Casasnovas, J.; Peñalvo, J. Design and development of an instrument to measure overall lifestyle habits for epidemiological research: The Mediterranean Lifestyle (MEDLIFE) index. *Public Health Nutr.* **2015**, *18*, 959–967. [CrossRef] [PubMed]

45. Martínez-González, M.A.; Fernández-Jarne, E.; Serrano-Martínez, M.; Wright, M.; Gomez-Gracia, E. Development of a short dietary intake questionnaire for the quantitative estimation of adherence to a cardioprotective Mediterranean diet. *Eur. J. Clin. Nutr.* **2004**, *58*, 1550–1552. [CrossRef] [PubMed]

46. Estruch, R.; Ros, E.; Salas-Salvadó, J.; Covas, M.-I.; Corella, D.; Arós, F.; Gómez-Gracia, E.; Ruiz-Gutiérrez, V.; Fiol, M.; Lapetra, J.; et al. Primary Prevention of Cardiovascular Disease with a Mediterranean Diet. *N. Engl. J. Med.* **2013**, *368*, 1279–1290. [CrossRef] [PubMed]

47. McCullough, M.L.; Feskanich, D.; Stampfer, M.J.; Giovannucci, E.L.; Rimm, E.B.; Hu, F.B.; Spiegelman, D.; Hunter, D.J.; Colditz, G.A.; Willett, W.C. Diet quality and major chronic disease risk in men and women: Moving toward improved dietary guidance. *Am. J. Clin. Nutr.* **2002**, *76*, 1261–1271. [PubMed]

48. Fung, T.T.; McCullough, M.L.; Newby, P.K.; Manson, J.E.; Meigs, J.B.; Rifai, N.; Willett, W.C.; Hu, F.B. Diet-quality scores and plasma concentrations of markers of inflammation and endothelial dysfunction. *Am. J. Clin. Nutr.* **2005**, *82*, 163–173. [PubMed]

49. Sevilla-Villanueva, B.; Gibert, K.; Sanchez-Marre, M.; Fito, M.; Covas, M.-I. Evaluation of Adherence to Nutritional Intervention through Trajectory Analysis. *IEEE J. Biomed. Heal. Inform.* **2017**, *21*, 628–634. [CrossRef] [PubMed]

50. Sevilla-Villanueva, B.; Gibert, K.; Sànchez-Marrè, M. Identifying Nutritional Patterns through Integrative Multiview Clustering. *Artif. Intell. Res. Dev.* **2015**, *277*, 185.

51. Konstantinidou, V.; Covas, M.-I.; Munoz-Aguayo, D.; Khymenets, O.; de la Torre, R.; Saez, G.; Tormos, M.d.C.; Toledo, E.; Marti, A.; Ruiz-Gutierrez, V.; et al. In vivo nutrigenomic effects of virgin olive oil polyphenols within the frame of the Mediterranean diet: A randomized controlled trial. *FASEB J.* **2010**, *24*, 2546–2557. [CrossRef] [PubMed]

52. Dhurandhar, N.V.; Schoeller, D.; Brown, A.W.; Heymsfield, S.B.; Thomas, D.; Sørensen, T.I.A.; Speakman, J.R.; Jeansonne, M.; Allison, D.B. Energy balance measurement: When something is not better than nothing. *Int. J. Obes.* **2015**, *39*, 1109–1113. [CrossRef] [PubMed]

53. Nybacka, S.; Bertéus Forslund, H.; Wirfält, E.; Larsson, I.; Ericson, U.; Warensjö Lemming, E.; Bergström, G.; Hedblad, B.; Winkvist, A.; Lindroos, A.K. Comparison of a web-based food record tool and a food-frequency questionnaire and objective validation using the doubly labelled water technique in a Swedish middle-aged population. *J. Nutr. Sci.* **2016**, *5*, e39. [CrossRef] [PubMed]

54. Bergström, G.; Berglund, G.; Blomberg, A.; Brandberg, J.; Engström, G.; Engvall, J.; Eriksson, M.; de Faire, U.; Flinck, A.; Hansson, M.G.; et al. The Swedish CArdioPulmonary BioImage Study: Objectives and design. *J. Intern. Med.* **2015**, *278*, 645–659. [CrossRef]

55. Martin, C.K.; Han, H.; Coulon, S.M.; Allen, H.R.; Champagne, C.M.; Anton, S.D. A novel method to remotely measure food intake of free-living individuals in real time: The remote food photography method. *Br. J. Nutr.* **2009**, *101*, 446. [CrossRef] [PubMed]

56. Martín, C.K.; Correa, J.B.; Han, H.; Allen, H.R.; Rood, J.C.; Champagne, C.M.; Gunturk, B.K.; Bray, G.A. Validity of the Remote Food Photography Method (RFPM) for Estimating Energy and Nutrient Intake in Near Real-Time. *Obesity* **2012**, *20*, 891–899. [CrossRef] [PubMed]

57. Dong, Y.; Hoover, A.; Scisco, J.; Muth, E. A New Method for Measuring Meal Intake in Humans via Automated Wrist Motion Tracking. *Appl. Psychophysiol. Biofeedback* **2012**, *37*, 205–215. [CrossRef] [PubMed]

58. Schoeller, D.A.; Thomas, D.; Archer, E.; Heymsfield, S.B.; Blair, S.N.; Goran, M.I.; Hill, J.O.; Atkinson, R.L.; Corkey, B.E.; Foreyt, J.; et al. Self-report-based estimates of energy intake offer an inadequate basis for scientific conclusions. *Am. J. Clin. Nutr.* **2013**, *97*, 1413–1415. [CrossRef] [PubMed]

59. Mattfeld, R.S.; Muth, E.R.; Hoover, A. Measuring the consumption of individual solid and liquid bites using a table embedded scale during unrestricted eating. *IEEE J. Biomed. Heal. Informatics* **2016**. [CrossRef] [PubMed]

60. Fontana, J.M.; Farooq, M.; Sazonov, E. Automatic Ingestion Monitor: A Novel Wearable Device for Monitoring of Ingestive Behavior. *IEEE Trans. Biomed. Eng.* **2014**, *61*, 1772–1779. [CrossRef] [PubMed]

61. Potter, G.D.M.; Cade, J.E.; Grant, P.J.; Hardie, L.J. Nutrition and the circadian system. *Br. J. Nutr.* **2016**, *116*, 434–442. [CrossRef] [PubMed]

62. Garaulet, M.; Vera, B.; Bonnet-Rubio, G.; Gómez-Abellán, P.; Lee, Y.-C.; Ordovás, J.M. Lunch eating predicts weight-loss effectiveness in carriers of the common allele at PERILIPIN1: The ONTIME (Obesity, Nutrigenetics, Timing, Mediterranean) study. *Am. J. Clin. Nutr.* **2016**, *104*, 1160–1166. [CrossRef] [PubMed]

63. Garaulet, M.; Corbalán-Tutau, M.D.; Madrid, J.A.; Baraza, J.C.; Parnell, L.D.; Lee, Y.-C.; Ordovas, J.M. PERIOD2 Variants Are Associated with Abdominal Obesity, Psycho-Behavioral Factors, and Attrition in the Dietary Treatment of Obesity. *J. Am. Diet. Assoc.* **2010**, *110*, 917–921. [CrossRef] [PubMed]

64. Gomez-Delgado, F.; Garcia-Rios, A.; Alcala-Diaz, J.F.; Rangel-Zuñiga, O.; Delgado-Lista, J.; Yubero-Serrano, E.M.; Lopez-Moreno, J.; Tinahones, F.J.; Ordovas, J.M.; Garaulet, M.; et al. Chronic consumption of a low-fat diet improves cardiometabolic risk factors according to the CLOCK gene in patients with coronary heart disease. *Mol. Nutr. Food Res.* **2015**, *59*, 2556–2564. [CrossRef] [PubMed]

65. Dashti, H.S.; Smith, C.E.; Lee, Y.-C.; Parnell, L.D.; Lai, C.-Q.; Arnett, D.K.; Ordovás, J.M.; Garaulet, M. CRY1 circadian gene variant interacts with carbohydrate intake for insulin resistance in two independent populations: Mediterranean and North American. *Chronobiol. Int.* **2014**, *31*, 660–667. [CrossRef] [PubMed]

66. Asher, G.; Sassone-Corsi, P. Time for Food: The Intimate Interplay between Nutrition, Metabolism, and the Circadian Clock. *Cell* **2015**, *161*, 84–92. [CrossRef] [PubMed]

67. Oike, H.; Oishi, K.; Kobori, M. Nutrients, Clock Genes, and Chrononutrition. *Curr. Nutr. Rep.* **2014**, *3*, 204–212. [CrossRef] [PubMed]

68. Hill, J.O.; Wyatt, H.R.; Peters, J.C. Energy balance and obesity. *Circulation* **2012**, *126*, 126–132. [CrossRef] [PubMed]

69. Bouchard, C.; Blair, S.N.; Church, T.S.; Earnest, C.P.; Hagberg, J.M.; H?kkinen, K.; Jenkins, N.T.; Karavirta, L.; Kraus, W.E.; Leon, A.S.; et al. Adverse Metabolic Response to Regular Exercise: Is It a Rare or Common Occurrence? *PLoS ONE* **2012**, *7*, e37887. [CrossRef] [PubMed]

70. de Lannoy, L.; Clarke, J.; Stotz, P.J.; Ross, R.; Senn, S.; Meyer, T. Effects of intensity and amount of exercise on measures of insulin and glucose: Analysis of inter-individual variability. *PLoS ONE* **2017**, *12*, e0177095. [CrossRef] [PubMed]

71. Atkinson, G.; Batterham, A.M. True and false interindividual differences in the physiological response to an intervention. *Exp. Physiol.* **2015**, *100*, 577–588. [CrossRef] [PubMed]

72. Qi, Q.; Li, Y.; Chomistek, A.K.; Kang, J.H.; Curhan, G.C.; Pasquale, L.R.; Willett, W.C.; Rimm, E.B.; Hu, F.B.; Qi, L. Television Watching, Leisure Time Physical Activity, and the Genetic Predisposition in Relation to Body Mass Index in Women and Men. *Circulation* **2012**, *126*, 1821–1827. [CrossRef] [PubMed]

73. Loos, R.J.F.; Yeo, G.S.H. The bigger picture of FTO: The first GWAS-identified obesity gene. *Nat. Rev. Endocrinol.* **2014**, *10*, 51–61. [CrossRef] [PubMed]

74. Frayling, T.M.; Timpson, N.J.; Weedon, M.N.; Zeggini, E.; Freathy, R.M.; Lindgren, C.M.; Perry, J.R.B.; Elliott, K.S.; Lango, H.; Rayner, N.W.; et al. A common variant in the FTO gene is associated with body mass index and predisposes to childhood and adult obesity. *Science* **2007**, *316*, 889–894. [CrossRef] [PubMed]

75. Vimaleswaran, K.S.; Li, S.; Zhao, J.H.; Luan, J.; Bingham, S.A.; Khaw, K.-T.; Ekelund, U.; Wareham, N.J.; Loos, R.J. Physical activity attenuates the body mass index-increasing influence of genetic variation in the FTO gene. *Am. J. Clin. Nutr.* **2009**, *90*, 425–428. [CrossRef] [PubMed]

76. Li, S.; Zhao, J.H.; Luan, J.; Ekelund, U.; Luben, R.N.; Khaw, K.T.; Wareham, N.J.; Loos, R.J.F. Physical activity attenuates the genetic predisposition to obesity in 20,000 men and women from EPIC-Norfolk prospective population study. *PLoS Med.* **2010**, *7*, e1000332. [CrossRef] [PubMed]

77. Ahmad, S.; Rukh, G.; Varga, T. V.; Ali, A.; Kurbasic, A.; Shungin, D.; Ericson, U.; Koivula, R.W.; Chu, A.Y.; Rose, L.M.; et al. Gene × Physical Activity Interactions in Obesity: Combined Analysis of 111,421 Individuals of European Ancestry. *PLoS Genet.* **2013**, *9*, e1003607. [CrossRef] [PubMed]

78. Graff, M.; Scott, R.A.; Justice, A.E.; Young, K.L.; Feitosa, M.F.; Barata, L.; Winkler, T.W.; Chu, A.Y.; Mahajan, A.; Hadley, D.; et al. Genome-wide physical activity interactions in adiposity—A meta-analysis of 200,452 adults. *PLoS Genet.* **2017**, *13*, e1006528. [CrossRef] [PubMed]

79. Scott, R.A.; Chu, A.Y.; Grarup, N.; Manning, A.K.; Hivert, M.-F.; Shungin, D.; Tönjes, A.; Yesupriya, A.; Barnes, D.; Bouatia-Naji, N.; et al. No Interactions Between Previously Associated 2-h Glucose Gene Variants and Physical Activity or BMI on 2-Hour Glucose Levels. *Diabetes* **2012**, *61*, 1291–1296. [CrossRef] [PubMed]

80. Moon, J.-Y.; Wang, T.; Sofer, T.; North, K.E.; Isasi, C.R.; Cai, J.; Gellman, M.D.; Moncrieft, A.E.; Sotres-Alvarez, D.; Argos, M.; et al. Gene-environment Interaction Analysis Reveals Evidence for Independent Influences of Physical Activity and Sedentary Behavior on Obesity: Results From the Hispanic Community Health Study/study of Latinos (HCHS/SOL). *Circulation* **2017**, *135*, AMP027.

81. Celis-Morales, C.; Marsaux, C.F.M.; Livingstone, K.M.; Navas-Carretero, S.; San-Cristobal, R.; O'donovan, C.B.; Forster, H.; Woolhead, C.; Fallaize, R.; Macready, A.L.; et al. Physical activity attenuates the effect of the *FTO* genotype on obesity traits in European adults: The Food4Me study. *Obesity* **2016**, *24*, 962–969. [CrossRef] [PubMed]

82. Andreasen, C.H.; Stender-Petersen, K.L.; Mogensen, M.S.; Torekov, S.S.; Wegner, L.; Andersen, G.; Nielsen, A.L.; Albrechtsen, A.; Borch-Johnsen, K.; Rasmussen, S.S.; et al. Low physical activity acentuates the effect of rs9939609 polymorphism. *Diabetes* **2008**, *57*, 95–101. [CrossRef] [PubMed]

83. Goodman, E.; Evans, W.D.; DiPietro, L. Preliminary Evidence for School-Based Physical Activity Policy Needs in Washington, DC. *J. Phys. Act. Heal.* **2012**, *9*, 124–128. [CrossRef]

84. Cadenas-Sanchez, C.; Ruiz, J.R.; Labayen, I.; Huybrechts, I.; Manios, Y.; Gonz??lez-Gross, M.; Breidenassel, C.; Kafatos, A.; De Henauw, S.; Vanhelst, J.; et al. Prevalence of Metabolically Healthy but Overweight/Obese Phenotype and Its Association With Sedentary Time, Physical Activity, and Fitness. *J. Adolesc. Heal.* **2016**. [CrossRef] [PubMed]

85. Cameron, N.; Godino, J.; Nichols, J.F.; Wing, D.; Hill, L.; Patrick, K. Associations between physical activity and BMI, body fatness, and visceral adiposity in overweight or obese Latino and non-Latino adults. *Int. J. Obes.* **2017**. [CrossRef] [PubMed]

86. Jeran, S.; Steinbrecher, A.; Pischon, T. Prediction of activity-related energy expenditure using accelerometer-derived physical activity under free-living conditions: A systematic review. *Int. J. Obes.* **2016**, *40*, 1187–1197. [CrossRef] [PubMed]

87. Westerterp, K.R. Reliable assessment of physical activity in disease. *Curr. Opin. Clin. Nutr. Metab. Care* **2014**, *17*, 401–406. [CrossRef] [PubMed]

88. Ross, R.; Hudson, R.; Stotz, P.J.; Lam, M. Effects of Exercise Amount and Intensity on Abdominal Obesity and Glucose Tolerance in Obese Adults. *Ann. Intern. Med.* **2015**, *162*, 325. [CrossRef] [PubMed]

89. Livingstone, K.M.; Celis-Morales, C.; Navas-Carretero, S.; San-Cristoba, R.; MacReady, A.L.; Fallaize, R.; Forster, H.; Woolhead, C.; O'Donovan, C.B.; Marsaux, C.F.M.; et al. Effect of an Internet-based, personalized nutrition randomized trial on dietary changes associated with the Mediterranean diet: The Food4Me Study. *Am. J. Clin. Nutr.* **2016**, *104*, 288–297. [CrossRef] [PubMed]

90. Prince, S.A.; Adamo, K.B.; Hamel, M.; Hardt, J.; Connor Gorber, S.; Tremblay, M.; O'Brien, W.; Bassett, D.; Schmitz, K.; Emplaincourt, P. A comparison of direct versus self-report measures for assessing physical activity in adults: A systematic review. *Int. J. Behav. Nutr. Phys. Act.* **2008**, *5*, 56. [CrossRef] [PubMed]

91. Thompson, D.; Peacock, O.; Western, M.; Batterham, A.M. Multidimensional physical activity: An opportunity, not a problem. *Exerc. Sport Sci. Rev.* **2015**, *43*, 67–74. [CrossRef] [PubMed]

92. Tracy, R.P. "Deep phenotyping": Characterizing populations in the era of genomics and systems biology. *Curr. Opin. Lipidol.* **2008**, *19*, 151–157. [CrossRef] [PubMed]

93. Kramer, C.K.; Zinman, B.; Retnakaran, R. Are metabolically healthy overweight and obesity benign conditions?: A systematic review and meta-analysis. *Ann. Intern. Med.* **2013**, *159*, 758–769. [CrossRef] [PubMed]

94. Tchernof, A.; Després, J.-P. Pathophysiology of human visceral obesity: An update. *Physiol. Rev.* **2013**, *93*, 359–404. [CrossRef] [PubMed]

95. Sam, S.; Haffner, S.; Davidson, M.H.E. AI Predicts Increased Visceral Fat in Subjects With Type 2 Diabetes. *Diabetes* **2009**, *32*, 1916–1920. [CrossRef]

96. Lemieux, I.; Poirier, P.; Bergeron, J.; Alméras, N.; Lamarche, B.; Cantin, B.; Dagenais, G.R.; Després, J.-P. Hypertriglyceridemic waist: A useful screening phenotype in preventive cardiology? *Can. J. Cardiol.* **2007**, *23* Suppl B, 23B–31B. [CrossRef]

97. Arsenault, B.J.; Lemieux, I.; Despres, J.-P.; Wareham, N.J.; Kastelein, J.J.P.; Khaw, K.-T.; Boekholdt, S.M. The hypertriglyceridemic-waist phenotype and the risk of coronary artery disease: Results from the EPIC-Norfolk Prospective Population Study. *Can. Med. Assoc. J.* **2010**, *182*, 1427–1432. [CrossRef] [PubMed]

98. Guénard, F.; Tchernof, A.; Deshaies, Y.; Pérusse, L.; Biron, S.; Lescelleur, O.; Biertho, L.; Marceau, S.; Vohl, M.-C. Differential methylation in visceral adipose tissue of obese men discordant for metabolic disturbances. *Physiol. Genomics* **2014**, *46*, 216–222. [CrossRef]

99. Macartney-Coxson, D.; Benton, M.C.; Blick, R.; Stubbs, R.S.; Hagan, R.D.; Langston, M.A. Genome-wide DNA methylation analysis reveals loci that distinguish different types of adipose tissue in obese individuals. *Clin. Epigenetics* **2017**, *9*, 48. [CrossRef] [PubMed]

100. Guénard, F.; Deshaies, Y.; Hould, F.-S.; Lebel, S.; Tchernof, A.; Marceau, P.; Vohl, M.-C. Use of Blood as a Surrogate Model for the Assessment of Visceral Adipose Tissue Methylation Profiles Associated with the Metabolic Syndrome in Men. *J. Mol. Genet. Med.* **2016**, *10*, 1–8. [CrossRef]

101. Rönn, T.; Volkov, P.; Gillberg, L.; Kokosar, M.; Perfilyev, A.; Jacobsen, A.L.; Jørgensen, S.W.; Brøns, C.; Jansson, P.-A.; Eriksson, K.-F.; et al. Impact of age, BMI and HbA1c levels on the genome-wide DNA methylation and mRNA expression patterns in human adipose tissue and identification of epigenetic biomarkers in blood. *Hum. Mol. Genet.* **2015**, *24*, 3792–3813. [CrossRef]

102. Moleres, A.; Campion, J.; Milagro, F.I.; Marcos, A.; Campoy, C.; Garagorri, J.M.; Gomez-Martinez, S.; Martinez, J.A.; Azcona-Sanjulian, M.C.; Marti, A.; et al. Differential DNA methylation patterns between high and low responders to a weight loss intervention in overweight or obese adolescents: The EVASYON study. *FASEB J.* **2013**, *27*, 2504–2512. [CrossRef] [PubMed]

103. Milagro, F.I.; Campión, J.; Cordero, P.; Goyenechea, E.; Gómez-Uriz, A.M.; Abete, I.; Zulet, M.A.; Martínez, J.A. A dual epigenomic approach for the search of obesity biomarkers: DNA methylation in relation to diet-induced weight loss. *FASEB J.* **2011**, *25*, 1378–1389. [CrossRef] [PubMed]

104. Bouchard, L.; Rabasa-Lhoret, R.; Faraj, M.; Lavoie, M.-E.; Mill, J.; Pérusse, L.; Vohl, M.-C. Differential epigenomic and transcriptomic responses in subcutaneous adipose tissue between low and high responders to caloric restriction. *Am. J. Clin. Nutr.* **2010**, *91*, 309–320. [CrossRef] [PubMed]

105. Nicoletti, C.F.; Nonino, C.B.; de Oliveira, B.A.P.; Pinhel, M.A.; de Souza Pinhel, M.A.; Mansego, M.L.; Milagro, F.I.; Zulet, M.A.; Martinez, J.A. DNA Methylation and Hydroxymethylation Levels in Relation to Two Weight Loss Strategies: Energy-Restricted Diet or Bariatric Surgery. *Obes. Surg.* **2016**, *26*, 603–611. [CrossRef] [PubMed]

106. Robinson, P.N. Deep phenotyping for precision medicine. *Hum. Mutat.* **2012**, *33*, 777–780. [CrossRef] [PubMed]

107. Delude, C.M. Deep phenotyping: The details of disease. *Nature* **2015**, *527*, S14–S15. [CrossRef] [PubMed]

108. Schram, M.T.; Sep, S.J.S.; van der Kallen, C.J.; Dagnelie, P.C.; Koster, A.; Schaper, N.; Henry, R.M.A.; Stehouwer, C.D.A. The Maastricht Study: An extensive phenotyping study on determinants of type 2 diabetes, its complications and its comorbidities. *Eur. J. Epidemiol.* **2014**, *29*, 439–451. [CrossRef] [PubMed]

109. Lanktree, M.B.; Hassell, R.G.; Lahiry, P.; Hegele, R.A. Phenomics: Expanding the role of clinical evaluation in genomic studies. *J. Investig. Med.* **2010**, *58*, 700–706. [CrossRef] [PubMed]

110. Sébédio, J.L. Metabolomics, Nutrition, and Potential Biomarkers of Food Quality, Intake, and Health Status. *Adv. Food Nutr. Res.* **2017**, *82*, 83–116. [CrossRef] [PubMed]

111. Trabado, S.; Al-Salameh, A.; Croixmarie, V.; Masson, P.; Corruble, E.; Fève, B.; Colle, R.; Ripoll, L.; Walther, B.; Boursier-Neyret, C.; et al. The human plasma-metabolome: Reference values in 800 French healthy volunteers; impact of cholesterol, gender and age. *PLoS ONE* **2017**, *12*, e0173615. [CrossRef] [PubMed]

112. Edmands, W.M.; Ferrari, P.; Rothwell, J.A.; Rinaldi, S.; Slimani, N.; Barupal, D.K.; Biessy, C.; Jenab, M.; Clavel-Chapelon, F.; Fagherazzi, G.; et al. Polyphenol metabolome in human urine and its association with intake of polyphenol-rich foods across European countries. *Am. J. Clin. Nutr.* **2015**, *102*, 905–913. [CrossRef] [PubMed]

113. Garg, R.; Brennan, L.; Price, R.K.; Wallace, J.M.W.; Strain, J.J.; Gibney, M.J.; Shewry, P.R.; Ward, J.L.; Garg, L.; Welch, R.W. Using NMR-Based Metabolomics to Evaluate Postprandial Urinary Responses Following Consumption of Minimally Processed Wheat Bran or Wheat Aleurone by Men and Women. *Nutrients* **2016**, *8*, 96. [CrossRef] [PubMed]

114. Gibbons, H.; McNulty, B.A.; Nugent, A.P.; Walton, J.; Flynn, A.; Gibney, M.J.; Brennan, L. A metabolomics approach to the identification of biomarkers of sugar-sweetened beverage intake. *Am. J. Clin. Nutr.* **2015**, *101*, 471–477. [CrossRef] [PubMed]

115. Garcia-Aloy, M.; Llorach, R.; Urpi-Sarda, M.; Tulipani, S.; Estruch, R.; Martínez-González, M.A.; Corella, D.; Fitó, M.; Ros, E.; Salas-Salvadó, J.; et al. Novel Multimetabolite Prediction of Walnut Consumption by a Urinary Biomarker Model in a Free-Living Population: The PREDIMED Study. *J. Proteome Res.* **2014**, *13*, 3476–3483. [CrossRef] [PubMed]

116. Playdon, M.C.; Moore, S.C.; Derkach, A.; Reedy, J.; Subar, A.F.; Sampson, J.N.; Albanes, D.; Gu, F.; Kontto, J.; Lassale, C.; et al. Identifying biomarkers of dietary patterns by using metabolomics. *Am. J. Clin. Nutr.* **2017**, *105*, 450–465. [CrossRef] [PubMed]

117. Garcia-Perez, I.; Posma, J.M.; Gibson, R.; Chambers, E.S.; Hansen, T.H.; Vestergaard, H.; Hansen, T.; Beckmann, M.; Pedersen, O.; Elliott, P.; et al. Objective assessment of dietary patterns by use of metabolic phenotyping: A randomised, controlled, crossover trial. *Lancet Diabetes Endocrinol.* **2017**, *5*, 184–195. [CrossRef]

118. Bhupathiraju, S.N.; Hu, F.B. One (small) step towards precision nutrition by use of metabolomics. *Lancet Diabetes Endocrinol.* **2017**, *5*, 154–155. [CrossRef]

119. Rådjursöga, M.; Karlsson, G.B.; Lindqvist, H.M.; Pedersen, A.; Persson, C.; Pinto, R.C.; Ellegård, L.; Winkvist, A. Metabolic profiles from two different breakfast meals characterized by 1H NMR-based metabolomics. *Food Chem.* **2017**, *231*, 267–274. [CrossRef] [PubMed]

120. Brennan, L. Metabolomics in nutrition research–a powerful window into nutritional metabolism. *Essays Biochem.* **2016**, *60*, 451–458. [CrossRef] [PubMed]

121. Allam-Ndoul, B.; Guénard, F.; Garneau, V.; Cormier, H.; Barbier, O.; Pérusse, L.; Vohl, M.-C. Association between Metabolite Profiles, Metabolic Syndrome and Obesity Status. *Nutrients* **2016**, *8*, 324. [CrossRef] [PubMed]

122. Bakker, G.C.; van Erk, M.J.; Pellis, L.; Wopereis, S.; Rubingh, C.M.; Cnubben, N.H.; Kooistra, T.; van Ommen, B.; Hendriks, H.F. An antiinflammatory dietary mix modulates inflammation and oxidative and metabolic stress in overweight men: A nutrigenomics approach. *Am. J. Clin. Nutr.* **2010**, *91*, 1044–1059. [CrossRef] [PubMed]

123. Paquette, M.; Medina Larqué, A.S.; Weisnagel, S.J.; Desjardins, Y.; Marois, J.; Pilon, G.; Dudonné, S.; Marette, A.; Jacques, H. Strawberry and cranberry polyphenols improve insulin sensitivity in insulin-resistant, non-diabetic adults: A parallel, double-blind, controlled and randomised clinical trial. *Br. J. Nutr.* **2017**, *117*, 519–531. [CrossRef] [PubMed]

124. Riedl, A.; Gieger, C.; Hauner, H.; Daniel, H.; Linseisen, J. Metabotyping and its application in targeted nutrition: An overview. *Br. J. Nutr.* **2017**, *117*, 1631–1644. [CrossRef] [PubMed]

125. Connaugton, R.M.; Mcmorrow, A.M.; Healy, M.L.; Mcgillicuddy, F.C.; Lithander, F.E.; Roche, H.M. An anti-inflammatory nutritional intervention selectively improves insulin sensitivity in overweight and obese adolescents wherein baseline metabotype predicts response. *Proc. Nutr. Soc.* **2017**, *73*, E84. [CrossRef]

126. Kang, J.X. Gut microbiota and personalized nutrition. *J. Nutrigenet. Nutrigenomics* **2013**, *6*, 6–7. [CrossRef] [PubMed]

127. Ridaura, V.K.; Faith, J.J.; Rey, F.E.; Cheng, J.; Alexis, E.; Kau, A.L.; Griffin, N.W.; Lombard, V.; Henrissat, B.; Bain, J.R.; et al. Cultured gut microbiota from twins discordant for obesity modulate adiposity and metabolic phenotypes in mice. *Science* **2014**, *341*, 1241214. [CrossRef] [PubMed]

128. Famodu, O.A.; Cuff, C.F.; Cockburn, A.; Downes, M.T.; Murray, P.J.; McFadden, J.W.; Colby, S.E.; Morrell, J.S.; Olfert, I.M. Impact of free-living nutrition intervention on microbiome in college students at risk for Disease: FRUVEDomic pilot study. *FASEB J.* **2016**, *30*, 146–147.

129. Olfert, M.D.; Cuff, C.; Cockburn, A.; Olfert, M.; McFadden, J.W.; Downes, M.; Murray, P.J.; Holaskova, I.; Barr, M.L.; Colby, S.E.; et al. Nutrition Intervention to Profile Microbiome and Behaviors in Young Adults at Risk for Metabolic Syndrome: FRUVEDomic Pilot Study. *J. Nutr. Educ. Behav.* **2016**, *48*, S145. [CrossRef]

130. Mathews, A.T.; Famodu, O.A.; Olfert, M.D.; Murray, P.J.; Cuff, C.F.; Downes, M.T.; Haughey, N.J.; Colby, S.E.; Olfert, I.M.; McFadden, J.W. Fruit and Vegetable Intervention Lowers Circulating Ceramide Levels and Improves Estimated Insulin Sensitivity in Young Adults at Risk of Developing Metabolic Syndrome: A FRUVEDomic Pilot Study. *FASEB J.* **2016**, *30*, 1260.3.

131. Bonder, M.J.; Kurilshikov, A.; Tigchelaar, E.F.; Mujagic, Z.; Imhann, F.; Vila, A.V.; Deelen, P.; Vatanen, T.; Schirmer, M.; Smeekens, S.P.; et al. The effect of host genetics on the gut microbiome. *Nat. Genet.* **2016**, *48*, 1407–1412. [CrossRef] [PubMed]

132. Corella, D.; Arregui, M.; Coltell, O.; Portolés, O.; Guillem-Sáiz, P.; Carrasco, P.; Sorlí, J.V.; Ortega-Azorín, C.; González, J.I.; Ordovás, J.M. Association of the LCT-13910C>T Polymorphism With Obesity and Its Modulation by Dairy Products in a Mediterranean Population. *Obesity* **2011**, *19*, 1707–1714. [CrossRef] [PubMed]

133. Heianza, Y.; Qi, L. Gene-diet interaction and precision nutrition in obesity. *Int. J. Mol. Sci.* **2017**, *18*, 787. [CrossRef] [PubMed]

134. Koeth, R.A.; Wang, Z.; Levison, B.S.; Buffa, J.A.; Org, E.; Sheehy, B.T.; Britt, E.B.; Fu, X.; Wu, Y.; Li, L.; et al. Intestinal microbiota metabolism of L-carnitine, a nutrient in red meat, promotes atherosclerosis. *Nat. Med.* **2013**, *19*, 576–585. [CrossRef] [PubMed]

135. Tang, W.H.W.; Wang, Z.; Levison, B.S.; Koeth, R.A.; Britt, E.B.; Fu, X.; Wu, Y.; Hazen, S.L. Intestinal Microbial Metabolism of Phosphatidylcholine and Cardiovascular Risk. *N. Engl. J. Med.* **2013**, *368*, 1575–1584. [CrossRef] [PubMed]

136. Zmora, N.; Zeevi, D.; Korem, T.; Segal, E.; Elinav, E. Taking it Personally: Personalized Utilization of the Human Microbiome in Health and Disease. *Cell Host Microbe* **2016**, *19*, 12–20. [CrossRef] [PubMed]

137. Rohrmann, S.; Overvad, K.; Bueno-de-Mesquita, H.B.; Jakobsen, M.U.; Egeberg, R.; Tjønneland, A.; Nailler, L.; Boutron-Ruault, M.-C.; Clavel-Chapelon, F.; Krogh, V.; et al. Meat consumption and mortality - results from the European Prospective Investigation into Cancer and Nutrition. *BMC Med.* **2013**, *11*, 63. [CrossRef] [PubMed]

138. Suez, J.; Korem, T.; Zeevi, D.; Zilberman-Schapira, G.; Thaiss, C.A.; Maza, O.; Israeli, D.; Zmora, N.; Gilad, S.; Weinberger, A.; et al. Artificial sweeteners induce glucose intolerance by altering the gut microbiota. *Nature* **2014**, *514*, 181–186. [CrossRef] [PubMed]

139. Bokulich, N.A.; Blaser, M.J. A Bitter Aftertaste: Unintended Effects of Artificial Sweeteners on the Gut Microbiome. *Cell Metab.* **2014**, *20*, 701–703. [CrossRef] [PubMed]

140. Feehley, T.; Nagler, C.R. Health: The weighty costs of non-caloric sweeteners. *Nature* **2014**, *514*, 176–177. [CrossRef] [PubMed]

141. Nettleton, J.E.; Reimer, R.A.; Shearer, J. Reshaping the gut microbiota: Impact of low calorie sweeteners and the link to insulin resistance? *Physiol. Behav.* **2016**, *164*, 488–493. [CrossRef] [PubMed]

142. Frankenfeld, C.L.; Sikaroodi, M.; Lamb, E.; Shoemaker, S.; Gillevet, P.M. High-intensity sweetener consumption and gut microbiome content and predicted gene function in a cross-sectional study of adults in the United States. *Ann. Epidemiol.* **2015**, *25*, 736–742. [CrossRef] [PubMed]

143. Locke, A.E.; Kahali, B.; Berndt, S.I.; Justice, A.E.; Pers, T.H.; Day, F.R.; Powell, C.; Vedantam, S.; Buchkovich, M.L.; Yang, J.; et al. Genetic studies of body mass index yield new insights for obesity biology. *Nature* **2015**, *518*, 197–206. [CrossRef] [PubMed]

144. Fall, T.; Ingelsson, E. Genome-wide association studies of obesity and metabolic syndrome. *Mol. Cell. Endocrinol.* **2014**, *382*, 740–757. [CrossRef] [PubMed]

145. Go, M.J.; Hwang, J.-Y.; Park, T.-J.; Kim, Y.J.; Oh, J.H.; Kim, Y.-J.; Han, B.-G.; Kim, B.-J. Genome-wide association study identifies two novel Loci with sex-specific effects for type 2 diabetes mellitus and glycemic traits in a korean population. *Diabetes Metab. J.* **2014**, *38*, 375–387. [CrossRef] [PubMed]

146. Winkler, T.W.; Justice, A.E.; Graff, M.; Barata, L.; Feitosa, M.F.; Chu, S.; Czajkowski, J.; Esko, T.; Fall, T.; Kilpeläinen, T.O.; et al. The Influence of Age and Sex on Genetic Associations with Adult Body Size and Shape: A Large-Scale Genome-Wide Interaction Study. *PLoS Genet.* **2015**, *11*, e1005378. [CrossRef] [PubMed]

147. Loos, R.J.F.; Lindgren, C.M.; Li, S.; Wheeler, E.; Zhao, J.H.; Prokopenko, I.; Inouye, M.; Freathy, R.M.; Attwood, A.P.; Beckmann, J.S.; et al. Common variants near MC4R are associated with fat mass, weight and risk of obesity. *Nat. Genet.* **2008**, *40*, 768–775. [CrossRef] [PubMed]

148. Schierding, W.; O'Sullivan, J.M. Connecting SNPs in Diabetes: A Spatial Analysis of Meta-GWAS Loci. *Front. Endocrinol. (Lausanne)* **2015**, *6*, 102. [CrossRef] [PubMed]

149. Belsky, D.W.; Moffitt, T.E.; Sugden, K.; Williams, B.; Houts, R.; McCarthy, J.; Caspi, A. Development and Evaluation of a Genetic Risk Score for Obesity. *Biodemography Soc. Biol.* **2013**, *59*, 85–100. [CrossRef] [PubMed]

150. Welter, D.; MacArthur, J.; Morales, J.; Burdett, T.; Hall, P.; Junkins, H.; Klemm, A.; Flicek, P.; Manolio, T.; Hindorff, L.; et al. The NHGRI GWAS Catalog, a curated resource of SNP-trait associations. *Nucleic Acids Res.* **2014**, *42*, D1001–D1006. [CrossRef] [PubMed]

151. Claussnitzer, M.; Dankel, S.N.; Kim, K.-H.; Quon, G.; Meuleman, W.; Haugen, C.; Glunk, V.; Sousa, I.S.; Beaudry, J.L.; Puviindran, V.; et al. FTO Obesity Variant Circuitry and Adipocyte Browning in Humans. *N. Engl. J. Med.* **2015**, *373*, 895–907. [CrossRef] [PubMed]

152. Sofi, F.; Abbate, R.; Gensini, G.F.; Casini, A. Accruing evidence on benefits of adherence to the Mediterranean diet on health: An updated systematic review and meta-analysis. *Am. J. Clin. Nutr.* **2010**, *92*, 1189–1196. [CrossRef] [PubMed]

153. Mente, A.; de Koning, L.; Shannon, H.S.; Anand, S.S. A Systematic Review of the Evidence Supporting a Causal Link Between Dietary Factors and Coronary Heart Disease. *Arch. Intern. Med.* **2009**, *169*, 659. [CrossRef] [PubMed]

154. Martínez-González, M.A.; García-Arellano, A.; Toledo, E.; Salas-Salvadó, J.; Buil-Cosiales, P.; Corella, D.; Covas, M.I.; Schröder, H.; Arós, F.; Gómez-Gracia, E.; et al. A 14-Item Mediterranean Diet Assessment Tool and Obesity Indexes among High-Risk Subjects: The PREDIMED Trial. *PLoS ONE* **2012**, *7*, e43134. [CrossRef] [PubMed]

155. Fito, M.; Melander, O.; Martinez, J.A.; Toledo, E.; Carpene, C.; Corella, D. Advances in integrating traditional and omic biomarkers when analyzing the effects of the mediterranean diet intervention in cardiovascular prevention. *Int. J. Mol. Sci.* **2016**, *17*, 1469. [CrossRef] [PubMed]

156. Ortega-Azorin, C.; Sorli, J. V.; Estruch, R.; Asensio, E.M.; Coltell, O.; Gonzalez, J.I.; Martinez-Gonzalez, M.A.; Ros, E.; Salas-Salvado, J.; Fito, M.; et al. Amino Acid Change in the Carbohydrate Response Element Binding Protein Is Associated With Lower Triglycerides and Myocardial Infarction Incidence Depending on Level of Adherence to the Mediterranean Diet in the PREDIMED Trial. *Circ. Cardiovasc. Genet.* **2014**, *7*, 49–58. [CrossRef] [PubMed]

157. Rudkowska, I.; Guenard, F.; Julien, P.; Couture, P.; Lemieux, S.; Barbier, O.; Calder, P.C.; Minihane, A.M.; Vohl, M.-C. Genome-wide association study of the plasma triglyceride response to an *n*-3 polyunsaturated fatty acid supplementation. *J. Lipid Res.* **2014**, *55*, 1245–1253. [CrossRef] [PubMed]

158. Ortega-Azorín, C.; Sorlí, J.V.; Asensio, E.M.; Coltell, O.; Martínez-González, M.; Salas-Salvadó, J.; Covas, M.-I.; Arós, F.; Lapetra, J.; Serra-Majem, L.; et al. Associations of the FTO rs9939609 and the MC4R rs17782313 polymorphisms with type 2 diabetes are modulated by diet, being higher when adherence to the Mediterranean diet pattern is low. *Cardiovasc. Diabetol.* **2012**, *11*, 137. [CrossRef]

159. Garcia-Aloy, M.; Llorach, R.; Urpi-Sarda, M.; Jáuregui, O.; Corella, D.; Ruiz-Canela, M.; Salas-Salvadó, J.; Fitó, M.; Ros, E.; Estruch, R.; et al. A metabolomics-driven approach to predict cocoa product consumption by designing a multimetabolite biomarker model in free-living subjects from the PREDIMED study. *Mol. Nutr. Food Res.* **2015**, *59*, 212–220. [CrossRef] [PubMed]

160. Ryan, N.M.; O'Donovan, C.B.; Forster, H.; Woolhead, C.; Walsh, M.C. New tools for personalised nutrition: The Food4Me project. *Nutr. Bull.* **2015**, *40*, 134–139. [CrossRef]

161. Livingstone, K.M.; Celis-Morales, C.; Mathers, J. Who Benefits Most from Personalized Nutrition? Findings from the Pan-European Food4Me Randomized Controlled Trial. *FASEB J.* **2017**, *31*, 963.4.

162. Celis-Morales, C.; Livingstone, K.M.; Marsaux, C.F.M.; Forster, H.; O'Donovan, C.B.; Woolhead, C.; Macready, A.L.; Fallaize, R.; Navas-Carretero, S.; San-Cristobal, R.; et al. Design and baseline characteristics of the Food4Me study: A web-based randomised controlled trial of personalised nutrition in seven European countries. *Genes Nutr.* **2015**, *10*, 450. [CrossRef] [PubMed]

163. Fallaize, R.; Forster, H.; Macready, A.L.; Walsh, M.C.; Mathers, J.C.; Brennan, L.; Gibney, E.R.; Gibney, M.J.; Lovegrove, J.A. Online dietary intake estimation: Reproducibility and validity of the Food4Me food frequency questionnaire against a 4-day weighed food record. *J. Med. Internet Res.* **2014**, *16*, e190. [CrossRef] [PubMed]

164. Forster, H.; Fallaize, R.; Gallagher, C.; O'Donovan, C.B.; Woolhead, C.; Walsh, M.C.; Macready, A.L.; Lovegrove, J.A.; Mathers, J.C.; Gibney, M.J.; et al. Online Dietary Intake Estimation: The Food4Me Food Frequency Questionnaire. *J. Med. Internet Res.* **2014**, *16*, e150. [CrossRef] [PubMed]

165. Baecke, J.A.H.; Burema, J.; Frijters, J.E.R. A short questionnaire for the measurement of habitual physical activity in epidemiological studies. *Am. J. Clin. Nutr.* **1982**, *36*, 936–942. [CrossRef] [PubMed]

166. Nielsen, D.E.; El-Sohemy, A. Disclosure of Genetic Information and Change in Dietary Intake: A Randomized Controlled Trial. *PLoS ONE* **2014**, *9*, e112665. [CrossRef] [PubMed]

167. Celis-Morales, C.; Livingstone, K.M.; Marsaux, C.F.M.; Macready, A.L.; Fallaize, R.; O'Donovan, C.B.; Woolhead, C.; Forster, H.; Walsh, M.C.; Navas-Carretero, S.; et al. Effect of personalized nutrition on health-related behaviour change: Evidence from the Food4me European randomized controlled trial. *Int. J. Epidemiol.* **2016**. [CrossRef] [PubMed]

168. Guenther, P.M.; Casavale, K.O.; Reedy, J.; Kirkpatrick, S.I.; Hiza, H.A.B.; Kuczynski, K.J.; Kahle, L.L.; Krebs-Smith, S.M. Update of the Healthy Eating Index: HEI-2010. *J. Acad. Nutr. Diet.* **2013**, *113*, 569–580. [CrossRef] [PubMed]

169. Kirwan, L.; Walsh, M.C.; Celis-Morales, C.; Marsaux, C.F.M.; Livingstone, K.M.; Navas-Carretero, S.; Fallaize, R.; O'Donovan, C.B.; Woolhead, C.; Forster, H.; et al. Phenotypic factors influencing the variation in response of circulating cholesterol level to personalised dietary advice in the Food4Me study. *Br. J. Nutr.* **2016**, *116*, 2011–2019. [CrossRef] [PubMed]

170. Celis-Morales, C.; Marsaux, C.F.; Livingstone, K.M.; Navas-Carretero, S.; San-Cristobal, R.; Fallaize, R.; Macready, A.L.; O'Donovan, C.; Woolhead, C.; Forster, H.; et al. Can genetic-based advice help you lose weight? Findings from the Food4Me European randomized controlled trial. *Am. J. Clin. Nutr.* **2017**, *105*, 1204–1213. [CrossRef] [PubMed]

171. Livingstone, K.M.; Celis-Morales, C.; Papandonatos, G.D.; Erar, B.; Florez, J.C.; Jablonski, K.A.; Razquin, C.; Marti, A.; Heianza, Y.; Huang, T.; et al. FTO genotype and weight loss: Systematic review and meta-analysis of 9563 individual participant data from eight randomised controlled trials. *BMJ* **2016**, *354*, i4707. [CrossRef] [PubMed]

172. Ramos-Lopez, O.; Milagro, F.I.; Allayee, H.; Chmurzynska, A.; Choi, M.S.; Curi, R.; De Caterina, R.; Ferguson, L.R.; Goni, L.; Kang, J.X.; et al. Guide for Current Nutrigenetic, Nutrigenomic, and Nutriepigenetic Approaches for Precision Nutrition Involving the Prevention and Management of Chronic Diseases Associated with Obesity. *J. Nutrigenet. Nutrigenomics* **2017**, *10*, 43–62. [CrossRef] [PubMed]

173. Abrahams, M.; Frewer, L.J.; Bryant, E.; Stewart-Knox, B. Factors determining the integration of nutritional genomics into clinical practice by registered dietitians. *Trends Food Sci. Technol.* **2017**, *59*, 139–147. [CrossRef]

174. Cormier, H.; Tremblay, B.L.; Paradis, A.-M.; Garneau, V.; Desroches, S.; Robitaille, J.; Vohl, M.-C. Nutrigenomics-perspectives from registered dietitians: A report from the Quebec-wide e-consultation on nutrigenomics among registered dietitians. *J. Hum. Nutr. Diet.* **2014**, *27*, 391–400. [CrossRef] [PubMed]

175. Kohlmeier, M.; De Caterina, R.; Ferguson, L.R.; Görman, U.; Allayee, H.; Prasad, C.; Kang, J.X.; Nicoletti, C.F.; Martinez, J.A. Guide and Position of the International Society of Nutrigenetics/Nutrigenomics on Personalized Nutrition: Part 2-Ethics, Challenges and Endeavors of Precision Nutrition. *J. Nutrigenet. Nutrigenomics* **2016**, *9*, 28–46. [CrossRef] [PubMed]

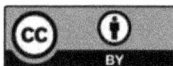

nutrients

MDPI

Review

Bariatric Surgery and Precision Nutrition

Carolina F. Nicoletti [1], Cristiana Cortes-Oliveira [1], Marcela A. S. Pinhel [1,2] and Carla B. Nonino [1,*]

[1] Internal Medicine Department, Ribeirão Preto Medical School, University of São Paulo, Ribeirão Preto, São Paulo 14049-900, Brazil; carol_nicolettif@yahoo.com.br (C.F.N.); cristiana.cortes@outlook.com (C.C.-O.); marcelapinhel@yahoo.com.br (M.A.S.P.)
[2] Molecular Biology Department, São Jose do Rio Preto Medical School, São José do Rio Preto, São Paulo 15090-000, Brazil
*   Correspondence: carla@fmrp.usp.br; Tel.: +55-16-3315-4810

Received: 24 July 2017; Accepted: 18 August 2017; Published: 6 September 2017

Abstract: This review provides a literature overview of new findings relating nutritional genomics and bariatric surgery. It also describes the importance of nutritional genomics concepts in personalized bariatric management. It includes a discussion of the potential role bariatric surgery plays in altering the three pillars of nutritional genomics: nutrigenetics, nutrigenomics, and epigenetics. We present studies that show the effect of each patient's genetic and epigenetic variables on the response to surgical weight loss treatment. We include investigations that demonstrate the association of single nucleotide polymorphisms with obesity phenotypes and their influence on weight loss after bariatric surgery. We also present reports on how significant weight loss induced by bariatric surgery impacts telomere length, and we discuss studies on the existence of an epigenetic signature associated with surgery outcomes and specific gene methylation profile, which may help to predict weight loss after a surgical procedure. Finally, we show articles which evidence that bariatric surgery may affect expression of numerous genes involved in different metabolic pathways and consequently induce functional and taxonomic changes in gut microbial communities. The role nutritional genomics plays in responses to weight loss after bariatric surgery is evident. Better understanding of the molecular pathways involved in this process is necessary for successful weight management and maintenance.

Keywords: obesity; bariatric surgery; gene; polymorphism; gene expression; epigenetics; DNA methylation; microbiota; biomarkers

1. Introduction

Bariatric surgery, including gastric bypass, has emerged as the most effective strategy to treat obesity and its associated comorbidities [1,2]. Non-surgical treatments generally fail to provide substantial and long-term weight loss in severe obesity cases [3]. Every year, about 500,000 bariatric surgical procedures are performed worldwide; sleeve gastrectomy (SG, 49%) and Roux-en Y gastric bypass procedure (RYGB, 43%) are the most commonly performed techniques [4–6].

Long-term excess body weight reduction is a major goal of bariatric surgery. Excess weight loss is about 62%, 68%, and 48% for RYGB, vertical-banded gastroplasty (VBG), and laparoscopic adjustable gastric banding (LAGB), respectively [7]. Despite the positive effects of bariatric surgery, weight regain; that is, recovery of 10 to 20% of the minimum weight achieved by the patient [8], occurs in between 30% and 50% of the patients at the late postoperative period (between one and a half and two years after the surgical procedure) [9,10].

Just as genetic and epigenetic signatures influence the obesity phenotype [11], genetics recognizably underlies weight loss percentage, resistance, and maintenance after surgical treatment [11,12]. Different surgical techniques (restrictive, malabsortive, or a combination of both) [13] and genetic background [14] account for the wide variation in responses to bariatric surgery.

In the last decades, many efforts have been made to understand the variations in inter-individual responses to the same obesity treatment strategy. In this context, "omics" sciences such as genomics, transcriptomics, proteomics, metabolomics, microbiomics, and epigenomics have emerged. Together, these sciences establish genomic nutrition [15]. Genetic variation among individuals underlies the variety of physiological responses in the same environment and explains why some individuals are more likely to gain/lose weight than others in the same environmental conditions [16], including weight gain/loss after bariatric surgery. However, the complex interactions between nutrients and genes have not been fully elucidated [17].

In this scenario, precision nutrition in bariatric surgery is an important tool in personalized medicine and may target specific guidelines based on interindividual differences (Figure 1). In this paper, we summarize the main literature findings relating nutritional genomics and bariatric surgery.

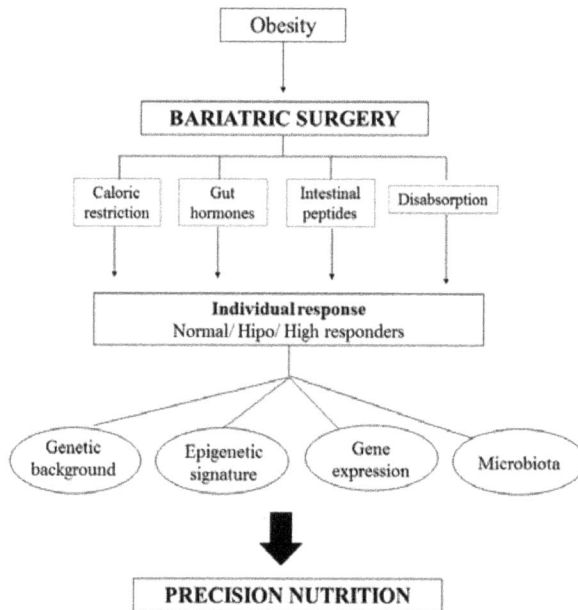

Figure 1. Algorithm of Personalized Nutrition in Bariatric Surgery. The individual responses of the surgery are due, in addition to the caloric restriction, alterations of the gut hormones and the malabsorption process, of the individuals' genetic information, as well as of the epigenetic signature, modifications in the gene expression and the microbiota.

2. Genetic Background and Bariatric Surgery Management

Nutrigenetics studies inborn genetic variants that predict an individual's risk for disease and explains the individual's nutritional requirements and nutrient absorption, metabolism, and excretion [18,19]. In this sense, it is possible to affirm that genetic factors partially determine susceptibility to obesity, and that an obesogenic environment is necessary for phenotypic obesity expression. Therefore, despite new evidence that genetics influences obesity, it is necessary to consider that biological and psychosocial factors interact in a complex way [19].

In the context of obesity treatment, different types of patients exist. Obese patients may be classified as normo-responders, hypo-responders, or hyper-responders, depending on their phenotypic response to diet or surgical treatment. This indicates that not only the environment but also genetic variations account for successful weight-loss therapy [20,21]. Several genes as well as single nucleotide polymorphisms (SNPs) are associated with obesity phenotypes and weight loss after bariatric surgery [21–25].

Novais et al. (2016) [24] evidenced that the *5-HT2C* gene polymorphism (rs3813929) is associated with a greater percentage of excess body weight after RYGB. Two SNPs in the *UCP2* gene (Ala55Pro and −866G > A) are considered as biomarkers of weight loss after bariatric surgery [22]. When Seip et al. (2016) [26] evaluated 330 SNPs of genes involved in metabolic regulation they identified many genes that could be potential markers to discriminate changes in body mass index (BMI) one year after surgical intervention (LAGB or RYGB). Other authors suggested that polymorphisms, like the SNP of the preproghrelin gene (rs696217), could mark a successful weight loss outcome [27]. Table 1 lists recent studies that associate SNPs and bariatric surgery outcomes.

Table 1. List of recent articles associating the outcomes of different types of bariatric surgery with single nucleotide polymorphisms (SNPs).

Genes	Polymorphism	Main Results	Surgery/Time	N° Patients	Ref.
MC4R	rs17782313	Women carrying this polymorphism present higher pre-surgical BMI and tend to maintain BMI > 35 kg/m^2, which characterizes treatment failure	60 months of RYGB	217	[21]
UCP2	Ala55Val −866G > A	Mutated alleles (T and A) could be biomarkers of weight loss	12 months of RYGB	150	[22]
FTO	rs9930506	Weight percentage is significantly higher in carriers of the AG and GG genotypes	Six months of sleeve gastrectomy	11	[28]
PNPLA3 *TM6SF2* *MBOAT7*	p.I148M p.E167E rs641738	Mutated allele might be associated with greater improvement of hepatic steatosis after bariatric surgery	One year of gastric bypass gastric sleeve	84	[29]
5-HT2C	rs3813929	The TT genotype predicts greater percentage of excess weight loss among female patients	12 months of RYGB	351	[24]
FKBP5	rs1360780	The T allele is associated with weight loss.	Bariatric surgery	42	[25]
UCP2	Ala55Val −866G > A	Patients with at least one rare allele for polymorphisms and with at least one rare allele for both polymorphisms together (haplotype) present greater energy and carbohydrate intake even after adjustment for gender, age, and weight.	12 months of RYGB	150	[30]
32 SNPs	-	The LYPLAL1 genotype is associated with different eating behavior and loss of extensive body weight	Two years of RYGB	251	[31]
330 SNPs	-	Information derived from patient DNA may be useful to predict surgical weight loss outcomes and to guide selection of surgical approach.	One year of RYGB or LAGB	161	[26]
FTO	rs9939609	Weight loss progresses differently in obese carriers of the FTO gene variant rs9939609 after bariatric surgery	Two months of RYGB	146	[32]

MC4R: melanocortin 4 receptor; *UCP2*: uncoupling protein 2; *FTO*: alpha-ketoglutarate-dependent dioxygenase or fat mass and obesity-associated protein; *PNPLA3*: patatin-like phospholipase domain containing 3; *TM6SF2*: transmembrane 6 superfamily member 2; *MBOAT7*: membrane-bound O-acyltransferase domain containing 7; *5-HT2C*: 5-hydroxytryptamine receptor 2C; *FKBP5*: FK506 binding protein 5; *n*: number of individuals; RYGB: Roux-en-Y gastric by-pass; LAGB: laparoscopic adjustable gastric banding; BMI: body mass index.

Algorithms that predict the chances of treatment failure or that even help to identify guidelines to prevent body weight recovery are critical to obesity management [24]. Nicoletti et al. (2016) [30] proposed a genetic predisposition score to estimate the contribution of seven obesity-related polymorphisms to the weight loss process after one year of RYGB. The authors found that lower score is associated with higher weight and BMI values, which shows that the higher the number of effect alleles, the lower the severity of obesity and the better the metabolic outcomes after the surgical procedure. Moreover, weight regain in the late postoperative period is more frequent and occurs sooner in individuals that carries a polymorphism in the *FTO* gene (rs9939609) [32].

It is noteworthy that the genetic variants reported in the literature are located in genes associated with obesity development per se, thermogenesis, adipogenisis, and eating behavior/appetite control.

However, the mechanisms through which these variants influence weight loss are largely unknown. Some authors investigated variants of genes associated with eating behavior in obese individuals before and after bariatric surgery. Bandstein et al. (2016) [31] demonstrated that the rs4846567 SNP in lysophospholipase-like 1 gene is associated with the hunger score, a factor that can determine therapeutic success. Likewise, a haplotype of the *UCP2* gene is associated with dietary consumption after RYGB. Nicoletti et al. (2016) [30] showed that carriers of at least one rare haplotype present greater energy and carbohydrate intake [30].

Located at the end of eukaryotic chromosomes, telomeres are special structures characterized by a TTAGGG sequence [33], which ensures stable genetic material inheritance [34]. Telomeres shorten progressively at each cellular division, and they can serve as a cellular aging marker [35]. Several large studies show that telomere length (TL), adiposity, and BMI are inversely associated [36,37].

Knowing that oxidative stress and chronic inflammation are related to weight gain, and that obesity is associated with telomere shortening [38,39], studies associate shorter telomeres with obesity comorbidities such as diabetes and hypertension [40,41]. On the other hand, published works show that diet components (e.g., fiber) and caloric restriction with significant weight loss influence TL and possibly have a preventive effect on telomere shortening [42,43].

The fact that weight loss induced by bariatric surgery does not restore short TL after one year was one of the first signs that bariatric surgery impact TL [43]. Formich et al. (2014) [44] discussed that the immediate postoperative period is characterized by a catabolic state, which accelerates telomere erosion [44,45]. In contrast, Dersham et al. (2017) [37] evaluated subjects between three and five years after gastric bypass. The latter authors observed increased TL and emphasized that significant lengthening occurs in patients with the shortest baseline TL. Nevertheless, TL does not correlate with weight loss percentage. In the late postoperative period (10 years), some authors also verified increased TL [46]. These changes in TL may stem from weight loss itself and from an improved metabolic condition, which reduce telomere attrition [46]. Interestingly, a study that investigated subjects before and six months after bioenteric intragastric balloon found that individuals who present greater weight loss show greater telomere lengthening [47].

Further studies are necessary to assess and to establish interactions between these genetic variants and bariatric surgery outcome, so that biomarkers can be determined for more personalized weight loss management.

3. Epigenetic Signatures Related to Bariatric Surgery Outcomes

DNA is a highly dynamic biomolecule, which is reflected in its diverse and complex regulation [48]. Epigenetics is defined as an inheritable process during which reversible changes in the chromatin structure take place without involving the underlying DNA sequence, to impact transcriptional control and cellular function [49,50]. Epigenetic alterations include DNA methylation, histone modification (such as histone acetylation and methylation), and noncoding RNAs (e.g., microRNAs) [51–53].

In this context, epigenome dysregulation may modify an individual's phenotype and lead to numerous chronic diseases, like obesity [54,55]. In a recent guide paper, authors discussed interactions among dietary components and epigenetic alterations involved in disease risk [56]. For example, high-fat and high-sugar diet is related to leptin and fatty acid synthase methylation, which consequently contributes to the obesity phenotype in Wistar rats [57,58]. Other studies describe the role epigenetic markers play in the anthropometric and metabolic outcomes of obesity treatment [59,60]. Methylation patterns of appetite-regulatory genes are related to weight loss and regain after eight-week nutritional intervention [61]. Indeed, Nicoletti et al. (2016) [62] showed that DNA methylation patterns behave differently according to the adopted weight loss strategies.

In the bariatric surgery context, genome-wide DNA methylation analysis shows that weight loss is associated with changes in methylation at CpG and exonic regions close to transcription start sites [63]. Numerous mechanisms are likely to contribute to metabolic improvements after RYGB surgery; for example, restricted calorie ingestion, rapid influx of undigested complex nutrients, and altered gut and intestinal hormone secretion [64,65]. However, authors have recently reported that changes in DNA methylation could be another mechanism that contributes to the metabolic outcomes observed after gastric bypass and to postoperative metabolic homeostasis [63,66]. Table 2 summarizes the main recent studies that evaluate epigenetic modifications after bariatric surgery. Epigenetic changes related to bariatric surgery may be due to weight loss per se or to other factors related to the surgical procedure, such as the daily use of vitamin-mineral supplements and alterations in hormone secretion and dietary intake after the procedure [62].

Table 2. Recent studies evaluating epigenetics modifications after bariatric surgery.

Target Gene	Type of Material	Modification Type	Surgery/Time	Ref.
IL-6	Whole blood	Decrease	six months after RYGB	[62]
PDK4, IL-6, and *TNF*	Whole blood	Increase	12 months after RYGB	[66]
SCD-1	Whole blood	Increase	six months after RYGB	[67]
PGC-1a and *PDK4*	Skeletal muscle	-	six months after RYGB	[63]
ADK	-	Decrease	six months after RYGB	[68]
PTPRE	Liver	Increase	-	[69]
ETP, FOXP2, HDAC4 and *DNMT3B*	Adipose tissue	Decrease	-	[70]
Global *LINE-1*	Whole blood	Not modified	six months after RYGB	[71]

IL-6: interleukin 6; *PDK4*: pyruvate dehydrogenase kinase 4; *TNF*: tumor necrosis fator; *SCD-1*: stearoyl CoA desaturase-1; *PGC-1a*: proliferator-activated receptor g coactivator-1 a; *ADK*: adenosine kinase; *PTPRE*: protein tyrosine phosphatase, receptor type E; *ETP*: early T-cell precursor; *FOXP2*: forkhead box protein P2; *HDAC4*: histone deacetylase 4; *DNMT3B*: DNA methyltransferase 3 beta; *LINE-1*: long interspersed nuclear elements; RYGB: Roux-em Y gastric bypass.

Furthermore, a specific gene methylation profile can be used to predict weight loss after RYGB. Nicoletti et al. (2016) [62] evidenced that high responders have lower *SERPINE-1* methylation levels six months after RYGB. There is evidence that the methylation profiles in promoter gene regions of postoperative obese patients presenting weight loss become similar to the methylation profiles of normal-weight individuals [72]. Barres et al. (2013) [63] compared obese women before and six months after RYGB. These authors found increased and decreased promoter methylation of pyruvate dehydrogenase kinase, isoenzyme 4 *(PDK4)* and proliferator-activated receptor g coactivator-1 a *(PGC-1a)*, respectively, and observed that surgery normalized this pattern to the levels in control women [63]. Methylation profile normalization occurs at the same time that metabolic parameters such as fasting glucose, total cholesterol, and triglycerides concentrations normalize [63].

Remarkably, studies demonstrate that bariatric surgery promotes durable and detectable changes in subsequent offspring methylome and transcriptome [73]. When Guénarda et al. (2013) [73] compared methylation profiles in siblings born before and after the surgical procedure, these authors found that 3% of the probes are differentially methylated, and they identified differences in genes that underlie improved cardiometabolic risk profile. Moreover, the sperm methylome is changed in morbidly obese men submitted to RYGB, and these gametic epigenetic modifications modify the metabolic profile [74].

DNA methylome studies hold enormous promise for personalized medicine and nutrition, but technological challenges like cost-effective sample analysis impair such studies [75].

4. Bariatric Surgery and Gene Expression Profile

Nutrigenomics is the science that studies how nutrients and food components influence gene expression profile [76]. This science also examines how a nutritional strategy affects gene expression and uses the gene expression pattern as a tool to predict responsiveness to nutritional treatments [56,77]. Dietary caloric restriction is sufficient to alter the expression of different genes related to resting energy expenditure and lipid metabolism and contributes to the development of strategies for obesity and weight control [78–80].

In this sense, bariatric surgery may affect the expression of various genes involved in different metabolic pathways [80]. Table 3 depicts some interactions between bariatric surgery and the gene expression profile. A recent study on whole transcriptome analysis evidenced that about 1366 genes are differentially expressed (1188 upregulated and 178 downregulated genes) in the postoperative period as compared to the preoperative period of RYGB, and that these genes are associated with gene transcription, lipid and energetic metabolism, immunological processes, cell differentiation, oxidative stress, substrate oxidation, and adipocyte differentiation [81].

Table 3. Some interactions between bariatric surgery and the gene expression profile.

Gene	Modification Type	Related Metabolic Pathways	Surgery/Time	Ref.
GGT1, CAMP, DEFA1, LCN2, TP53, PDSS1, OLR1, CNTNAP5, DHCR24, and HHAT	-	Lipid metabolism and obesity development	Six to twelve months after bariatric surgery (SG and RYGB)	[82]
IL-6, IL-8, and TNF-alpha	Increase	Inflammation	Acutely postoperative RYGB	[83]
GLUT4, IRS1, and adiponectin	Decrease	Glucose metabolism		
CIDEA	Increase	Lipid droplet formation in the adipose tissue	12 months after bariatric surgery (SG and RYGB)	[84]
Glutathione		Glutathione metabolism		
UCP2	Increase	Thermogenesis	Six months after RYGB	[85]
PLIN1	Unchanged	Lipolysis		
TNF, CASP3	Increase	Inflammation	12 months after bariatric surgery	[86]
Leptin	Decrease			
PPARg1	Increase	Insulin metabolism	12 months after RYGB	[87]
PPARg2	Unchanged			
UCP1	Unchanged	Thermogenesis	Six months after RYGB	[88]
UCP3				

GGT1: gamma-glutamyltransferase; CAMP: cathelicidin antimicrobial peptide; DEFA1: defensin alpha 1; LCN2: lipocalin 2; TP53: tumor protein p53; PDSS1: decaprenyl diphosphate synthase subunit 1; ORL1: oxidized low-density lipoprotein receptor 1; CNTNAP5: contactin- associated protein like 5; DHCR24: 24-dehydrocholesterol reductase; HHAT: hedgehog acyltransferase; IL-6: interleukin 6; IL-8: interleukin 8; TNF: tumor necrosis factor; GLUT4: glucose transport; IRS1: insulin receptor substrate 1; CIDEA: cell death-inducing DFFA-like effector A; UCP2: uncoupling protein 2; PLIN1: perilipin 1; CASP3: caspase 3; PPARg1: peroxisome proliferator activated receptor gamma 1; PPARg2: peroxisome proliferator activated receptor gamma 2; UCP1: uncoupling protein 1; UCP3: uncoupling protein 3.

Ortega et al. (2016) [83] observed that acutely postoperative RYGB changes insulin receptor substrate 1 (*IRS1*) expression in the subcutaneous adipose tissue. Concomitantly, RYGB increases expression of inflammatory (interleukin (IL) 6 (*IL-6*), *IL-8*, and tumor necrosis factor alpha (*TNF-alpha*)) and lipogenic (lipopolysaccharide binding protein, *LBP*) genes. Moreover, a recent study showed that gene expression patterns in subcutaneous adipose tissue one year postoperatively are characteristic of a reduced inflammatory profile [86]. In contrast, cytokine expression in adipose tissue does not change one and 12 months after the surgical procedure [89].

Expression of the gene*UCP2*, a gene that participates in thermogenesis and body weight regulation, affects weight loss after bariatric surgery. A study conducted with obese women revealed increased *UCP2* expression six months after the surgical procedure and a positive association between baseline gene expression and weight loss percentage [85].

Eutrophic individuals and obese patients have different gene expression profile, and bariatric surgery modulates this default [87]. Knowledge of the metabolic pathways affected by this surgical procedure is important when bariatric surgery is indicated and ensures successful obesity treatment [85].

5. The Role of Bariatric Surgery on Microbiota

According to several studies, bariatric surgery as a strategy to achieve weight loss plays a crucial part in functional and taxonomic changes observed in the gut microbial communities after surgery [90–92]. Gut microbiota is associated with an individual's metabolic health, so it is essential that these microorganisms be taken into consideration during development of new personalized treatments and identification of biomarkers of different metabolic diseases [90,93]. Given that bariatric surgery elicits significant anatomical and physiological alterations in the gastrointestinal tract regardless of the surgical technique, there is growing interest in understanding intestinal microbiota modification and in establishing how these changes contribute to improving the metabolic profile and the weight loss process.

Liou et al. (2013) [92] evaluated germ-free mice that received intestinal microbiota from other animals that had undergone RYGB surgery. These authors found that the former animals had reduced diet caloric intake, increased resting energy expenditure, and higher fatty acid concentrations, which proved transmission of these characteristics. Moreover, Tremaroli et al. (2015) [91] verified that germ-free mice that received fecal microbiota collected from humans nine years after RYGB or SG had lower body fat accumulation (46% and 26%, respectively) two weeks after transplantation as compared to rats that received microbiota from obese individuals that had not undergone any surgical procedure. In addition, the test animals used more fat as energy substrate, but energy expenditure at rest remained unaltered.

In a more recent study, Palleja et al. (2017) [94] compared patients before and after bariatric surgery. These authors verified not only weight loss and improved glycemic profile, but also alterations in the intestinal microbiota, including changes in microbiota diversity and composition within three months after the surgical procedure. In addition, more than half of the altered microbiota species were maintained in the long term, which indicated that bariatric surgery could lead to rapid and sustained changes in the patients' gut microbiota.

Human feces microbial composition analysis showed that six main phyla are present therein: Bacteroidetes, Firmicutes, Proteobacteria, Actinobacteria, Fusobacteria, and Verrucomicrobia [95]. Some studies compared patients' pre- and postoperative (RYGB) microbiota to non-operated control individuals' microbiota, to detect alterations in intestinal bacteria after surgery; more specifically, increased Proteobacteria and Bacteroidetes and decreased Firmicutes (Table 4).

Table 4. Alterations of bacterial phyla after bariatric surgery.

Phylum	Changes	Ref.
Firmicutes	Decrease	[91,96–98]
Bacteroidetes	Decrease	[96]
Actinobacteria	Decrease	[96–98]
Chloroflexi	Decrease	[96]
Fibrobacteres	Decrease	[96]
Verrucomicrobia	Increase	[95,96]
Proteobacteria	Increase	[91,95]
Spirochaetes	Decrease	[96]
Fusobacteria	Decrease	[95,96]

New studies aiming at better understanding the interactions between microbiota and obesity and the possible ways to modulate gut microbiota could benefit bariatric surgery patients in the future.

6. Conclusions

Surgical management of obesity requires understanding the genetic and epigenetic factors that play a crucial key role in obesity development and weight loss response. Given the concepts of nutritional genomics, defining a "nutrigenomic risk score" or a "nutrigenomic profile" for each individual may represent a novel therapeutic approach for the management of obese patients submitted to bariatric surgery. We believe that nutritional genomics will soon enable the delivery of precise nutrition recommendations to patients undergoing bariatric surgery, to provide high-risk individuals with personalized treatment and to prevent complications.

Acknowledgments: This work was supported by grant #2016/05638-1; #2015/18669-0 and #2013/12819-4 from the São Paulo Research Foundation (FAPESP).

Author Contributions: C.F.N., C.C.-O., M.A.S.P. and C.B.N. have been contributed to entire manuscript's development and writing.

Conflicts of Interest: The authors declare no conflict of interest.

References

1. Hao, Z.; Mumphrey, M.B.; Morrison, C.D.; Münzberg, H.; Ye, J.; Berthoud, H.R. Does gastric bypass surgery change body weight set point? *Int. J. Obes. Suppl.* **2016**, *6*, S37–S43. [CrossRef] [PubMed]
2. Schauer, P.R.; Nor Hanipah, Z.; Rubino, F. Metabolic surgery for treating type 2 diabetes mellitus: Now supported by the world's leading diabetes organizations. *Clevel. Clin. J. Med.* **2017**, *84*, S47–S56. [CrossRef] [PubMed]
3. Busetto, L.; Dixon, J.; De Luca, M.; Shikora, S.; Pories, W.; Angrisani, L. Bariatric surgery in class I obesity: A position statement from the international federation for the surgery of obesity and metabolic disorders (IFSO). *Obes. Surg.* **2014**, *24*, 487–519. [CrossRef] [PubMed]
4. Angrisani, L.; Santonicola, A.; Iovino, P.; Formisano, G.; Buchwald, H.; Scopinaro, N. Bariatric surgery world wide 2013. *Obes. Surg.* **2015**, *25*, 1822–1832. [CrossRef] [PubMed]
5. Schauer, P.R.; Mingrone, G.; Ikramuddin, S.; Wolfe, B. Clinical outcomes of metabolic surgery: Efficacy of glycemic control, weight loss, and remission of diabetes. *Diabetes Care* **2016**, *39*, 902–911. [CrossRef] [PubMed]
6. Khorgami, Z.; Andalib, A.; Corcelles, R.; Aminian, A.; Brethauer, S.; Schauer, P. Recent national trends in the surgical treatment of obesity: Sleeve gastrectomy dominates. *Surg. Obes. Relat. Dis.* **2015**, *11*, S1–S34. [CrossRef]
7. Buchwald, H.; Avidor, Y.; Braunwald, E.; Jensen, M.D.; Pories, W.; Fahrbach, K.; Schoelles, K. Bariatric surgery: A systematic review and meta-analysis. *JAMA* **2004**, *292*, 1724–1737. [CrossRef] [PubMed]
8. Nicoletti, C.F.; de Oliveira, B.A.P.; Pinhel, M.A.S.; Donati, B.; Marchini, J.S.; Salgado-Junior, W.; Nonino, C.B. Influence of excess weight loss and weight regain on biochemical indicators during a 4-year follow-up after Roux-en-Y gastric bypass. *Obes. Surg.* **2015**, *25*, 279–284. [CrossRef] [PubMed]
9. Cooper, T.C.; Simmons, E.B.; Webb, K.; Burns, J.L.; Kushner, R.F. Trends in weight regain following Rouxen-Y gastric bypass (RYGB) bariatric surgery. *Obes. Surg.* **2015**, *25*, 1474–1481. [CrossRef] [PubMed]
10. Magro, D.O.; Geloneze, B.; Delfini, R.; Pareja, B.C.; Callejas, F.; Pareja, J.C. Long-term weight regain after gastric bypass: A 5-year prospective study. *Obes. Surg.* **2008**, *18*, 648–651. [CrossRef] [PubMed]
11. Still, C.D.; Wood, G.C.; Chu, X.; Erdman, R.; Manney, C.H.; Benotti, P.N.; Petrick, A.T.; Strodel, W.E.; Mirshahi, U.L.; Mirshahi, T.; et al. High allelic burden of four obesity SNPs is associated with poorer weight loss outcomes following gastric bypass surgery. *Obesity* **2011**, *19*, 1676–1683. [CrossRef] [PubMed]
12. Hainer, V.; Zamrazilova, H.; Spalova, J.; Hainerova, I.; Kunesova, M.; Aldhoon, B.; Bendlová, B. Role of hereditary factors in weight loss and its maintenance. *Phys. Res.* **2008**, *57*, S1–S15.
13. Kashyap, S.R.; Gatmaitan, P.; Brethauer, S.; Schauer, P. Bariatric surgery for type 2 diabetes: Weighing the impact for obese patients. *Clevel. Clin. J. Med.* **2010**, *77*, 468–476. [CrossRef] [PubMed]
14. De Luis, D.A.; Sagrado, M.G.; Pacheco, D.; Terroba, M.C.; Martin, T.; Cuellar, L.; Ventosa, M. Effect of C358A missense polymorphism of the endocannabinoid degrading enzyme fatty acid hydrolase on weight loss and cardiovascular risk factors 1 year after biliopancreatic diversion surgery. *Surg. Obes. Relat. Dis.* **2010**, *6*, 516–520. [CrossRef] [PubMed]
15. Ferguson, L.R.; De Caterina, R.; Görman, U.; Allayee, H.; Kohlmeier, M.; Prasad, C.; Choi, M.S.; Curi, R.; de Luis, D.A.; Gil, Á.; et al. Guide and position of the International Society of Nutrigenetics/Nutrigenomics on personalised nutrition: Part 1—Fields of precision nutrition. *J. Nutrigenet. Nutrigenom.* **2016**, *9*, 12–27. [CrossRef] [PubMed]
16. Kaput, J.; Astley, S.; Renkema, M.; Ordovas, J.; van Ommen, B. Harnessing Nutrigenomics: Development of web-based communication, databases, resources, and tools. *Genes Nutr.* **2006**, *1*, 5–11. [CrossRef] [PubMed]
17. Peña-Romero, A.C.; Navas-Carrillo, D.; Marín, F.; Orenes-Piñero, E. The future of nutrition: nutrigenomics and nutrigenetics in obesity and cardiovascular diseases. *Crit. Rev. Food Sci. Nutr.* **2017**, *5*. [CrossRef] [PubMed]
18. Simopoulos, A.P. Nutrigenetics/nutrigenomics. *Annu. Rev. Public Health* **2010**, *31*, 53–68. [CrossRef] [PubMed]
19. Martínez, J.A. Perspectives on personalized nutrition for obesity. *Nutrigenet. Nutrigenom.* **2014**, *7*. [CrossRef] [PubMed]

Nutrients **2017**, *9*, 974

20. Kovolou, G.D.; Kolovou, V.; Papadopoulou, A.; Watts, G.F. MTP gene variants and response to lomitapide in patients with homozygous familial hypercholesterolemia. *J. Atheroscler. Thromb.* **2016**, *23*, 878–883. [CrossRef] [PubMed]

21. Resende, C.M.M.; Durso, D.F.; Borges, K.B.G.; Pereira, R.M.; Rodrigues, G.K.D.; Rodrigues, K.F.; Silva, J.L.P.; Rodrigues, E.C.; Franco, G.R.; Alvarez-Leite, J.I. The polymorphism rs17782313 near MC4R gene is related with anthropometric changes in women submitted to bariatric surgery over 60 months. *Clin. Nutr.* **2017**. [CrossRef] [PubMed]

22. Nicoletti, C.F.; de Oliveira, A.P.; Brochado, M.J.; Pinhel, M.A.; de Oliveira, B.A.; Marchini, J.S.; Dos Santos, J.E.; Salgado, W., Jr.; Cury, N.M.; de Araújo, L.F.; et al. The Ala55Val and −866G > A polymorphisms of the UCP2 gene could be biomarkers for weight loss in patients who had Roux-en-Y gastric bypass. *Nutrition* **2017**, *33*, 326–330. [CrossRef] [PubMed]

23. De Luis, D.A.; Izaola, O.; Primo, D.; Pacheco, D. Effect of the rs10767664 Variant of the brain-derived neurotrophic factor gene on weight change and cardiovascular risk factors in morbidly obese patients after biliopancreatic diversion surgery. *J. Nutrigenet. Nutrigenom.* **2016**, *9*, 116–122. [CrossRef] [PubMed]

24. Novais, P.F.; Weber, T.K.; Lemke, N.; Verlengia, R.; Crisp, A.H.; Rasera-Junior, I.; de Oliveira, M.R. Gene polymorphisms as a predictor of body weight loss after Roux-en-Y gastric bypass surgery among obese women. *Obes. Res. Clin. Pract.* **2016**, *10*, 724–727. [CrossRef] [PubMed]

25. Hartmann, I.B.; Fries, G.R.; Bücker, J.; Scotton, E.; von Diemen, L.; Kauer-Sant'Anna, M. The FKBP5 polymorphism rs1360780 is associated with lower weight loss after bariatric surgery: 26 months of follow-up. *Surg. Obes. Relat. Dis.* **2016**, *12*, 1554–1560. [CrossRef] [PubMed]

26. Seip, R.L.; Papasavas, P.; Stone, A.; Thompson, S.; Ng, J.; Tishler, D.S.; Ruaño, G. Comparative physiogenomic analyses of weight loss in response to 2 modes of bariatric surgery: Demonstration with candidate neuropsychiatric and cardiometabolic genes. *Surg. Obes. Relat. Dis.* **2016**, *12*, 369–377. [CrossRef] [PubMed]

27. Vitolo, E.; Santini, E.; Seghieri, M.; Giannini, L.; Coppedè, F.; Rossi, C.; Dardano, A.; Solini, A. Heterozygosity for the rs696217 SNP in the preproghrelin gene predicts weight loss after bariatric surgery in severely obese individuals. *Obes. Surg.* **2017**, *27*, 961–967. [CrossRef] [PubMed]

28. Figueroa-Veja, N.; Jordán, B.; Pérez-Luque, E.L.; Parra-Laporte, L.; Garnelo, S.; Malacara, J.M. Effects of sleeve gastrectomy and rs9930506 FTO variants on angiopoietin/Tie-2 system in fat expansion and M1 macrophages recruitment in morbidly obese subjects. *Endocrine* **2016**, *54*, 700–713. [CrossRef] [PubMed]

29. Krawczyk, M.; Jiménez-Agüero, R.; Alustiza, J.M.; Emparanza, J.I.; Perugorria, M.J.; Bujanda, L.; Lammert, F.; Banales, J.M. PNPLA3 p.I148M variant is associated with greater reduction of liver fat content after bariatric surgery. *Surg. Obes. Relat. Dis.* **2016**, *12*, 1838–1846. [CrossRef] [PubMed]

30. Nicoletti, C.F.; Pinhel, M.A.; de Oliveira, B.A.; Marchini, J.S.; Salgado Junior, W.; Silva Junior, W.A.; Nonino, C.B. The genetic predisposition score of seven obesity-related single nucleotide polymorphisms is associated with better metabolic outcomes after Roux-en-Y gastric bypass. *J. Nutrigenet. Nutrigenom.* **2016**, *9*, 222–230. [CrossRef] [PubMed]

31. Bandstein, M.; Mwinyi, J.; Ernst, B.; Thurnheer, M.; Schultes, B.; Schiöth, H.B. A genetic variant in proximity to the gene LYPLAL1 is associated with lower hunger feelings and increased weight loss following Roux-en-Y gastric bypass surgery. *Scand. J. Gastroenterol.* **2016**, *51*, 1050–1055. [CrossRef] [PubMed]

32. Rodrigues, G.K.; Resende, C.M.; Durso, D.F.; Rodrigues, L.A.; Silva, J.L.; Reis, R.C.; Pereira, S.S.; Ferreira, D.C.; Franco, G.R.; Alvarez-Leite, J. A single FTO gene variant rs9939609 is associated with body weight evolution in a multiethnic extremely obese population that underwent bariatric surgery. *Nutrition* **2015**, *31*, 1344–1350. [CrossRef] [PubMed]

33. Jia, P.; Her, C.; Chai, W. DNA excision repair at telomeres. *DNA Repair* **2015**, *36*, 137–145. [CrossRef] [PubMed]

34. Blackburn, E.H. Telomeres and telomerase: The means to the end (Nobel lecture). *Angew. Chem. Int. Ed. Eng.* **2010**, *49*, 7405–7421. [CrossRef] [PubMed]

35. Barceló, A.; Piérola, J.; López-Escribano, H.; de la Peña, M.; Soriano, J.B.; Alonso-Fernández, A.; Ladaria, A.; Agustí, A. Telomere shortening in sleep apnea syndrome. *Respir. Med.* **2010**, *104*, 1225–1229. [CrossRef] [PubMed]

36. Lee, M.; Martin, H.; Firpo, M.A.; Demerath, E.W. Inverse association between adiposity and telomere length: The fels longitudinal study. *Am. J. Hum. Biol.* **2010**, *23*, 100–106. [CrossRef] [PubMed]

37. Dersham, R.; Chu, X.; Wood, G.C.; Benotti, P.; Still, C.D.; Rolston, D.D. Changes in telomere length 3–5 years after gastric bypass surgery. *Int. J. Obes.* **2017**. [CrossRef] [PubMed]
38. Wong, J.M.; Collins, K. Telomere maintenance and disease. *Lancet* **2003**, *362*, 983–988. [CrossRef]
39. Rode, L.; Nordestgaard, B.G.; Weischer, M.; Bojesen, S.E. Increased body mass index, elevated C-reactive protein, and short telomere length. *J. Clin. Endocrinol. Metab.* **2014**, *99*, E1671–E1675. [CrossRef] [PubMed]
40. Harte, A.L.; da Silva, N.F.; Miller, M.A.; Cappuccio, F.P.; Kelly, A.; O'Hare, J.P.; Barnett, A.H.; Al-Daghri, N.M.; Al-Attas, O.; Alokail, M.; et al. Telomere length attrition, a marker of biological senescence, is inversely correlated with triglycerides and cholesterol in south Asian males with type 2 dibates mellitus. *Exp. Diabetes Res.* **2012**, 895185. [CrossRef] [PubMed]
41. Salpea, K.D.; Humphries, S.E. Telomeres length in atherosclerosis and diabetes. *Atherosclerosis* **2010**, *209*, 35–38. [CrossRef] [PubMed]
42. Cassidy, A.; De Vivo, I.; Liu, Y.; Han, J.; Prescott, J.; Hunter, D.J.; Rimm, E.B. Associations between diet, lifestyle factors, and telomere length in women. *Am. J. Clin. Nutr.* **2010**, *91*, 1273–1280. [CrossRef] [PubMed]
43. O'Callaghan, N.J.; Clifton, P.M.; Noakes, M.; Fenech, M. Weight loss in obese men is associated with increased telomere length and decreased abasic sites in rectal mucosa. *Rejuvenation Res.* **2009**, *12*, 169–176. [CrossRef] [PubMed]
44. Formichi, C.; Cantara, S.; Ciuoli, C.; Neri, O.; Chiofalo, F.; Selmi, F.; Tirone, A.; Colasanto, G.; Di Cosmo, L.; Vuolo, G.; et al. Weight loss associated with bariatric surgery does not restore short telomere length of severe obese patients after 1 Year. *Obes. Surg.* **2014**, *24*, 2089–2093. [CrossRef] [PubMed]
45. Epel, E.S. Psychological and metabolic stress: A recipe for accelerated cellular aging? *Hormones* **2009**, *8*, 7–22. [CrossRef] [PubMed]
46. Laimer, M.; Melmer, A.; Lamina, C.; Raschenberger, J.; Adamovski, P.; Engl, J.; Ress, C.; Tschoner, A.; Gelsinger, C.; Mair, L.; et al. Telomere length increase after weight loss induced by bariatric surgery: Results from a 10 year prospective study. *Int. J. Obes.* **2016**, *40*, 773–778. [CrossRef] [PubMed]
47. Carulli, L.; Anzivino, C.; Baldelli, E.; Zenobii, M.F.; Rocchi, M.B.; Bertolotti, M. Telomere length elongation after weight loss intervention in obese adults. *Mol. Genet. Metab.* **2016**, *118*, 138–142. [CrossRef] [PubMed]
48. Bernstein, B.E.; Meissner, A.; Lander, E.S. The mammalian epigenome. *Cell* **2007**, *128*, 669–681. [CrossRef] [PubMed]
49. Fan, S.; Zhang, X. CpG island methylation pattern in different human tissues and its correlation with gene expression. *Biochem. Biophys. Res. Commun.* **2009**, *383*, 421–425. [CrossRef] [PubMed]
50. Franks, P.W.; Ling, C. Epigenetics and obesity: The devil is in the details. *BMC Med.* **2010**, *8*, 88. [CrossRef] [PubMed]
51. Udali, S.; Guarini, P.; Moruzzi, S.; Choi, S.W.; Friso, S. Cardiovascular epigenetics: From DNA methylation to microRNAs. *Mol. Asp. Med.* **2013**, *34*, 883–901. [CrossRef] [PubMed]
52. Choi, S.W.; Friso, S. Epigenetics: A new bridge between nutrition and health. *Adv. Nutr.* **2010**, *1*, 8–16. [CrossRef] [PubMed]
53. Saetrom, P.; Snove O., Jr.; Rossi, J.J. Epigenetics and microRNAs. *Pediatr. Res.* **2007**, *61*, 17R–23R. [CrossRef] [PubMed]
54. Campión, J.; Milagro, F.; Martínez, J.A. Epigenetics and obesity. *Prog. Mol. Biol. Transl. Sci.* **2010**, *94*, 291–347. [CrossRef] [PubMed]
55. Duthie, S.J. Epigenetic modifications and human pathologies: Cancer and CVD. *Proc. Nutr. Soc.* **2011**, *70*, 47–56. [CrossRef] [PubMed]
56. Ramos-Lopez, O.; Milagro, F.I.; Allayee, H.; Chmurzynska, A.; Choi, M.S.; Curi, R.; De Caterina, R.; Ferguson, L.R.; Goni, L.; Kang, J.X.; et al. Guide for current nutrigenetic, nutrigenomic, and nutriepigenetic approaches for precision nutrition involving the prevention and management of chronic diseases associated with obesity. *J. Nutrigenet. Nutrigenom.* **2017**, *10*, 43–62. [CrossRef] [PubMed]
57. Boqué, N.; de la Iglesia, R.; de la Garza, A.L.; Milagro, F.I.; Olivares, M.; Bañuelos, O.; Soria, A.C.; Rodríguez-Sánchez, S.; Martínez, J.A.; Campión, J. Prevention of diet-induced obesity by apple polyphenols in Wistar rats through regulation of adipocyte gene expression and DNA methylation patterns. *Mol. Nutr. Food Res.* **2013**, *57*, 1473–1478. [CrossRef] [PubMed]
58. Uriarte, G.; Paternain, L.; Milagro, F.I.; Martínez, J.A.; Campion, J. Shifting to a control diet after a high-fat, highsucrose diet intake induces epigenetic changes in retroperitoneal adipocytes of Wistar rats. *J. Physiol. Biochem.* **2013**, *69*, 601–611. [CrossRef] [PubMed]

59. Milagro, F.I.; Campión, J.; Cordero, P.; Goyenechea, E.; Gómez-Uriz, A.M.; Abete, I.; Zulet, M.A.; Martínez, J.A. A dual epigenomic approach for the search of obesity biomarkers: DNA methylation in relation to diet-induced weight loss. *FASEB J.* **2011**, *25*, 1378–1389. [CrossRef] [PubMed]

60. Cordero, P.; Campion, J.; Milagro, F.I.; Goyenechea, E.; Steemburgo, T.; Javierre, B.M.; Martinez, J.A. Leptin and TNF-alpha promoter methylation levels measured by MSP could predict the response to a low-calorie diet. *J. Physiol. Biochem.* **2011**, *67*, 463–470. [CrossRef] [PubMed]

61. Crujeiras, A.B.; Campion, J.; Díaz-Lagares, A.; Milagro, F.I.; Goyenechea, E.; Abete, I.; Casanueva, F.F.; Martínez, J.A. Association of weight regain with specific methylation levels in the NPY and POMC promoters in leukocytes of obese men: A translational study. *Regul. Pept.* **2013**, *186*, 1–6. [CrossRef] [PubMed]

62. Nicoletti, C.F.; Nonino, C.B.; de Oliveira, B.A.; Pinhel, M.A.; Mansego, M.L.; Milagro, F.I.; Zulet, M.A.; Martinez, J.A. DNA methylation and hydroxymethylation levels in relation to two weight loss strategies: Energy-restricted diet or bariatric surgery. *Obes. Surg.* **2016**, *26*, 603–611. [CrossRef] [PubMed]

63. Barres, R.; Kirchner, H.; Rasmussen, M.; Yan, J.; Kantor, F.R.; Krook, A.; Näslund, E.; Zierath, J.R. Weight loss after gastric bypass surgery in human obesity remodels promoter methylation. *Cell Rep.* **2013**, *3*, 1020–1027. [CrossRef] [PubMed]

64. Falken, Y.; Hellstrom, P.M.; Holst, J.J.; Naslund, E. Changes in glucose homeostasis after Roux-en-Y gastric bypass surgery for obesity at day three, two months, and one year after surgery: Role of gut peptides. *J. Clin. Endocrinol. Metab.* **2011**, *96*, 2227–2235. [CrossRef] [PubMed]

65. Rubino, F.; Forgione, A.; Cummings, D.E.; Vix, M.; Gnuli, D.; Mingrone, G.; Castagneto, M.; Marescaux, J. The mechanism of diabetes control after gastrointestinal bypass surgery reveals a role of the proximal small intestine in the pathophysiology of type 2 diabetes. *Ann. Surg.* **2006**, *244*, 741–749. [CrossRef] [PubMed]

66. Kirchner, H.; Nylen, C.; Laber, S.; Barrès, R.; Yan, J.; Krook, A.; Zierath, J.R.; Näslund, E. Altered promoter methylation of PDK4, IL1 B, IL6, and TNF after Roux-en Y gastric bypass. *Surg. Obes. Relat. Dis.* **2014**, *10*, 671–678. [CrossRef] [PubMed]

67. Morcillo, S.; Martín-Núñez, G.M.; García-Serrano, S.; Gutierrez-Repiso, C.; Rodriguez-Pacheco, F.; Valdes, S.; Gonzalo, M.; Rojo-Martinez, G.; Moreno-Ruiz, F.J.; Rodriguez-Cañete, A.; et al. Changes in SCD gene DNA methylation after bariatric surgery in morbidly obese patients are associated with free fatty acids. *Sci. Rep.* **2017**, *7*, 46292. [CrossRef] [PubMed]

68. Nilsson, E.K.; Ernst, B.; Voisin, S.; Almén, M.S.; Benedict, C.; Mwinyi, J.; Fredriksson, R.; Schultes, B.; Schiöth, H.B. Rouxen-Y gastric bypass surgery induces genome-wide promoter-specific changes in DNA methylation in whole blood of obese patients. *PLoS ONE* **2015**, *10*, e0115186. [CrossRef] [PubMed]

69. Ahrens, M.; Ammerpohl, O.; von Schönfels, W.; Kolarova, J.; Bens, S.; Itzel, T.; Teufel, A.; Herrmann, A.; Brosch, M.; Hinrichsen, H.; et al. DNA methylation analysis in nonalcoholic fatty liver disease suggests distinct disease-specific and remodeling signatures after bariatric surgery. *Cell Metab.* **2013**, *18*, 296–302. [CrossRef] [PubMed]

70. Benton, M.C.; Johnstone, A.; Eccles, D.; Harmon, B.; Hayes, M.T.; Lea, R.A.; Griffiths, L.; Hoffman, E.P.; Stubbs, R.S.; Macartney-Coxson, D. An analysis of DNA methylation in human adipose tissue reveals differential modification of obesity genes before and after gastric bypass and weight loss. *Genome Biol.* **2015**, *16*, 8. [CrossRef] [PubMed]

71. Martín-Núñez, G.M.; Cabrera-Mulero, A.; Alcaide-Torres, J.; García-Fuentes, E.; Tinahones, F.J.; Morcillo, S. No effect of different bariatric surgery procedures on LINE-1 DNA methylation in diabetic and nondiabetic morbidly obese patients. *Surg. Obes. Relat. Dis.* **2017**, *13*, 442–450. [CrossRef] [PubMed]

72. Van Dijk, S.J.; Molloy, P.L.; Varinli, H.; Morrison, J.L.; Muhlhausler, B.S. Epigenetics and human obesity. *Int. J. Obes.* **2015**, *39*, 85–97. [CrossRef] [PubMed]

73. Guénarda, F.; Deshaiesb, Y.; Cianfloneb, K.; Krald, J.G.; Marceauc, P.; Vohla, M.C. Differential methylation in glucoregulatory genes of offspring born before vs. after maternal gastrointestinal bypass surgery. *Proc. Natl. Acad. Sci. USA* **2013**, *110*, 11439–11444. [CrossRef] [PubMed]

74. Donkin, I.; Versteyhe, S.; Ingerslev, L.R.; Qian, K.; Mechta, M.; Nordkap, L.; Mortensen, B.; Appel, E.V.; Jørgensen, N.; Kristiansen, V.B.; et al. Obesity and bariatric surgery drive epigenetic variation of spermatozoa in humans. *Cell Metab.* **2016**, *23*, 369–378. [CrossRef] [PubMed]

75. Dedeurwaerder, S.; Defrance, M.; Calonne, E.; Denis, H.; Sotiriou, C.; Fuks, F. Evaluation of the infinium methylation 450K technology. *Epigenomics* **2011**, *3*, 771–784. [CrossRef] [PubMed]

76. Ferguson, L.R. Nutrigenomics approaches to functional foods. *J. Am. Diet. Assoc.* **2009**, *109*, 452–458. [CrossRef] [PubMed]

77. Mutch, D.M.; Temanni, M.R.; Henegar, C.; Combes, F.; Pelloux, V.; Holst, C.; Sørensen, T.I.; Astrup, A.; Martinez, J.A.; Saris, W.H.; et al. Adipose gene expression prior to weight loss can differentiate and weakly predict dietary responders. *PLoS ONE* **2007**, *2*, e1344. [CrossRef] [PubMed]

78. Cortes-Oliveira, C.; Nicoletti, C.F.; Pinhel, M.A.S.; Oliveira, B.A.P.; Quinhoneiro, D.C.G.; Noronha, N.Y.; Marchini, J.S.; da Silva Júnior, W.A.; Júnior, W.S.; Nonino, C.B. UCP2 expression is associated with weight loss after hypocaloric diet intervention. *Eur. J. Clin. Nutr.* **2016**, 1–5. [CrossRef] [PubMed]

79. Cortes-Oliveira, C.; Nicoletti, C.F.; Pinhel, M.A.S.; Oliveira, B.A.P.; Quinhoneiro, D.C.G.; Noronha, N.Y.; Fassini, P.G.; Marchini, J.S.; da Silva Júnior, W.A.; Salgado Júnior, W.; et al. Influence of expression of UCP3, PLIN1 and PPARG2 on the oxidation of substrates after hypocaloric dietary intervention. *Clin. Nutr.* **2017**, 1–6. [CrossRef]

80. Ordovás, J.M.; Robertson, R.; Cléirigh, E.N. Gene–gene and gene–environment interactions defining lipid-related traits. *Curr. Opin. Lipidol.* **2011**, *22*, 129–136. [CrossRef] [PubMed]

81. Pinhel, M.A.S.; Nicoletti, C.F.; Noronha, N.Y.; Oliveira, B.A.P.; Quinhoneiro, D.C.G.; Cortes-Oliveira, C.; Salgado, W., Jr.; Salgado Junior, W.; Machry, A.J.; da Silva Junior, W.A.; Souza, D.R.S.; et al. Changes in global transcriptional profiling of women following obesity surgery bypass. *Obes. Surg.* **2017**. [CrossRef] [PubMed]

82. Berisha, S.Z.; Serre, D.; Schauer, P.; Kashyap, S.R.; Smith, J.D. Changes in whole blood gene expression in obese subjects with type 2 diabetes following bariatric surgery: A pilot study. *PLoS ONE* **2011**, *6*, e16729. [CrossRef] [PubMed]

83. Ortega, F.J.; Vilallonga, R.; Xifra, G.; Sabater, M.; Ricart, W.; Fernández-Real, J.M. Bariatric surgery acutely changes the expression of inflammatory and lipogenic genes in obese adipose tissue. *Surg. Obes. Relat. Dis.* **2016**, *12*, 357–362. [CrossRef] [PubMed]

84. Mardinoglu, A.; Heiker, J.T.; Gärtner, D.; Björnson, E.; Schön, M.R.; Flehmig, G.; Klöting, N.; Krohn, K.; Fasshauer, M.; Stumvoll, M.; et al. Extensive weight loss reveals distinct gene expression changes in human subcutaneous and visceral adipose tissue. *Sci. Rep.* **2015**, *5*, 14841. [CrossRef] [PubMed]

85. Oliveira, B.A.P.; Pinhel, M.A.S.; Nicoletti, C.F.; Cortes-Oliveira, C.; Quinhoneiro, D.C.G.; Noronha, N.Y.; Fassini, P.G.; da Silva Júnior, W.A.; Junior, W.S.; Nonino, C.B. UCP2 and PLIN1 expression affects the resting metabolic rate and weight loss on obese patients. *Obes. Surg.* **2016**, *27*, 343–348. [CrossRef] [PubMed]

86. Jürets, A.; Itariu, B.K.; Keindl, M.; Prager, G.; Langer, F.; Grablowitz, V.; Zeyda, M.; Stulnig, T.M. Upregulated TNF expression 1 year after bariatric surgery reflects a cachexia-like state in subcutaneous adipose tissue. *Obes. Surg.* **2017**, *27*, 1514–1523. [CrossRef] [PubMed]

87. Leyvraz, C.; Verdumo, C.; Suter, M.; Paroz, A.; Calmes, J.M.; Marques-Vidal, P.M.; Giusti, V. Changes in gene expression profile in human subcutaneous adipose tissue during significant weight loss. *Obes. Facts* **2012**, *5*, 440–451. [CrossRef] [PubMed]

88. Oliveira, B.A.P.; Pinhel, M.A.S.; Nicoletti, C.F.; Cortes-Oliveira, C.; Quinhoneiro, D.C.G.; Noronha, N.Y.; Marchini, J.S.; Marchry, A.J.; Junior, W.S.; Nonino, C.B. UCP1 and UCP3 expression is associated with lipid and carbohydrate oxidation and body composition. *PLoS ONE* **2016**. [CrossRef] [PubMed]

89. Hagman, D.K.; Larson, I.; Kuzma, J.N.; Cromer, G.; Makar, K.; Rubinow, K.B.; Foster-Schubert, K.E.; van Yserloo, B.; Billing, P.S.; Landerholm, R.W.; et al. The short-term and long-term effects of bariatric/metabolic surgery on subcutaneous adipose tissue inflammation in humans. *Metabolism* **2017**, *70*, 12–22. [CrossRef] [PubMed]

90. Anhê, F.F.; Varin, T.V.; Schertzer, J.D.; Marette, A. The gut microbiota as a mediator of metabolic benefits after bariatric surgery. *Can. J. Diabetes* **2017**, 30521–30524. [CrossRef] [PubMed]

91. Tremaroli, V.; Karlsson, F.; Werling, M.; Ståhlman, M.; Kovatcheva-Datchary, P.; Olbers, T.; Fändriks, L.; le Roux, C.W.; Nielsen, J.; Bäckhed, F. Roux-en-Y gastric bypass and verticalbandedgastroplasty induce long-term changes on the human gutmicrobiome contributing to fat mass regulation. *Cell Metab.* **2015**, *22*, 228–238. [CrossRef] [PubMed]

92. Liou, A.P.; Paziuk, M.; Luevano, J.M., Jr.; Machineni, S.; Turnbaugh, P.J.; Kaplan, L.M. Conserved shifts in the gut microbiotadue to gastric bypass reduce host weight and adiposity. *Sci. Transl. Med.* **2013**, *5*. [CrossRef] [PubMed]

93. Qin, J.; Li, Y.; Cai, Z.; Li, S.; Zhu, J.; Zhang, F.; Liang, S.; Zhang, W.; Guan, Y.; Shen, D.; et al. A metagenome-wide association study of gut microbiota in type 2 diabetes. *Nature* **2012**, *490*, 55–60. [CrossRef] [PubMed]

94. Palleja, A.; Kashani, A.; Allin, K.H.; Nielsen, T.; Zhang, C.; Li, Y.; Brach, T.; Liang, S.; Feng, Q.; Jørgensen, N.B.; et al. Roux-en-Y gastric bypass surgery of morbidly obese patients induces swift and persistent changes of the individual gut microbiota. *Genome Med.* **2016**, *8*, 67. [CrossRef] [PubMed]

95. Zhang, H.; DiBaise, J.K.; Zuccolo, A.; Kudrna, D.; Braidotti, M.; Yu, Y.; Parameswarana, P.; Crowellb, M.D.; Wingc, R.; Rittmann, B.E.; et al. Human gutmicrobiota in obesity and after gastric bypass. *Proc. Natl. Acad. Sci. USA* **2009**, *106*, 2365–2370. [CrossRef] [PubMed]

96. Graessler, J.; Qin, Y.; Zhong, H.; Zhang, J.; Licinio, J.; Wong, M.L.; Xu, A.; Chavakis, T.; Bornstein, A.B.; Ehrhart-Bornstein, M.; et al. Metagenomic sequencing of the human gut microbiome before and after bariatric surgery in obese patients with type 2 diabetes: Correlation with inflammatory and metabolic parameters. *Pharmacogenom. J.* **2013**, *13*, 514–522. [CrossRef] [PubMed]

97. Kong, L.C.; Tap, J.; Aron-Wisnewsky, J.; Pelloux, V.; Basdevant, A.; Bouillot, J.L.; Zucker, J.D.; Doré, J.; Clément, K. Gut microbiota after gastric bypass in human obesity: Increased richness and associations of bacterial genera with adipose tissue genes. *Am. J. Clin. Nutr.* **2013**, *98*, 16–24. [CrossRef] [PubMed]

98. Furet, J.P.; Kong, L.C.; Tap, J.; Poitou, C.; Basdevant, A.; Bouillot, J.L.; Mariat, D.; Corthier, G.; Doré, J.; Henegar, C.; et al. Differential adaptation of human gut microbiota to bariatric surgery-induced weight loss: Links with metabolic and lowgrade inflammation markers. *Diabetes* **2010**, *59*, 3049–3057. [CrossRef] [PubMed]

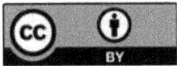

nutrients

MDPI

Article

Developmental Programming of Obesity and Liver Metabolism by Maternal Perinatal Nutrition Involves the Melanocortin System

Paul Cordero [1,*], Jiawei Li [1], Vi Nguyen [1], Joaquim Pombo [2], Nuria Maicas [2], Marco Novelli [3], Paul D. Taylor [2], Anne-Maj Samuelsson [2], Manlio Vinciguerra [1,4] and Jude A. Oben [1,5,*]

1 Institute for Liver and Digestive Health, University College London, London NW3 2PF, UK; jiawei.li.10@ucl.ac.uk (J.L.); v.nguyen@ucl.ac.uk (V.N.); manlio.vinciguerra@fnusa.cz (M.V.)
2 Division of Women's Health, Faculty of Life Sciences & Medicine, King's College London, London SE1 7EH, UK; joaquim.1.pombo@kcl.ac.uk (J.P.); nuriamaicas82@gmail.com (N.M.); paul.taylor@kcl.ac.uk (P.D.T.); anne-maj.samuelsson@kcl.ac.uk (A.-M.S.)
3 Department of Pathology, University College London, London WC1E 6JJ, UK; m.novelli@ucl.ac.uk
4 Center for Translational Medicine, International Clinical Research Center (FNUSA-ICRC), Brno 65691, Czech Republic
5 Department of Gastroenterology and Hepatology, Guy's and St Thomas' Hospital, NHS Foundation Trust, London SE1 7EH, UK
* Correspondence: paul.sanchez@ucl.ac.uk (P.C.); j.oben@ucl.ac.uk (J.A.O.); Tel.: +44-207-433-2875 (P.C. & J.A.O.)

Received: 30 July 2017; Accepted: 15 September 2017; Published: 20 September 2017

Abstract: Maternal obesity predisposes offspring to metabolic dysfunction and Non-Alcoholic Fatty Liver Disease (NAFLD). Melanocortin-4 receptor (Mc4r)-deficient mouse models exhibit obesity during adulthood. Here, we aim to determine the influence of the Mc4r gene on the liver of mice subjected to perinatal diet-induced obesity. Female mice heterozygous for Mc4r fed an obesogenic or a control diet for 5 weeks were mated with heterozygous males, with the same diet continued throughout pregnancy and lactation, generating four offspring groups: control wild type (C_wt), control knockout (C_KO), obese wild type (Ob_wt), and obese knockout (Ob_KO). At 21 days, offspring were genotyped, weaned onto a control diet, and sacrificed at 6 months old. Offspring phenotypic characteristics, plasma biochemical profile, liver histology, and hepatic gene expression were analyzed. Mc4r_ko offspring showed higher body, liver and adipose tissue weights respect to the wild type animals. Histological examination showed mild hepatic steatosis in offspring group C_KO. The expression of hepatic genes involved in regulating inflammation, fibrosis, and immune cell infiltration were upregulated by the absence of the Mc4r gene. These results demonstrate that maternal obesogenic feeding during the perinatal period programs offspring obesity development with involvement of the Mc4r system.

Keywords: obesity; developmental programming; Non-Alcoholic Fatty Liver Disease; maternal nutrition; intra-abdominal fat

1. Introduction

Obesity is a chronic, multifactorial and pro-inflammatory disease defined as a disproportionate increase of body weight with excessive adipose tissue accumulation [1]. The prevalence of obesity is rising alarmingly worldwide, with more than 640 million obese patients and an estimated 1.5 billion overweight people according to the World Health Organization (WHO) [2]. This increase in adiposity is associated with all causes of mortality, a significant decrease in lifespan of up to 20 years, and a tremendous fiscal burden [3,4]. Obesity is associated with multiple comorbidities representing the main causes of illness and death in affluent societies, especially cardiovascular and cerebrovascular illnesses, type 2 diabetes mellitus, many cancers, and Non-Alcoholic Fatty Liver Disease (NAFLD) [1,5]. NAFLD is now the most common cause of liver disease in these affluent countries; it may progress through steatosis, inflammation and injury (non-alcoholic steatohepatitis, NASH), fibrosis, cirrhosis, and hepatocellular carcinoma [6–8]. Considering that the prevalence of obesity and NAFLD in Western countries ranges between 20–30%, these alterations in liver morphology and functionality secondary to NAFLD are a major concern for national health policies [6].

The increase in global obesity rate affects all populations, including women in their reproductive age. As a result, the risk of pregnancy loss, maternal gestational diabetes, fetal malformations, and other complications during pregnancy has increased in obese women [9]. Interestingly, retrospective epidemiological human studies and animal interventions have recently highlighted that, during early development, an adverse pro-obesogenic in utero environment plays an important role in promoting offspring obesity and metabolic diseases in later life [10]. Our previous studies have demonstrated that maternal obesogenic diet during perinatal periods programs the development of obesity and NAFLD in the offspring [11–13], although the precise involved mechanism remains uncertain.

The etiology of obesity is mostly thought of, perhaps simplistically, as higher caloric intake greater than energy expenditure. However, the underlying mechanisms are much more complex and include genetic predisposition, epigenetic regulation, environmental factors, and/or interactions with the gut microbiota [1,14]. Indeed, current Genome Wide Association Studies (GWAS) point to several key genes with very important influences on the origin and development of obesity: these include Fat-Associated Obesity (FTO), Leptin, Leptin Receptor, Pro-Opiomelanocortin (Pomc), or Melanocortin Receptor 4 (Mc4r) [15]. Importantly, multiple meta-analyses and GWAS studies have confirmed the association between Mc4r polymorphisms and obesity and its associated comorbidities [16–18]. Mc4r is a critical mediator in energy homeostasis, regulating both food intake and energy expenditure as well as affecting blood pressure homeostasis [19,20]. Interestingly, a novel study in rats by Tabachnik et al. demonstrated that perinatal obesogenic environment increased in the offspring histone acetylation marks at the Mc4r promoter. This epigenetic regulation was also associated with thyroid hormones metabolism as well as with the inhibition of Mc4r transcription [21]. The aim of this study, therefore, was to investigate ab initio whether the Mc4r gene plays a role in the maternal programming of offspring obesity and consequent NAFLD.

2. Materials and Methods

2.1. Animals and Experimental Design

All experiments were approved by the Local Ethics Committee of the University of King's College London, and were conducted in accordance with the Home Office Animals (Scientific Procedures) Act of 1986 guidelines (United Kingdom). Mice were housed under controlled conditions (light-dark cycle 12 h, 21 ± 2 °C, 40–50% humidity) with food and water available ad libitum. Adult female mice heterozygous for Mc4r with C57BL/6J background were fed an obesogenic diet (824053, Special Dietary Services, Wittam, UK) [22] supplemented with sweetened condensed milk (Nestlé, Vevey, Switzerland) and fortified with 3.5% (AIN 93G; Special Diets Services) mineral mix and 1% vitamin mix or a control standard laboratory diet (RM1, Special Diets Services) for 5 weeks (dietary composition in Table 1). Then, as previously described, obesogenic-fed heterozygous females were around 50% heavier than control-fed females [23]. The female mice were mated with control-fed heterozygous males from the same litter. Conception was determined by vaginal plug formation. The female animals were maintained on their allocated diets throughout gestation and lactation, as previously described [11]. Litter sizes from both maternal feeding groups were similar [23]. After birth, litters were standardized to six pups each with an equal number of males and females when possible. At day 21 postnatally, offspring were genotyped and weaned onto a control diet until 6 months old. They were then killed by schedule 1 method after an overnight fast. Blood samples were collected, centrifuged ($10,000\times$ *g*,

10 min at 4 °C), and stored at −80 °C until further analysis. Liver and inguinal adipose depots were harvested, weighted, and stored at −80 °C. A representative sample of each liver was fixed in 10% formalin for histological analysis.

Table 1. Macronutrient composition of the diets.

Dietary Composition (g/Kg)	Control	Obesogenic	Condensed Milk
Protein	144	230	80
Amino Acids			
Glutamic Acid	31.7	45.5	16.6
Proline	12	24.8	7.7
Leucine	9.8	20.5	7.8
Aspartic Acid	6.7	15.4	6
Serine	5.6	12.9	4.3
Valine	6.9	14.5	5.3
Lysine	6.6	18.9	6.3
Glycine	11.1	4.1	1.7
Arginine	9.1	8.1	2.9
Others	44.5	65.3	20.5
Carbohydrates			
Polysaccharides	500	283	0
Simple sugars	40	105	550
Cellulose	43.2	61.7	
Hemicellulose	101.7		
Lipid	27	226	90
Saturated Fatty Acids	5.1	76.2	59.4
Monounsaturated Fatty Acids	8.8	85.2	24.3
Polyunsaturated Fatty Acids	8.8	39.1	3.4
Mineral content	35		
Vitamin content	4.1		
AIN-93G mineral mix			1.68
AIN-93M mineral mix		43	
Vitamin mix		12	
Energy (kcal/g)	3.52	4.54	3.22

2.2. Liver Histology

Offspring liver samples at 6 months of age (n = 5–6 per experiment group) were fixed in formalin (10%), dehydrated, and subsequently embedded in paraffin. Liver samples were cut into 4-µm sections, mounted, and dried overnight at 37 °C. The liver sections were then stained with hematoxylin and eosin (H&E), and the extent of steatosis assessed by an expert liver pathologist blinded to the group identities, as previously described [24].

2.3. Plasma Analysis

Plasma glucose, triglycerides, alanine aminotransferase (ALT), and aspartate aminotransferase (ALT) concentrations were assayed by the Royal Free Hospital Clinical Biochemistry Department (London, UK).

2.4. mRNA Extraction and Real-Time qPCR

Frozen liver samples (n = 5–6 per experiment group) were homogenized using TRIzol Reagent (Invitrogen, Carlsbad, CA, USA) and mRNA was extracted by following the suppliers' protocol. Sample quality and concentrations were measured using a NanoDrop ND-1000 Spectrometer (Thermo Scientific, Waltham, MA, USA). DNase treatment and retrotranscription to cDNA were carried out using the Qiagen QuantiTect Reverse Transcriptase kit (Qiagen, Hilden, Germany). Quantitative real-time PCR (rt-qPCR) was performed by triplicate using the ABI PRISM 7500 HT Fast real-time PCR system (Applied Biosystems, Austin, TX, USA) with QuantiFast SYBR Green PCR

(Qiagen, Hilden, Germany). 18S was used as a control for cDNA quality and Gapdh was used as the control housekeeping reference gene. All designed primers were obtained from Sigma-Aldrich (St. Louis, MO, USA) and a melting curve analysis confirmed the amplification of specific PCR products and the absence of non-specific amplification or primer-dimers. Gene-specific primer sequences for 18S ribosomal RNA (18S), glyceraldehyde-3-phosphate dehydrogenase (Gapdh), alpha-smooth muscle actin (α-SMA), tumor necrosis factor alpha (TNF-α), collagen type I alpha 1 (Col-1α), interleukin 6 (IL6), chemokine (C-C motif) ligand 2 (MCP1), interleukin 1 beta (IL-1β), and transforming growth factor beta (TGF-β) are listed in Table 2. Fold changes between groups were calculated using the $2^{-\Delta\Delta ct}$ method.

Table 2. Rt-qPCR primer sequences.

Gene	Primer Sequence
18S	sense: AGTCCCTGCCCTTTGTACACA antisense: CGATCCGAGGGCCTCACTA
Gapdh	sense: CGTCCCGTAGACAAAATGGT antisense: TCAATGAAGGGGTCGTTGAT
α-SMA	sense: CTCTTGCTCTGGGCTTCATC antisense: GGCTGTTTTCCCATCCATC
TNF-α	sense: CCACCACGCTCTTCTGTCTA antisense: AGGGTCTGGGCCATAGAACT
Col-1α	sense: GTCCCCGAGGCAGAGATG antisense: GTCCAGGGCCAGATGAAACT
IL6	sense: TCAATTCCAGAAACCGCTATG antisense: GTCTCCTCTCCGGACTTGTG
MCP1	sense: CCCACTCACCTGCTGCTACT antisense: TCTGGACCCATTCCTTCTTG
IL-1β	sense: CAACCAACAAGTGATATTCTCCATG antisense: GATCCACACTCTCCAGCTGCA
TGF-β	sense: AAAATCAAGTGTGGAGCAAC antisense: CCACGTGGAGTTTGTTATCT

18S: 18S ribosomal RNA; Gapdh: glyceraldehyde-3-phosphate dehydrogenase; α-SMA: alpha-smooth muscle actin; TNF-α: tumor necrosis factor alpha; Col-1α: collagen type I alpha 1; IL6: interleukin 6; MCP1: chemokine (C-C motif) ligand 2; IL-1β: interleukin 1 beta; TGF-β: transforming growth factor beta.

2.5. Statistical Analysis

All data are expressed as the mean ± standard error of the mean (SEM). Two-way ANOVA was applied for studying the effect of maternal obesogenic feeding (C vs. Ob) and offspring genotype (wt vs. knockout). Comparison of the means was carried out by Tukey post-hoc test. The statistical unit used throughout the analysis was the number of dams. Statistical significance was accepted with a *p* value of less than 0.05. IBM SPSS 24 software (24.0, SPSS Statistics, IBM, Chicago, IL, USA) was used for the statistical analysis.

3. Results

3.1. Phenotypic and Histological Characteristics

We firstly analyzed the effect of maternal obesogenic feeding on phenotypical parameters and hepatic morphology (Figure 1). As we have previously reported, at 6 months of age, body weight of Mc4rko and wild type mice from control- and obesogenic-fed dams had already reached a plateau [23]. Thus, at this age, there was a marked genotype effect independent of maternal nutrition, with increased body mass (+0.37-fold, *p* < 0.001) (Figure 1a), inguinal fat mass (+1.59-fold, *p* < 0.001) (Figure 1b), and liver weight (+1.51-fold, $p < 0.01$) (Figure 1c) in KO mice compared to the wild type animals. Furthermore, maternal obesogenic feeding during perinatal periods predisposed the offspring to higher body weight (+0.27-fold, $p < 0.05$) and inguinal fat deposition (+1.19-fold, $p < 0.05$). In offspring subjected to maternal control diet, C_KO mice presented a marked obesity phenotype compared to C_wt animals, with higher body mass (+0.29-fold, $p < 0.01$), inguinal fat mass (+1.96-fold, $p < 0.01$), and liver weight (+0.47-fold, $p < 0.05$). Finally, the combination of maternal obesity and Mc4r gene deletion strongly influenced offspring phenotype when compared to the C_wt group, showing a marked increase in body mass (+0.48-fold, $p < 0.001$), inguinal fat mass (+2.47-fold, $p < 0.001$), and liver weight (+0.60-fold, $p < 0.001$). According to the hepatic morphology (Figure 1d), there was a mild steatosis in C_KO animals with no changes in the general liver architecture.

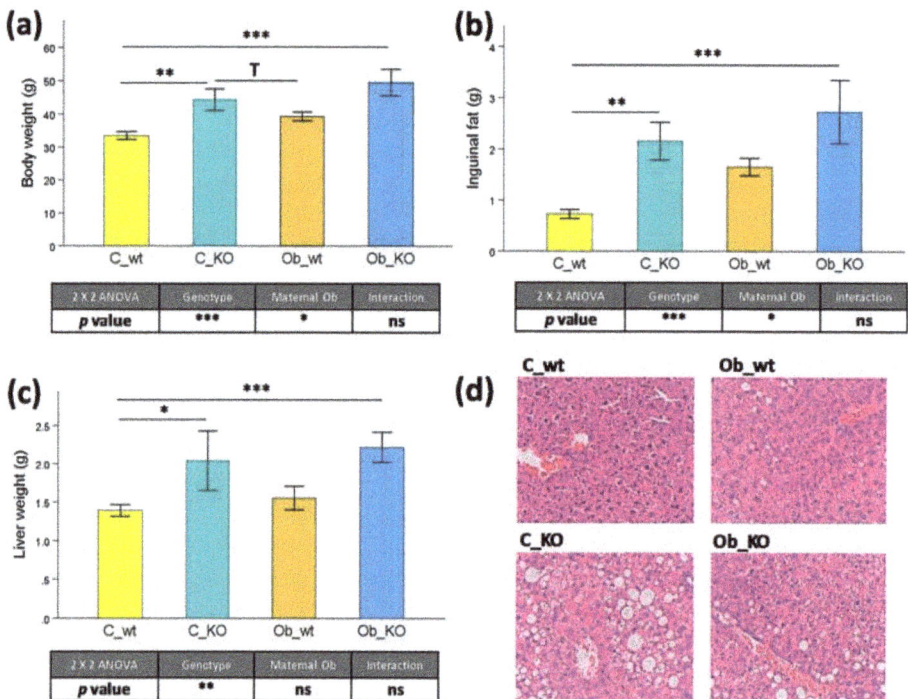

Figure 1. Phenotypic and histological parameters. Effects of Mc4r gene deletion and maternal obesogenic feeding on (**a**) body weight, (**b**) inguinal fat weight, (**c**) liver weight as well as (**d**) hepatic representative histological Hematoxylin and Eosin stained sections. Mc4r, melanocortin 4 receptor; C_wt, control wild type; C_KO, control knockout; Ob_wt, obese wild type; Ob_KO, obese knockout; n.s., non-significant; * $p < 0.05$; ** $p < 0.01$; *** $p < 0.001$; T $p > 0.05$ and $p < 0.1$.

3.2. Plasma Biochemical Features

Plasma glucose concentration (Figure 2a) showed a tendency to be increased (+0.38-fold, $p < 0.1$) in the offspring subjected to maternal obesity compared to control-fed dams. However, the absence of the Mc4r gene had no effect on this parameter. Furthermore, there was a decrease in plasma triglyceride concentration (Figure 2b) in offspring from obese mothers (−0.30-fold, $p < 0.05$) compared to the controls. However, this effect was mainly caused by the elevated TG levels in the C_KO group compared to the C_wt (+0.75-fold, $p < 0.05$), Ob_wt (+0.67-fold, $p < 0.1$), and Ob_KO groups (+1.05-fold, $p < 0.05$). With the hepatic transaminases (Figure 2c,d), there was a trend of increased ALT caused by maternal obesity (+0.74-fold, $p < 0.1$), which may be explained by the elevated concentrations of this transaminase in the Ob_KO with respect to the C_wt group (+1.68-fold, $p < 0.1$). Additionally, AST was markedly increased by the absence of the Mc4r gene in offspring from control-fed dams (+0.40-fold, $p < 0.05$) and partially increased in wild type animals subjected to maternal obesogenic feeding (+2.80-fold, $p < 0.1$).

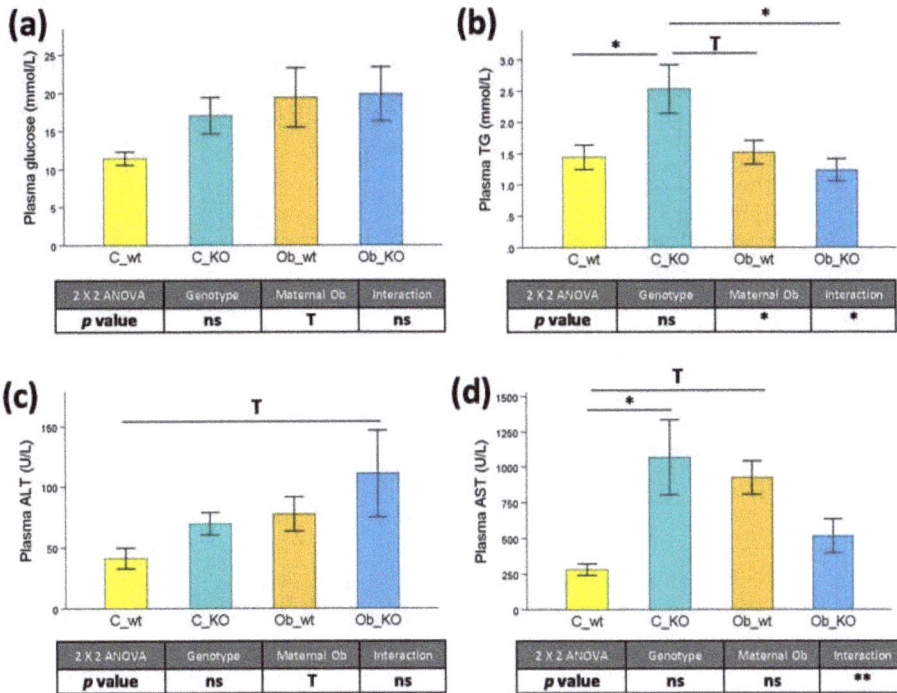

Figure 2. Plasma biochemical profile. Effects of Mc4r gene deletion and maternal obesogenic feeding on (**a**) Glucose, (**b**) Triglycerides, (**c**) ALT, and (**d**) AST concentrations. Mc4r, melanocortin 4 receptor; C_wt, control wild type; C_KO, control knockout; Ob_wt, obese wild type; Ob_KO, obese knockout; n.s., non-significant; * $p < 0.05$; T $p > 0.05$ and $p < 0.1$; TG: triglycerides; ALT: alanine aminotransferase; AST: aspartate aminotransferase.

3.3. Hepatic Transcriptomic Profile

We also studied the effect of maternal and obesogenic feeding on hepatic mRNA expression of genes associated with inflammation and immune mediation. As depicted in Figure 3, there was a marked effect of the genotype on the expression of α-SMA (+2.33-fold, $p < 0.05$) (Figure 3a), TNF-α (+1.85-fold, $p < 0.01$) (Figure 3b), Col-1α (+0.90-fold, $p < 0.05$) (Figure 3c), and TGF-β (+1.36-fold, $p < 0.01$) (Figure 3g) in KO mice independent of maternal feeding. On the other hand, maternal obesity compounded with the Mc4r KO genotype had decreased α-SMA (−0.73-fold, $p < 0.01$), TNF-α (−0.54-fold, $p < 0.05$), and IL6 (−0.56-fold, $p < 0.05$) (Figure 3d) hepatic mRNA levels in the offspring. These effects were mainly explained by the characteristic transcriptional profile of the C_KO group, which showed a consistent higher expression of α-SMA (from +3.19-fold to +6.61-fold, $p < 0.01$), TNF-α (from +1.59-fold to +3.37-fold, from $p < 0.05$ to $p < 0.01$,) and Col-1α (from +1.08-fold to +1.75-fold, from $p < 0.05$ to $p < 0.01$) with respect to the C_wt, Ob_wt, and Ob_KO groups.

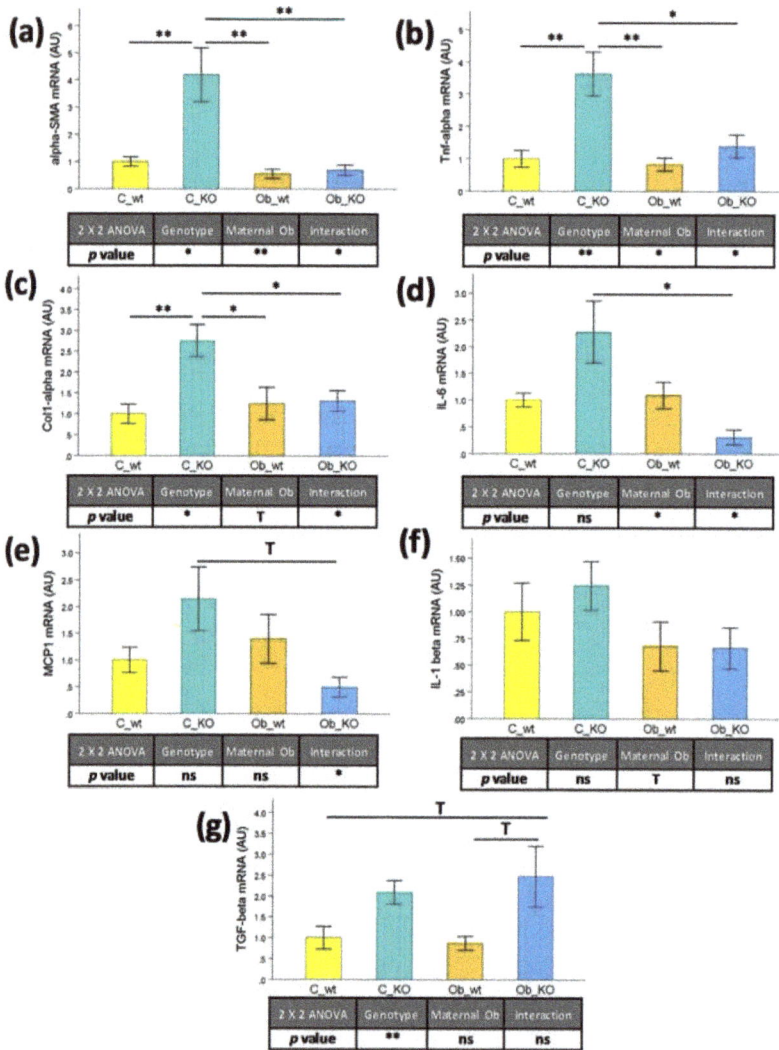

Figure 3. Liver mRNA levels by real-time qPCR. Effects of Mc4r gene deletion and maternal obesogenic feeding on (**a**) α-SMA, (**b**) TNF-α, (**c**) Col-1α, (**d**) IL6, (**e**) MCP1, (**f**) IL-1β, and (**g**) TGF-β expression. Mc4r, melanocortin 4 receptor; C_wt, control wild type; C_KO, control knockout; Ob_wt, obese wild type; Ob_KO, obese knockout; n.s., non-significant; * $p < 0.05$; ** $p < 0.01$; *** $p < 0.001$; T $p > 0.05$ and $p < 0.1$; α-SMA: alpha-smooth muscle actin; TNF-α: tumor necrosis factor alpha; Col-1α: collagen type I alpha 1; IL6: interleukin 6; MCP1: chemokine (C-C motif) ligand 2; IL-1β: interleukin 1 beta; TGF-β: transforming growth factor beta; AU: arbitrary units.

4. Discussion

Observations of human polymorphisms highlight the Mc4r gene as one of the key genes for understanding obesity risk and its associated comorbidities [16–18]. Mc4r is shown to be an energy balance modulator. Recently, a mouse study described that the activation of Mc4r reduces food intake and increases energy expenditure, preventing obesity-associated increased adiposity [25]. Additionally, the absence of Mc4r inhibits brown adipose tissue activity; therefore, the stimulation of the Mc4r pathway can be a potential target for increasing energy expenditure and accelerating weight loss [26]. Although melanocortin receptors are predominantly expressed in the brain, Mc4r is also known to be present in liver cells [27,28]. Therefore, the lack of this gene not only exerts systemic effects through the nervous system, but may also have a direct hepatic component. Evidence from liver regeneration after acute liver injury, where rats were subjected to partial hepatectomy, has shown that there is an overexpression of Mc4r in the hepatocytes [29]. Furthermore, NAFLD is the main hepatic manifestation of the metabolic syndrome, often accompanied by alterations in glucose homeostasis and waist circumference, and has been directly associated with genetic variations of Mc4r [30].

Itoh et al. reported that Mc4r_KO mice developed steatohepatitis when fed a high-fat diet, which was associated with an obese phenotype, insulin resistance, and dyslipidemia. Histologic analysis found enhanced inflammation, macrophage infiltration, hepatocyte ballooning, and, after a year of obesogenic feeding, hepatocellular carcinoma [31]. However, these results should be carefully compared with our experimental model because the direct, long-term effects of adult obesogenic feeding have greater impact on mice metabolism than maternally induced obesity. Probably due to this reason, our liver phenotypes did not present as marked of a proinflammatory stage. In the previous study, the authors also described obesity-related traits in Mc4r-silenced mice fed a control diet; similar to what we have showed here in our study, there was overexpression of TGF-β and Col-1α compared to wild type mice [31]. In vitro studies have also shown that the treatment of isolated liver cells with melanocortin agonists inhibits endotoxin-induced upregulation of the pro-inflammatory cytokines IL-6, IL1β, and TNF-α by Kupffer cells [28]. Thus, changes we described in liver gene expression in our Mcr4_ko offspring from control-fed dams may be the initial step for the apparition of later fibrotic markers in the liver, in addition to the detection of infiltrated macrophages and their polarization to different subpopulations. Indeed, there was a tendency to increase Mcp1 hepatic expression in these animals, which in turn may exacerbate, as we have shown, the hepatic expression of pro-inflammatory and immune system-related genes.

Maternal perinatal physiology and environmental insults predispose offspring to metabolic diseases in adult life. Thus, our previous studies with rodent models have demonstrated that a hypercaloric diet enriched in fat and simple sugars during peri-conception, pregnancy, and/or lactation periods affects offspring phenotype with increased body weights, visceral fat, liver and pancreas weights, plus a parallel accumulation of lipids in visceral organs [11–13,32]. Our previous results showed that maternal obesity programs development of a dysmetabolic and NAFLD phenotype, which is critically dependent on the early postnatal period involving alteration of hypothalamic appetite nuclei signaling by maternal breast milk and neonatal adipose tissue-derived leptin [12,32]. Furthermore, in a perinatal model of mice lacking the Mc4r gene, we demonstrated that maternal obesity (apparently through neonatal leptin exposure) permanently resets the responsiveness of the central sympathetic nervous system, specifically via the hypothalamic paraventricular nucleus melanocortin system, to initiate hypertension [23]. Moreover, in that study, we found increased food intake and leptin plasma levels influenced by maternal obesity and by the lack of the Mc4r gene. Surprisingly, in the current study, we found that the offspring phenotype was more influenced by the lack of the Mc4r gene, rather than by maternal obesity. Indeed, although maternal obesogenic feeding was associated with higher body and adipose depots, there was a lack of steatosis in liver histological samples. This may be partially explained by the age of these animals, as in our previous murine studies with similar feeding protocol, the steatotic effect induced by maternal obesity was well defined at 12 months and vague at 6 months of age [12,33]. Indeed, the age of these animals is directly proportional to their intra-abdominal adipose tissue accumulation and, therefore, to the abnormal fat infiltration in visceral organs. Interestingly, we did not find an additional effect of the lack of Mc4r on the maternal obesogenic feeding offspring. We may hypothesize that the molecular mechanisms affecting obesity and the associated liver fat accumulation and damage may be common for maternal-associated programming of obesity and for Mc4r pathways. For example,

Nutrients **2017**, *9*, 1041

there is appetite regulation in both situations as well as a decrease in energy expenditure induced by maternal obesity and Mc4r blockage [23,26]. Moreover, a study in rats with high-fat diet-induced maternal obesity recently described a downregulation of hypothalamic Mc4r mRNA expression at weaning in the offspring from obese dams [34]. Others have replicated these results, proposing an epigenetic mechanism for the decrease in Mc4r expression in the offspring of obese rats due to histone acetylation in the Mc4r promoter region, which may also be associated with the thyroid hormone receptor-β, a transcription inhibitor for this gene [21]. This research group has also described how other Mc4r-related genes involved in obesity through appetite regulation such as Pomc may be epigenetically regulated in the offspring because of maternal obesity [35,36].

As a limitation of this study, the use of animal models and, more specifically, knockout and perinatally-based designs makes the translation of the findings to the general population difficult. However, besides the ethical considerations of human interventions during pregnancy, rodent models shorten the experimental time, and also allow studying the effects during offspring adult life. Furthermore, the similar genetic and physiological background to humans and the control of external insults and confounding factors make necessary to perform experimental animal models in this field. Furthermore, although phenotypically the offspring were influenced by maternal obesity, from a metabolic and transcriptomic point of view the effect became partially diluted, which differs with our previously standardized developmental programing protocols [11–13,33,37]. This may be due to the Mc4r gene silencing; however, the lack of difference in some of the variables only due to maternal obesogenic feeding may be also due to a limited number of animals and the wide intra group differences. Finally, the lack of some interesting plasma and hepatic biochemical markers such as liver triglyceride content or food consumption may be a limitation for the explanation of the findings described in the current study.

5. Conclusions

In conclusion, these results emphasized the importance of the melanocortin system as a target for the development of new therapeutic tools against obesity and its associated implications in liver metabolism through obesogenic feeding and developmental programming. We showed that dietary changes during the perinatal period may follow an adaptive response of the offspring to be predisposed to long-term changes in metabolism and physiology. Although the lack of Mc4r induced an increase in body, fat, and liver weights, the interaction with maternal perinatal obesity suggested a protective effect in the Mc4r_ko mice. Thus, offspring from obese mothers did not show liver steatosis and presented lower hepatic expression of proinflammatory and profibrogenic genes. This interaction should warrant further research in this model, given the potential to elucidate new mechanistic pathways implicated in the developmental programing of obesity and NAFLD.

Acknowledgments: This work was supported by British Heart Foundation Grant FS/10/003/28163, Biotechnology and Biological Sciences Research Council Grant BBD5231861, Welcome Trust and Obesity Action Campaign (http://www.obesityac.org). This work was also supported by the European Social Fund and European Regional Development Fund-Project MAGNET (No. CZ.02.1.01/0.0/0.0/15 003/0000492) to Manlio Vinciguerra.

Author Contributions: A.M.S., P.D.T., J.A.O., P.C. and M.V. conceived and designed the experiments; P.C., A.M.S., J.P., M.N. and N.M.B. performed the experiments; P.C. analyzed the data; P.C., J.L., A.M.S., V.N., M.V. and J.A.O. wrote the paper. All authors participated in the manuscript preparation and approved the final version of the manuscript.

Conflicts of Interest: The authors declare no conflicts of interest.

References

1. Gonzalez-Muniesa, P.; Martinez-Gonzalez, M.A.; Hu, F.B.; Despres, J.P.; Matsuzawa, Y.; Loos, R.J.F.; Moreno, L.A.; Bray, G.A.; Martinez, J.A. Obesity. *Nat. Rev. Dis. Primers* **2017**, *3*, 17034. [CrossRef] [PubMed]
2. World Health Organization. Obesity and Overweight. Available online: Http://www.who.int/mediacentre/factsheets/fs311/en/ (accessed on 19 July 2017).

3. Fontaine, K.R.; Redden, D.T.; Wang, C.; Westfall, A.O.; Allison, D.B. Years of life lost due to obesity. *JAMA* **2003**, *289*, 187–193. [CrossRef] [PubMed]
4. Wang, Y.C.; McPherson, K.; Marsh, T.; Gortmaker, S.L.; Brown, M. Health and economic burden of the projected obesity trends in the USA and the UK. *Lancet* **2011**, *378*, 815–825. [CrossRef]
5. Shalitin, S.; Battelino, T.; Moreno, L.A. Obesity, Metabolic Syndrome and Nutrition. *World Rev. Nutr. Diet.* **2016**, *114*, 21–49. [PubMed]
6. Dietrich, P.; Hellerbrand, C. Non-alcoholic fatty liver disease, obesity and the metabolic syndrome. *Best Pract. Res. Clin. Gastroenterol.* **2014**, *28*, 637–653. [CrossRef] [PubMed]
7. Temple, J.L.; Cordero, P.; Li, J.; Nguyen, V.; Oben, J.A. A Guide to Non-Alcoholic Fatty Liver Disease in Childhood and Adolescence. *Int. J. Mol. Sci.* **2016**, *17*, 947. [CrossRef] [PubMed]
8. Vinciguerra, M. Protein intake, chronic liver diseases, and hepatocellular carcinoma. *Hepatology* **2015**, *61*, 730. [CrossRef] [PubMed]
9. Poston, L.; Caleyachetty, R.; Cnattingius, S.; Corvalan, C.; Uauy, R.; Herring, S.; Gillman, M.W. Preconceptional and maternal obesity: Epidemiology and health consequences. *Lancet Diabetes Endocrinol.* **2016**, *4*, 1025–1036. [CrossRef]
10. Martinez, J.A.; Cordero, P.; Campion, J.; Milagro, F.I. Interplay of early-life nutritional programming on obesity, inflammation and epigenetic outcomes. *Proc. Nutr. Soc.* **2012**, *71*, 276–283. [CrossRef] [PubMed]
11. Mouralidarane, A.; Soeda, J.; Sugden, D.; Bocianowska, A.; Carter, R.; Ray, S.; Saraswati, R.; Cordero, P.; Novelli, M.; Fusai, G.; et al. Maternal obesity programs offspring Non-Alcoholic Fatty Liver Disease through disruption of 24-h rhythms in mice. *Int. J. Obes.* **2015**, *39*, 1339–1348. [CrossRef] [PubMed]
12. Oben, J.A.; Mouralidarane, A.; Samuelsson, A.M.; Matthews, P.J.; Morgan, M.L.; McKee, C.; Soeda, J.; Fernandez-Twinn, D.S.; Martin-Gronert, M.S.; Ozanne, S.E.; et al. Maternal obesity during pregnancy and lactation programs the development of offspring Non-Alcoholic Fatty Liver Disease in mice. *J. Hepatol.* **2010**, *52*, 913–920. [CrossRef] [PubMed]
13. Soeda, J.; Cordero, P.; Li, J.; Mouralidarane, A.; Asilmaz, E.; Ray, S.; Nguyen, V.; Carter, R.; Novelli, M.; Vinciguerra, M.; et al. Hepatic rhythmicity of endoplasmic reticulum stress is disrupted in perinatal and adult mice models of high-fat diet-induced obesity. *Int. J. Food Sci. Nutr.* **2017**, *68*, 455–466. [CrossRef] [PubMed]
14. Pazienza, V.; Panebianco, C.; Rappa, F.; Memoli, D.; Borghesan, M.; Cannito, S.; Oji, A.; Mazza, G.; Tamburrino, D.; Fusai, G.; et al. Histone macroH2A1.2 promotes metabolic health and leanness by inhibiting adipogenesis. *Epigenet. Chromatin* **2016**, *9*, 45. [CrossRef] [PubMed]
15. Goni, L.; Milagro, F.I.; Cuervo, M.; Martinez, J.A. Single-nucleotide polymorphisms and DNA methylation markers associated with central obesity and regulation of body weight. *Nutr. Rev.* **2014**, *72*, 673–690. [CrossRef] [PubMed]
16. Loos, R.J.; Lindgren, C.M.; Li, S.; Wheeler, E.; Zhao, J.H.; Prokopenko, I.; Inouye, M.; Freathy, R.M.; Attwood, A.P.; Beckmann, J.S.; et al. Common variants near MC4R are associated with fat mass, weight and risk of obesity. *Nat. Genet.* **2008**, *40*, 768–775. [CrossRef] [PubMed]
17. Xi, B.; Chandak, G.R.; Shen, Y.; Wang, Q.; Zhou, D. Association between common polymorphism near the MC4R gene and obesity risk: A systematic review and meta-analysis. *PLoS ONE* **2012**, *7*, e45731. [CrossRef] [PubMed]
18. Xi, B.; Takeuchi, F.; Chandak, G.R.; Kato, N.; Pan, H.W.; Consortium, A.-T.D.; Zhou, D.H.; Pan, H.Y.; Mi, J. Common polymorphism near the MC4R gene is associated with type 2 diabetes: Data from a meta-analysis of 123,373 individuals. *Diabetologia* **2012**, *55*, 2660–2666. [CrossRef] [PubMed]
19. Krashes, M.J.; Lowell, B.B.; Garfield, A.S. Melanocortin-4 receptor-regulated energy homeostasis. *Nat. Neurosci.* **2016**, *19*, 206–219. [CrossRef] [PubMed]
20. Samuelsson, A.M. New perspectives on the origin of hypertension; the role of the hypothalamic melanocortin system. *Exp. Physiol.* **2014**, *99*, 1110–1115. [CrossRef] [PubMed]
21. Tabachnik, T.; Kisliouk, T.; Marco, A.; Meiri, N.; Weller, A. Thyroid Hormone-Dependent Epigenetic Regulation of Melanocortin 4 Receptor Levels in Female Offspring of Obese Rats. *Endocrinology* **2017**, *158*, 842–851. [CrossRef] [PubMed]
22. Pindjakova, J.; Sartini, C.; Lo Re, O.; Rappa, F.; Coupe, B.; Lelouvier, B.; Pazienza, V.; Vinciguerra, M. Gut Dysbiosis and Adaptive Immune Response in Diet-induced Obesity vs. Systemic Inflammation. *Front. Microbiol.* **2017**, *8*, 1157. [CrossRef] [PubMed]

23. Samuelsson, A.S.; Mullier, A.; Maicas, N.; Oosterhuis, N.R.; Eun Bae, S.; Novoselova, T.V.; Chan, L.F.; Pombo, J.M.; Taylor, P.D.; Joles, J.A.; et al. Central role for melanocortin-4 receptors in offspring hypertension arising from maternal obesity. *Proc. Natl. Acad. Sci. USA* **2016**, *113*, 12298–12303. [CrossRef] [PubMed]

24. Rappa, F.; Greco, A.; Podrini, C.; Cappello, F.; Foti, M.; Bourgoin, L.; Peyrou, M.; Marino, A.; Scibetta, N.; Williams, R.; et al. Immunopositivity for histone macroH2A1 isoforms marks steatosis-associated hepatocellular carcinoma. *PLoS ONE* **2013**, *8*, e54458. [CrossRef]

25. Balthasar, N.; Dalgaard, L.T.; Lee, C.E.; Yu, J.; Funahashi, H.; Williams, T.; Ferreira, M.; Tang, V.; McGovern, R.A.; Kenny, C.D.; et al. Divergence of melanocortin pathways in the control of food intake and energy expenditure. *Cell* **2005**, *123*, 493–505. [CrossRef] [PubMed]

26. Kooijman, S.; Boon, M.R.; Parlevliet, E.T.; Geerling, J.J.; van de Pol, V.; Romijn, J.A.; Havekes, L.M.; Meurs, I.; Rensen, P.C. Inhibition of the central melanocortin system decreases brown adipose tissue activity. *J. Lipid Res.* **2014**, *55*, 2022–2032. [CrossRef] [PubMed]

27. Barb, C.R.; Hausman, G.J.; Rekaya, R.; Lents, C.A.; Lkhagvadorj, S.; Qu, L.; Cai, W.; Couture, O.P.; Anderson, L.L.; Dekkers, J.C.; et al. Gene expression in hypothalamus, liver, and adipose tissues and food intake response to melanocortin-4 receptor agonist in pigs expressing melanocortin-4 receptor mutations. *Physiol. Genomics* **2010**, *41*, 254–268. [CrossRef] [PubMed]

28. Malik, I.A.; Triebel, J.; Posselt, J.; Khan, S.; Ramadori, P.; Raddatz, D.; Ramadori, G. Melanocortin receptors in rat liver cells: Change of gene expression and intracellular localization during acute-phase response. *Histochem. Cell Biol.* **2012**, *137*, 279–291. [CrossRef] [PubMed]

29. Xu, M.; Alwahsh, S.M.; Ramadori, G.; Kollmar, O.; Slotta, J.E. Upregulation of hepatic melanocortin 4 receptor during rat liver regeneration. *J. Surg. Res.* **2016**, *203*, 222–230. [CrossRef] [PubMed]

30. Chambers, J.C.; Elliott, P.; Zabaneh, D.; Zhang, W.; Li, Y.; Froguel, P.; Balding, D.; Scott, J.; Kooner, J.S. Common genetic variation near MC4R is associated with waist circumference and insulin resistance. *Nat. Genet.* **2008**, *40*, 716–718. [CrossRef] [PubMed]

31. Itoh, M.; Suganami, T.; Nakagawa, N.; Tanaka, M.; Yamamoto, Y.; Kamei, Y.; Terai, S.; Sakaida, I.; Ogawa, Y. Melanocortin 4 receptor-deficient mice as a novel Mouse model of nonalcoholic steatohepatitis. *Am. J. Pathol.* **2011**, *179*, 2454–2463. [CrossRef] [PubMed]

32. Soeda, J.; Mouralidarane, A.; Cordero, P.; Li, J.; Nguyen, V.; Carter, R.; Kapur, S.R.; Pombo, J.; Poston, L.; Taylor, P.D.; et al. Maternal obesity alters endoplasmic reticulum homeostasis in offspring pancreas. *J. Physiol. Biochem.* **2016**, *72*, 281–291. [CrossRef] [PubMed]

33. Mouralidarane, A.; Soeda, J.; Visconti-Pugmire, C.; Samuelsson, A.M.; Pombo, J.; Maragkoudaki, X.; Butt, A.; Saraswati, R.; Novelli, M.; Fusai, G.; et al. Maternal obesity programs offspring nonalcoholic fatty liver disease by innate immune dysfunction in mice. *Hepatology* **2013**, *58*, 128–138. [CrossRef] [PubMed]

34. Nguyen, L.T.; Saad, S.; Tan, Y.; Pollock, C.; Chen, H. Maternal high-fat diet induces metabolic stress response disorders in offspring hypothalamus. *J. Mol. Endocrinol.* **2017**, *59*, 81–92. [CrossRef] [PubMed]

35. Marco, A.; Kisliouk, T.; Tabachnik, T.; Meiri, N.; Weller, A. Overweight and CpG methylation of the Pomc promoter in offspring of high-fat-diet-fed dams are not "reprogrammed" by regular chow diet in rats. *FASEB J.* **2014**, *28*, 4148–4157. [CrossRef] [PubMed]

36. Marco, A.; Kisliouk, T.; Tabachnik, T.; Weller, A.; Meiri, N. DNA CpG Methylation (5-Methylcytosine) and Its Derivative (5-Hydroxymethylcytosine) Alter Histone Posttranslational Modifications at the Pomc Promoter, Affecting the Impact of Perinatal Diet on Leanness and Obesity of the Offspring. *Diabetes* **2016**, *65*, 2258–2267. [CrossRef] [PubMed]

37. Oben, J.A.; Patel, T.; Mouralidarane, A.; Samuelsson, A.M.; Matthews, P.; Pombo, J.; Morgan, M.; McKee, C.; Soeda, J.; Novelli, M.; et al. Maternal obesity programmes offspring development of non-alcoholic fatty pancreas disease. *Biochem. Biophys. Res. Commun.* **2010**, *394*, 24–28. [CrossRef] [PubMed]

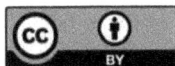

nutrients

MDPI

Review

Precision Nutrition for Targeting Lipid Metabolism in Colorectal Cancer

Cristina Aguirre-Portolés [†], Lara P. Fernández [†] and Ana Ramírez de Molina *

Molecular Oncology and Nutritional Genomics of Cancer Group, IMDEA Food Institute, CEI UAM + CSIC, Carretera de Cantoblanco 8, E-28049 Madrid, Spain; cristina.aguirre@imdea.org (C.A.-P.); lara.fernandez@imdea.org (L.P.F.)
* Correspondence: ana.ramirez@imdea.org; Tel.: +34-672-134-921
† These authors contributed equally to this work.

Received: 31 August 2017; Accepted: 25 September 2017; Published: 28 September 2017

Abstract: Cancer is a multistage and multifactorial condition with genetic and environmental factors modulating tumorogenesis and disease progression. Nevertheless, cancer is preventable, as one third of cancer deaths could be avoided by modifying key risk factors. Nutrients can directly affect fundamental cellular processes and are considered among the most important risk factors in colorectal cancer (CRC). Red and processed meat, poultry consumption, fiber, and folate are the best-known diet components that interact with colorectal cancer susceptibility. In addition, the direct association of an unhealthy diet with obesity and dysbiosis opens new routes in the understanding of how daily diet nutrients could influence cancer prognosis. In the "omics" era, traditional nutrition has been naturally evolved to precision nutrition where technical developments have contributed to a more accurate discipline. In this sense, genomic and transcriptomic studies have been extensively used in precision nutrition approaches. However, the relation between CRC carcinogenesis and nutrition factors is more complex than originally expected. Together with classical diet-nutrition-related genes, nowadays, lipid-metabolism-related genes have acquired relevant interest in precision nutrition studies. Lipids regulate very diverse cellular processes from ATP synthesis and the activation of essential cell-signaling pathways to membrane organization and plasticity. Therefore, a wide range of tumorogenic steps can be influenced by lipid metabolism, both in primary tumours and distal metastasis. The extent to which genetic variants, together with the intake of specific dietary components, affect the risk of CRC is currently under investigation, and new therapeutic or preventive applications must be explored in CRC models. In this review, we will go in depth into the study of co-occurring events, which orchestrate CRC tumorogenesis and are essential for the evolution of precision nutrition paradigms. Likewise, we will discuss the application of precision nutrition approaches to target lipid metabolism in CRC.

Keywords: precision nutrition; lipid metabolism; colorectal cancer; diet; genomics; transcriptomics; SNPs; obesity; microbiota

1. Introduction

Cancer is the second leading cause of mortality and is responsible for one sixth of deaths worldwide. During 2015, there were 17.5 million cancer cases and 8.8 million patient's deaths [1]. Particularly, colorectal cancer (CRC) ranks as the third leading cause of cancer-related deaths (data from The World Health Organization; WHO). In the course of this multifactorial condition, a cascade of alterations takes place, modifying the expression of both tumor suppressor genes and oncogenes. Together with this, when compared to quiescent cells, proliferating cells present a distinct metabolism characterized by high rates of glycolysis, lactate production, and the biosynthesis of lipids and other macromolecules. During the last decade, many laboratories focused their interest on understanding this metabolic switch that occurs during tumorogenesis [2,3]. In fact, several studies have demonstrated the importance of lipid metabolism regulation in the promotion of migration [4], invasion [5,6], and angiogenesis [7,8], three basic steps during metastasis [9]. Regarding CRC, key enzymes involved in lipid-metabolic pathways have been found differentially expressed in normal and tumoral tissues. Some of them were associated with cancer survival and were individually proposed as prognosis markers [6,10,11]. Furthermore, one of the transcriptomic consensus molecular subtypes (CMS) of CRC described by Guinney and colleagues [12], the "metabolic subtype 3" (CMS3), exhibits a clear enrichment for multiple metabolism signatures along with KRAS (Kirsten Rat Sarcoma Viral Oncogene Homolog)-activating mutations that have been described as inducing metabolic reprogramming [12].

The majority of the primary tumours initially respond to chemotherapy and regress, but frequently and due to minimal residual diseases, they relapse and are no longer sensitive to therapy [13]. The genetic alterations that directly affect the genome of tumoral cells before diagnosis and during treatment are the most studied factors implicated in resistance acquisition. However, not only gene expression but the interaction between genetic factors and environment plays a crucial role in the causality of cancer progression [14,15] (Figure 1). In this direction, epigenetic changes that could be originated by environmental factors can provide tumour heterogeneity and an ineffective response to chemotherapy [16].

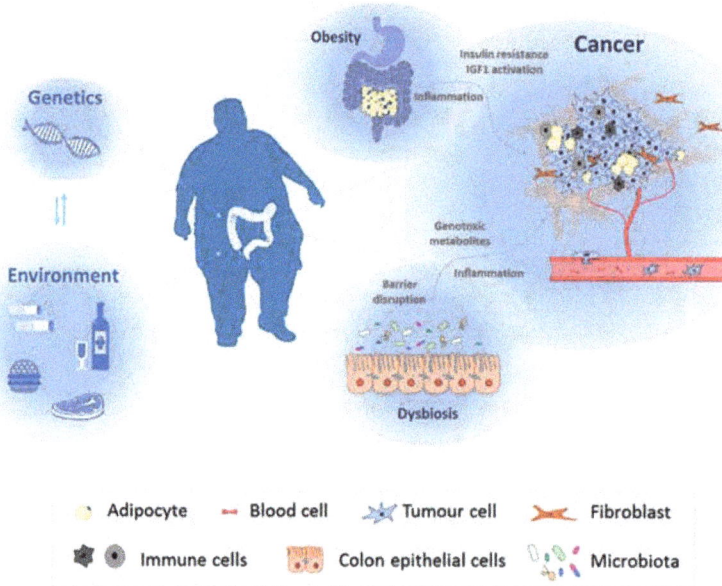

Figure 1. Colorectal cancer malignancy relays on genetic factors, environmental factors, and their interaction between each other. Together with patient genome, environmental factors associated with lifestyle (alcohol consumption, smoking, unhealthy diet, or reduced physical activity) influence colorectal cancer initiation and malignancy. They can alter specific target tissues or affect human physiology, giving rise to pathologies that can promote tumour progression such as obesity or dysbiosis.

Tumours cannot be considered as simple bulks of cells with an altered cell cycle control. Neoplastic cells interact with each other and, more importantly, with the healthy tissue that surrounds them, the tumour microenvironment (TME) [17]. Thus, during the neoplastic progression, a co-evolution takes place between malignant cells, the extracellular matrix (ECM), cancer associated fibroblasts (CAF), the immune system, and the vascular endothelial cells. Tumor heterogeneity not only relies on intratumoral variability derived from Darwinian evolution [18], but also on the different types of immune cells that infiltrate the primary tumor, the plasticity of the CAFs and the tissue of origin responsible for the neo-vascularization [19]. Distant metastases are responsible for 90% of cancer deaths, making it essential to consider its phenotypic variability in cancer malignancy (reviewed by Marusyk et al. [18]). Based on this intra-tumoral, TME and distant metastasis heterogeneity, basic research together with translation medicine and oncologists in the clinic, are gathering strength to identify patient subpopulations and designing new targeted therapies for personalized treatment.

Current evidence demonstrates that one third of cancer deaths could be prevented by modifying key risk factors such as smoking, assessment of infection-related risk factors, or alcohol consumption. Moreover, physical activity, nutrition, and diet are also considered among the most important environmental risk factors for cancer development due to their association with obesity (Figure 1). Nutrient components can modulate cancer progression or even the risk of developing this disease by regulating, directly or indirectly, gene expression.

In the early seventies, red meat and fat consumption were already proposed to increase the incidence and mortality of colon cancer [20,21]. Furthermore, in the last decade, several studies based on meta-analyses demonstrated a link between obesity, risk of cancer, and disease prognosis [22].

The recent development of powerful "omics" technologies has opened new avenues towards nutritional sciences. The genomics, transcriptomics, proteomics, metabolomics, and lipidomics approaches lead to a new vision of the delivery of nutritional advice: the precision nutrition. Current views on precision nutrition consider this discipline at three stages: (1) conventional nutrition based on general guidelines for population groups; (2) individualized nutrition based on phenotypic information; and (3) genotype-directed nutrition focused on gene variation and its consequences [23].

Single nucleotide polymorphisms (SNPs) are the most common forms of sequence variation in the human genome [24]. The analysis of SNPs is a well-known tool for precision nutrition, and the recent development of next generation sequencing (NGS) techniques is highly improving genetic variation studies [23,25]. Likewise, transcriptomic studies and RNA sequencing analyses will also refine precision nutrition. So far, both genomic and transcriptomic studies have been extensively used in precision nutrition approaches. Finally, the future technical development of proteomics, metabolomics, and lipidomics will complete the full nutritional landscape [23].

In this review, we will discuss co-occurring events that take place in the course of tumorogenesis and that were essential for the evolution of precision nutrition paradigms. The importance of new "omics" technologies such as genomics and transcriptomics and their application to target lipid metabolism will also be detailed.

2. Lipid Metabolism, Diet and Colorectal Cancer

Metabolic alterations encountered in tumors are well described and considered as a hallmark of cancer [26]. Taking into account the importance of lipids at different levels in cellular physiology, alterations in fatty acids (FA) synthesis and lipid metabolism can interfere with very diverse cellular processes that go from plasmatic and organelles membrane organization and plasticity [27,28], substrate supply for ATP synthesis [29], to cell signaling activation [30].

It is important to mention that these alterations do not only affect the primary tumour in a cell autonomous manner, the exogenous lipids synthetized by tumour microenvironment could also influence malignancy [31–34]. For example, pro-inflammatory eicosanoids can directly promote cell proliferation, apoptosis, migration and invasion. More importantly, they are also associated with angiogenesis promotion [35].

Regarding the primary tumour, alterations in lipid metabolism-related genes are able to promote migration and invasion. TGFβ was shown to promote epithelial-to-mesenchymal transition (EMT) together with a lipogenesis suppression, favoring energy production [4]. While sphingosine 1-phosphate plays an inhibitory role, lysophosphatidic acid (LPA) is able to regulate Membrane-type matrix metalloproteinase 1 (MT1-MMP) and promote invasion [5]. In addition to that, a recent publication uncovered ACSL1 (an isozyme of Acyl-CoA synthetase) and SCD (Stearoyl-CoA-desaturase 1) as part of a metabolic network that increased energetic efficiency in CRC-derived cells together with the promotion of migratory and invasive capacity [6]. Moreover, both Sphingosine 1-phosphate signaling pathways [36] and CPT1A (Carnitine Palmitoyltransferase 1A), a rate-controlling enzyme in fatty acid β-oxidation [8], were associated with lymphangiogenesis.

Several categories of lipids have been studied regarding its association with CRC. Fatty acids are the building blocks for the formation of more complex lipids and they have also been associated with colorectal tumorogenesis. Importantly, not all FAs behave in the same direction. First, plasma concentration of saturated FA (SFA) as well as essential FAs were found to be significantly decreased in CRC patients when compared to healthy controls [37]. Moreover, while ω3 is associated with a protective role in CRC [38–40], other types of polyunsaturated FA (PUFA), ω6 present opposite effects [41]. Regarding dietary FAs, while intake of unsaturated FA (UFA) may be beneficial for health [42], SFAs were associated with tumorogenesis [41,43]. The steroids are essential components of membrane lipids and can act as signaling molecules. Very low-density lipoprotein cholesterol (VLDL) was shown to be positively correlated with adenoma frequency in colon. Importantly, triglycerides (TG) and LDL were associated CRC prognosis, as its significantly increased levels were found in patients with distant metastasis. Cholesterol is present in high-fat diets and, together with red meat and total fat, its consumption is strongly associated with colorectal tumorogenesis [44]. Other essential structural components of the cellular membrane are the sphingolipids. Among them, ceramide is known as a chemopreventive agent; in fact, used in combination with tamoxifen, it is able to arrest cell cycle progression and promote apoptosis [45]. Glycerophospholipids are the major lipid components of the cellular membrane. The expression of cyclic phosphatidic acid (cPA) was found to impair metastasis and invasion of cancer cells [46]. However, phosphatidylcholine (PC) was found significantly increased in CRC-derived cells [47]. The knowledge of how glycerolipids, key molecules for the synthesis of membrane lipids, and TG could influence CRC remains shallow, but a protective role was described for 1-*O*-octadecyl 2-*O*-methyl-sn-glycerophosphocholine [48].

In addition to genetic alterations in genes that regulate lipid metabolism, affecting directly colorectal tumorogenesis, an unhealthy diet would be able to modify the physiology of the patients, giving rise to comorbidities that promote tumour growth and invasion of distant tissues [49].

2.1. Diet, Obesity, and CRC

Obesity can appear as a result of an unbalanced diet where the caloric intake is higher than the energy expenditure. This pathology is defined by an excessive adipose tissue accumulation that associates with a risk to the health of an individual [22]. Importantly, the worldwide prevalence of this pathology has doubled between 1980 and 2014. Nowadays, 13% of the overall adult population worldwide suffer from obesity. Importantly, in 2014, 41 million children under the age of 5 years were overweight or obese (WHO) and, by 2030, the number of overweight and obese adults is projected to reach 2.16 billion. Therefore, an unquestionable cause of concern is the constant increase in childhood obesity. The dietary patterns of children from low- and middle-income countries together with the low levels of physical activity gave rise to a sharp increase in obesity (WHO) [17]. This pathology has been implicated in the development of cardiovascular diseases and type-2 diabetes [50] as well as in the initiation and dissemination of several types of cancer [51]. In fact, overall risk of death from cancer is 1.5–1.6-fold higher in men and women with a BMI > 40 kg/m [52]. The excess of visceral fat provokes alterations in the cellular composition of the adipose tissue and promotes the increased malignancy of tumors that develop in a microenvironment rich in adipocytes like breast, ovary, or colon tumors [53]. The main types of cancer whose increased risk has been associated with obesity are: prostate [54], postmenstrual endometrial [55] and breast [51], ovary [56], bladder [57], liver [58], colon [22], pancreas [51], esophageal [59], gallbladder [60], kidney [61], and thyroid cancer [62].

During the last decade, in parallel with a decreased physical activity, the caloric intake has constantly increased. The main environmental factors that interact with genetic variants and contribute to obesity are sugar-sweetened beverages, fried food consumption, and sedentary lifestyle [63]. As a direct consequence of this energetic imbalance, a metabolic shift takes place in the body, giving rise to hypertrophy and hyperplasia of the adipose tissue.

In the course of obesity, the excess of adipocytes accumulates in locations not classically associated with adipose tissue. This increase in systemic ectopic fat shows positive correlation with several types of cancer, CRC among them [64]. Currently, there are two wide-spread hypotheses describing the underlying molecular mechanisms that link obesity and colorectal cancer: (1) insulin resistance and the activation of insulin growth factor-1 (IGF1). A large volume of epidemiological studies as well as meta-analysis, driven independently by several groups, demonstrated that the total levels of this growth factor correlates to several types of cancer [62,65–67]; (2) systemic inflammation due to hypertrophy of adipose tissue [68] (Figure 1).

Both overweight and obesity are largely preventable, but social education for health promotion, the individual responsibility, as well as the food industry, together with basic research, need to team up to face this urgent global health challenge.

2.2. Diet, Dysbiosis, and Colorectal Cancer

The term human microbiota refers to the assemblage of microorganisms (bacteria, archaea, or lower eukaryotes) present in a defined environment, such as the gastrointestinal tract. It consists of the 10–100 trillion symbiotic microbial cells harbored by each person, primarily bacteria in the gut. A symbiotic association with microbiota exists in healthy individuals, offering protection from invading pathogens and preventing tumorogenesis (eubiosis). The pathological condition developed when the gut microbiota homeostasis is disturbed, due to an imbalance in the flora, changes in functional composition and metabolic activities or changes if their local distribution is defined as dysbiosis [69]. This pathological scenario is characterized by a decrease in microbial diversity and an increase in pro-inflammatory species. This imbalanced microbiota is unable to protect from pathogenic organisms that could successfully be established and trigger inflammation, as well as producing genotoxins and carcinogenic microbial metabolites (Figure 1).

Moreover, during obesity and along with its comorbidities, the composition of gut microbiota and the features of the intestinal epithelium are altered, affecting its barrier function. Among other diseases, microbial dysbiosis was associated with colorectal carcinogenesis and gastric and esophageal cancers [70,71]. Several diet components are known to influence microbiota and protect or cause detrimental metabolites that negatively affect the digestive tract. Therefore, CRC can be influenced not just by specific pathogens in the patient but also by the metabolic output of the entire microbiota [72]. Both high fat diets as well as low fiber intake can lead to dysbiosis [72]. Low-carbohydrate intake or an extreme change from vegetable-based to animal-based diet would drastically affect microbiota composition. In fact, variations in regular diet generate specific profiles of microbiota: the pathogens present in the microbiota of an individual with high consumption of fiber would be different if we compared them with the composition of patients with high protein and fat intake [72]. These profiles, indeed, determine CRC incidence in different populations due to changes in dietary patterns, as they occur when rural native Africans are compared with African Americans [73].

The etiology of CRC is partially dependent on microflora and diet, so nowadays there is increasing interest in the use of probiotics to modulate gut microbiota [74]. The Food and Agriculture Organization of the United Nations (FAO) defines "probiotics" as the only bacterial group classified as functional food which is intended to be consumed as part of a normal diet and that delivers biologically active components that have the potential of disease risk reduction. The exact mechanisms underlying this positive association between probiotics and health are not fully understood, but there are consistent epidemiological and experimental data supporting its positive association with CRC prevention and treatment [75]. There are several proposed effects that would explain the anticancer effects of probiotics: (1) lowering of intestinal pH; (2) inactivation of carcinogens; (3) modulation of immune cells populations; (4) modulation of the physical barrier by altering the intestinal microflora;

(5) modulation of apoptosis and cell proliferation [74]. Epidemiological studies have shown that the composition of CRC patients microbiota is different to the one present in healthy population [76]. Taking into account the effectiveness of probiotics in modulating microbiome composition, the design of microbiota-targeting therapies is now considered as a feasible strategy in the clinic, both as a preventive and a therapeutic approach [77].

3. Nutrition and Colorectal Cancer

Although the 5-year survival after CRC diagnosis when metastasis is already present has improved in the last decade, this decrease is still lower than 3% [78]. The sequential administration of three different chemotherapeutic drugs, along with vascular endothelial growth factor (VEGF) and epithelial growth factor receptor (EGFR) inhibitors, allowed the median survival of the patients to reach 30 months [79].

In most cases, early detection allows tumors to be successfully removed by surgery and increases treatment efficiency. Nowadays, great part of survival improvements rely on CRC screening programs that allow early diagnosis [12]. Thus, the main challenge in the clinic nowadays is the understanding and characterization of the CRC inter and intra-tumour heterogeneity originated by genomic, epigenomic, transcriptomic, and immune variability to stratify patients and shape the future clinical development of personalized treatments [80]. New technologies allowed the identification of new biomarkers and their co-evolution with drug discovery and targeted therapies design. Importantly, cancer susceptibility does not just depend on the genetic background of patients; environmental factors as well as lifestyle are determinants in the etiology of CRC [81]. Despite the improvements in early diagnosis and targeted therapies design for CRC, the rates of its incidence have been increasing for people younger than 40 years, pointing out the pressing needs for identifying the underlying environmental factors and providing preventive strategies for high-risk individuals [82]. In addition to alcohol consumption, smoking [83] or the presence of dysbiosis [84], diets rich in red, processed, and grilled meats were strongly associated with colorectal cancer [85,86]. Several studies published during the last two years supported the assessment published by the International Agency for Research on Cancer (IARC) in October 2015 (data summarized by Bouvard et al. [87]). The results gathered by IARC reached the final conclusion that the consumption of 50 g of red meat per day increased by 18% the risk of suffering CRC. The meta-analysis carried out by Carr and collaborators found that different red meat subtypes influence differently the diverse CRC subtypes [88]. Moreover, they demonstrated that, although poultry or pork intake was not associated with higher risk of CRC, beef and lamb consumption presented positive moderate association. Importantly, in a second publication by the same group, they analysed patients 5 years after diagnosis and they observed no increased mortality in those with higher red and processed meat intake [89]. When pre-diagnosed consumption of red, processed meat, and poultry was assessed, no relation to CRC survival was found for red meat, whereas positive association was demonstrated for processed meat and CRC mortality in females. An increased all-cause mortality was associated with poultry consumption. Finally, no changes in CRC mortality were found for dietary fiber [90].

Regarding the molecular mechanisms underlying this detrimental effect of red and processed meat, multiple components were implicated. First, an increase in N-nitroso components production is induced in the digestive tract by red and processed meat consumption. Moreover, two genotoxic compounds that cause DNA damage as heterocyclic aromatic amines and poly-cyclic aromatic hydrocarbons are present in high-temperature cooked meat and smoked or grilled meat, respectively. In 2013, results from Kentucky Colon Cancer Study established statistical correlations among total dietary intake of 2-amino-3,8-dimethylimidazo[4,5-f]quinoxaline, 2-amino-3,4,8-trimethylimidazo[4,5-f]quinoxaline, meat-derived mutagenic (a marker for meat mutagens combined) and colon cancer risk. Their analysis support estimated heterocyclic amines and polycyclic aromatic hydrocarbons exposure as being a possible mechanism to increase colon cancer risk in the context of red meat intake [91]. Besides, higher oxidative stress, as well as induction of *APC* gene mutations and its promoter methylation, were suggested to be triggered by increased red and processed meat intake, and therefore with CRC risk [86,87].

Fiber is also among the well-studied dietary factors associated with colorectal tumorogenesis. In this case, most of the epidemiological data defend the protective role of dietary fiber in CRC, but the data are still no conclusive and further research needs to be performed [83,90,92].

Considering specific nutrient components, folate has been deeply studied as a modulator of colorectal cancer prevention [93,94]. Plasma alterations of this water-soluble vitamin B_9 are associated with the hypermethylation of several tumour suppressor genes and with DNA hypomethylation [95]. The most consistent piece of data demonstrating that folate can be considered an independent risk factor for CRC was published in 2011 [96]. The authors performed the largest prospective cohort study in this regard and showed that those individuals with the highest folate intake presented a 30% reduction in the risk of developing CRC.

In addition, according to several epidemiologic studies, milk, calcium and dietary vitamin D are considered as protective factors against CRC development and are positively associated with survival [97,98].

Apart from specific nutrients, the direct association of diet with an excessive accumulation of adipose tissue and the subsequent development of obesity plays a role in tumor prognosis. During cancer progression, a bidirectional crosstalk is established between malignant cells and adipocytes [78]. Because of malignant cell proximity, the cancer associated adipocytes (CAA) suffer delipidation and acquire fibroblast-like features that will influence malignancy. The lipids secreted by adipocytes are transferred to cancer cells that can use them for energy production through β-oxidation. Moreover, the rapid expansion and hypertrophy of adipose tissue provokes oxygen deficiency, and compensatory mechanisms to promote angiogenesis are triggered, favoring tumor spreading [99].

Precision Nutrition in Colorectal Cancer

The relation between CRC carcinogenesis and nutrition factors is probably more complex than originally conceptualized. However, it is widely accepted in the field of precision nutrition that several genetics variants in diet-nutrition-related genes are clearly associated with CRC prevention (Table 1) [49]. The most representative example is the association between variants in genes related to folate synthesis and CRC risk. Folate is involved in the synthesis of nucleic acids and DNA methylation [100]. It has been described that genetic polymorphisms in methylenetetrahydrofolate reductase (MTHFR) enzyme are modulating their own activity. In addition, SNPs in *MTHFR* and levels of folate intake combine to regulate CRC risk [100,101]. Particularly, minor homozygous allele TT of Cys677Thr polymorphism in *MTHFR* gene reduces in vitro MTHFR enzymatic activity to 30%. The TT genotype is associated with CRC risk in the context of low folate intake, whereas it is protective for CRC when high intake of folate occurs [100–102].

Many other examples of polymorphisms in diet-nutrition and/or metabolism-related genes, that modulate CRC risk, have been described in the literature. Genetic variations in enzymes like glutathione S-transferases (GSTs) have been related to CRC risk. These proteins are involved in phase II detoxification process of drugs and endogenous compounds. *GSTM1* and *GSTT1* null genotypes increased risk of CRC in Caucasian populations [103–105]. Polymorphisms in vitamin D receptor (*VDR*) gene, in combination with dietary fat or calcium, seem to also modulate CRC risk, but controversial results have been found [106–109]. The common Thr1482Ile polymorphism in the transient receptor potential melastatin 7 (*TRPM7*), a ubiquitously expressed constitutive ion channel with higher affinity for Mg2+ than for Ca2+, was associated with an elevated risk of both adenomatous and hyperplastic polyps. Moreover, this polymorphism significantly interacted with the Ca:Mg intake in relation to both types of polyps [110]. SNPs in genes belonging to the base excision repair pathway (BER) have been associated with CRC risk. An association has been reported between Glu51His in *APEX1* (ascorbate peroxidase) with CRC risk and a modifier role for the Val762Ala SNP in *PARP* gene (poly ADP ribose polymerase) on the effect of diets higher in high-temperature cooked red meat [111]. Genes belonging to angiogenesis pathway have been interrogated for gene-environment interactions: SNPs and smoking, dietary protein, and alcohol exposures, as well as associations of these interactions with CRC risk and survival. Variants on *FLT1* (vascular endothelial growth factor receptor 1) interacted with smoking, animal protein intake, and CRC risk. Besides, *KDR* (vascular endothelial growth factor receptor 2) variants interacted with alcohol and CRC risk [112]. However, there is high inter-group variability in the results. Replication studies with accurate designs are needed in order to clarify the use of many of these markers before applying these results to clinical practices [113,114]. In this context, consortium studies arise in order to solve reproducibility and low sample size problems [24]. Huge collaborations among scientific groups, such as the Personal Genome Project, the International HapMap consortium, or the Human Variome Project have been established to obtain information on genetic variation with the goal of linking genetic variation to human disease risk and promoting the development of personalized medicine [25].

Table 1. Associations between genetic variants in diet-nutrition-related genes and colorectal cancer (CRC) risk.

Gene Symbol	Gene Name	SNP		CRC Risk	Interactors	Reference
MTHFR	Methylenetetrahydrofolate reductase enzyme	rs1801133	Cys677Thr	Reduced	High folate intake	[100–102]
GSTM1	Glutathione S -transferase M1	-	Null Phenotype	Increased	-	[103,104]
GSTT1	Glutathione S -transferase T1	-	Null Phenotype	Increased	-	[103,104]
APEX1	Ascorbate peroxidase	rs1048945	Glu51His	Reduced	-	[111]
PARP	Poly ADP ribose polymerase	rs1136410	Val762Ala	Modifier of rs1048945	High-temperature cooked red meat	[111]
FLT1	Vascular endothelial growth factor receptor 1	rs678714		Reduced	Smoking	[112]
		rs2387632		Reduced	Animal protein intake	
KDR	Vascular endothelial growth factor receptor 2	rs6838752		Increased	Alcohol	[112]
BMP4	Bone morphogenetic protein 4	rs17563		Reduced	Smoking	[112]

Together with genomic approaches, transcriptomic studies also have been used for precision nutrition in order to study responses to nutrients and/or bioactive products that can influence gene expression. In this transcriptomic scenario, a representative example of a metabolic gene whose expression is both dysregulated in CRC and modulated by bioactive compounds is *GCNT3* (Glucosaminyl (*N*-Acetyl) transferase 3, mucin type). It codifies for a glycosyltransferase enzyme implicated in glycosylation processes. *GCNT3* catalyzes the formation of core 2 *O*-glycan, core 4 *O*-glycan, and I branches in mucin-type glycoproteins biosynthesis [115]. *GCNT3* expression is altered in cancer [116–119] and its upregulation has been clearly associated with favorable CRC prognosis [116,117].

It has been established that rosemary extracts regulate *GCNT3* expression in CRC. Rosemary (*Rosmarinus officinalis* L.) is an evergreen shrub from Mediterranean region [120]. The rosemary leaves have been employed as seasoning as well as in traditional medicine for treating several disorders such as renal colic and respiratory diseases. In recent years, scientific investigations have been performed in order to elucidate the potential utility of rosemary extracts and/or their constituents with antioxidant activity in several diseases, including cancer [120,121]. The major components of rosemary extracts are carnosic acid, carnosol, ursolic acid, and rosmarinic acid. Some of them exhibit intrinsic antitumor properties; nevertheless, the efficacy of the complete extract is usually higher, due to a synergistic effect as well as the presence of additional antitumor components whose effect has not been demonstrated yet. Moreover, rosemary extract has also been used in combination with several antitumor agents and chemotherapeutic drugs [121].

Interestingly, it has been shown that rosemary was able to increase the expression of *GCNT3* gene. *GCNT3* upregulation is associated with better prognosis in CRC [116,117] and this upregulation correlated with the antiproliferative effect of different rosemary extracts in tumor cells [122]. Moreover, rosemary also regulates miR-15b expression, which was reported to target *GCNT3* by *in silico* analysis [122]. miR-15b has been found upregulated in CRC patients and, consequently, it has been considered as potential biomarker [123]. miR-15b expression was downregulated by rosemary in CRC cells. The rosemary component responsible for this modulation is carnosic acid. Since this regulation was also detected in plasma, miR-15b could be considered as a potential non-invasive biomarker to monitor in vivo responses [122].

4. Precision Nutrition and Lipid Metabolism in Colorectal Cancer

In 2015, consensus studies on transcriptomic data were successfully applied in order to solve the intrinsic heterogeneity and molecular complexity of CRC. Several international research groups shared large-scale data and they proposed a new CRC classification based on an unbiased approach to facilitate clinical translation [12]. They established four transcriptomic consensus molecular subtypes (CMS) of CRC: CMS1 or microsatellite instability (MSI) immune subtype, CMS2 or canonical, CMS3 or metabolic, and CMS4 or mesenchymal subtype.

Interestingly, metabolic CRC subtype tumours (CMS3) have been characterized as those which harbor *KRAS* mutations, a mixed MSI status, low somatic copy number alterations (SCNA), and low CpG island methylator phenotype (CIMP). Furthermore, CMS3 tumours exhibit a prominent metabolic activation with a clear enrichment for multiple metabolism signatures, in connection with the presence of *KRAS*-activating mutations that have been described as inducing metabolic reprogramming [12]. Although *KRAS* mutants are more prevalent among CMS3 tumours, they are present in every molecular subtype. *KRAS* mutations were more likely to be present in patients without a family history of colon cancer and never smokers [124,125]. In a meta-analysis performed in 2009, no association was observed between smoking and *KRAS* mutations in colorectal adenocarcinomas [126]. A recent study links alcohol intake with an increased risk of *KRAS*+ and *BRAF-/KRAS-* [127]. Furthermore, a positive association was reported between heme iron intake from red meat and the risk of CRC with activating G > A mutations in *KRAS* [128].

In this cancer-metabolic scenario, the examples of metabolism-related pathways that could be implicated in precision nutrition are currently increasing. Alterations in lipid metabolism also contribute to cancer-metabolic progression (Figure 2). Highly proliferative cancer cells display strong lipid and cholesterol avidity, which they satisfy by increasing the uptake of dietary or exogenous lipids and lipoproteins or activating lipogenesis or cholesterol synthesis [129].

Metabolic genes belonging to fatty acids synthesis pathway have been interrogated in CRC for precision nutrition uses (summarized in Table 2). In 2010, 43 fatty acid metabolism-related genes and 392 SNPs were analyzed in 1225 CRC cases and 2032 controls from the European Prospective Investigation into Cancer and Nutrition study (EPIC cohort) [130]. Authors found evidence for an association of hydroxyprostaglandin dehydrogenase 15-(NAD) (*HPGD*), phospholipase A2 group VI (*PLA2G6*), and transient receptor potential vanilloid 3 (*TRPV3*) with increased risk for CRC, while prostaglandin E receptor 2 (*PTGER2*) was associated with lower CRC risk. This work highlighted the role of prostanoid signaling in colon carcinogenesis and gave weight to the relevance of genetic variation in fatty acid metabolism-related genes and CRC risk [130]. After that, a different study analyzed a new set of 8 fatty acid biosynthesis-related genes (30 SNPs) in 1780 CRC cases and 1864 controls from the Molecular Epidemiology Cancer study [131]. They found an association of rs9652472 polymorphism of *LIPC* (hepatic triglyceride lipase) with increased risk of CRC. They also replicated previous associations of *LIPC* SNPs with higher serum HDL levels [131].

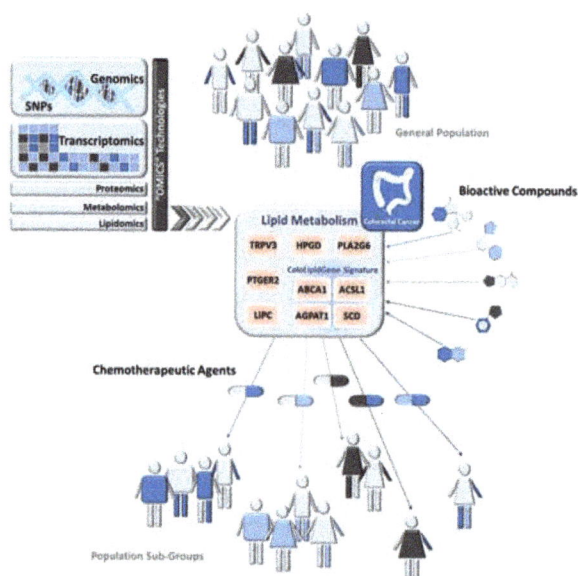

Figure 2. Modulation of Lipid Metabolism in Colorectal Cancer by Precision Nutrition Approaches. Genomics, transcriptomics, and other "omics" technologies have significantly contributed to the development of precision nutrition, which aims to identify patient subpopulations and design new targeted strategies for personalized treatment. Alterations in lipid metabolism have been implicated in cancer-metabolic progression. Examples of lipid-metabolic genes that have been interrogated for precision nutrition uses in colorectal cancer (CRC) are detailed. Bioactive compound could modulate lipid-metabolism-related gene expression. Their use together with classical chemotherapeutic agents, whose effect could be potentiated, is one of the current lines of research in CRC treatment. *HPGD*: hydroxyprostaglandin dehydrogenase 15-(NAD), *PLA2G6*: phospholipase A2 group VI, *TRPV3*: transient receptor potential vanilloid 3, *PTGER2*: prostaglandin E receptor 2, *LIPC*: hepatic triglyceride lipase, *ACSL1*: Acyl-CoA synthetase 1, *ABCA1*: ATP-Binding Cassette Subfamily-A Member 1, *AGPAT1*: 1-Acylglycerol-3-Phosphate *O*-Acyltransferase 1, *SCD*: Stearoyl-CoA-desaturase 1, SNPs: Single Nucleotide Polymorphisms.

Recently, genetic analysis of 57 SNPs located in 7 lipid-metabolism-related genes was performed in CRC patients in order to identify whether any genetic alteration might be related to overexpression of these enzymes and therefore constitute a biomarker of lipid metabolism-related alterations [11]. In a multivariate model, adjusting for clinical risk factors and multiple comparisons, the SNP rs8086 in *ACSL1* was associated with CRC disease-free survival (DFS), indicating that patients carrying the *ACSL1* rs8086 T/T genotype had significantly decreased DFS compared with patients carrying the C/T or C/C genotype, with 3-fold higher risk of relapse (Table 2). T/T genotype for rs8086 is associated with worse clinical outcome and simultaneously correlates with high ACSL1 mRNA levels, which, in turn, had already been associated with worse clinical outcome in these CRC patients [10,11]. Previous to this study, a lipid-metabolic signature (ColoLipidGene) was associated with CRC prognosis in stage II patients [10]. ColoLipidGene signature encompasses the transcriptional activation of four metabolic-related genes: *ACSL1*, *ABCA1* (ATP-Binding Cassette Subfamily-A Member 1), *AGPAT1* (1-Acylglycerol-3-Phosphate *O*-Acyltransferase 1), and *SCD*. Results from three different groups of patients, together with data from publicly available repository GEO (Gene Expression Omnibus Database), point out the activation of *ABCA1*, *ACSL1*, *AGPAT1*, and *SCD* as one of the main relevant metabolic factors in CRC malignant progression [10].

Table 2. Associations between polymorphisms in lipid-metabolism-related genes and colorectal cancer.

Gene Symbol	Gene Name	SNP	CRC Cases	Controls	Model	CRC Risk	Measure of Risk	(95% CI)	p-Value	Reference
HPGD	Hydroxyprostaglandin dehydrogenase 15-(NAD)	rs2612656	1225	2032	Dom.	Increased risk of developing CRC	OR: 1.24	(1.07–1.44)	0.005	[130]
		rs8752	1225	2032	Dom.	Increased risk of developing CRC	OR: 1.22	(1.05–1.43)	0.009	[130]
PLA2G6	Phospholipase A2 group VI	rs4821737	1225	2032	Rec.	Increased risk of developing CRC	OR: 1.26	(1.06–1.50)	0.009	[130]
TRPV3	Transient receptor potential vanilloid 3	rs11078458	1225	2032	Rec.	Increased risk of developing CRC	OR: 1.32	(1.10–1.59)	0.003	[130]
PTGER2	Prostaglandin E receptor 2	rs17831718	1225	2032	Dom.	Reduced risk of developing CRC	OR: 0.73	(0.58–0.91)	0.006	[130]
LIPC	Hepatic triglyceride lipase	rs9652472	1780	1864	Log-add.	Increased risk of developing CRC	OR: 1.52	(1.20–1.92)	0.0005	[131]
ACSL1	Acyl-CoA synthetase 1	rs8086	284	-	Rec.	Increased risk of CRC relapse	HR: 3.08	(1.69–5.63)	0.046	[11]

Dom.: Dominant model of inheritance; Rec.: Recessive model of inheritance; Log-add: Log-Additive model; OR: Odds ratio; HR: Hazzard ratio; Ref: Reference; SNP: Single Nucleotide Polymorphism; CRC: Colorectal cancer; CI: Confidence interval.

The extent to which genetic variants, together with intake of specific dietary components, affect risk of CRC in different populations is currently under investigation. Several natural compounds may modulate lipid metabolism [132] and, consequently, they could have a key role in the prevention and treatment of cancer [133–136]. Indeed, many anticancer agents employed clinically are natural compounds or their derivatives. Various in vitro studies pointed out an external regulation of lipid-metabolism-related genes whose expression could be modulated by bioactive products. Moreover, the use of bioactive compound together with classical chemotherapeutic agents, whose effect could be potentiated, constitutes an important line of development in CRC treatment with increasing number of clinical studies trying to address this point (Figure 2).

In the context of ColoLipiGene signature, few studies are focused on the transcriptional regulation of genes belonging to this signature by bioactive compounds that must be further explored for therapeutic or preventive application. For example, it is known that in THP-1 cells, eicosapentaenoic acid (EPA)-rich oil altered the expression of fatty acids metabolism genes including *SCD* and FA desaturase-1 and -2 (*FASDS1* and -2) [137].

Due in part to its relationship with cholesterol and cardiovascular disease, *ABCA1* is one of the most studied genes of ColoLipiGene signature. It is well known that curcumin enhanced cholesterol efflux by upregulating *ABCA1* expression through AMPK-SIRT1-LXRα signaling in THP-1 macrophage-derived foam cells [138]. It have been also described that hesperetin, a citrus flavonoid, increased *ABCA1* promoter and LXR enhancer activities in THP-1 macrophages [139]. Recently, dietary compounds from olive oil were tested for their capacity to enhance cellular ABCA1 protein level, and authors identified erythrodiol (Olean-12-ene-3b,28-diol) as an ABCA1 stabilizer [140]. Additionally, the mRNA and protein expression of LXRs and their target genes, including *ABCA1*, was significantly increased in macrophages stimulated with cineole [141]. The 1,8-Cineole (cineole), also known as eucalyptol or cajeputol, is a terpene oxide and a principal component of most eucalyptus oils, rosemary, and many other essential oils. Continuing in this line, other bioactive products like piperine (*Piper nigrum*) [142], silymarin (*Silybum marianum* L.) [143] and garlic-derived compounds [144], also modulate *ABCA1* expression. Nevertheless, studies in colorectal cancer models are needed in order to explore new therapeutic or preventive applications.

5. Concluding Remarks

Compelling evidence gained from epidemiological and experimental studies supports the crucial role of obesity, dietary patterns, gene-diet interactions and lipid metabolism in CRC prevention and prognosis.

Despite all advances in early cancer diagnosis and in the development of new targeted therapies, still many tumors continue to be untreatable. This is mainly due to inter and intra-heterogeneity, both in primary lesions and distal metastasis. The integration of basic and translational nutritional research into the clinic is contributing to identifying groups of patients and subsequent strategies for personalized treatment and diet recommendations.

Precision nutrition opens a window of opportunity to integrate omics technologies with clinical advice. In particular, lipid metabolism is gaining interest in the scientific community as a bona-fide target in CRC. The ultimate goal should be to identify or generate bioactive compounds that directly or indirectly modulate lipid metabolic processes. The design of clinical trials that combine classical chemotherapeutic agents with bioactive products targeting lipid metabolism constitutes an unquestionable line of research in CRC treatment.

Acknowledgments: This work has been supported by Ministerio de Economía y Competitividad del Gobierno de España (MINECO, Plan Nacional I+D+i AGL2016-76736-C3), Gobierno regional de la Comunidad de Madrid (P2013/ABI-2728, ALIBIRD-CM), EU Structural Funds, and AMAROUT-Marie Curie actions (COFUND2014-51539-04).

Author Contributions: C.A.-P. and L.P.F. wrote the paper. A.R.M. performed critical revision of the article.

Conflicts of Interest: The authors declare no conflict of interest.

References

1. Fitzmaurice, C.; Allen, C.; Barber, R.M.; Barregard, L.; Bhutta, Z.A.; Brenner, H.; Dicker, D.J.; Chimed-Orchir, O.; Dandona, R.; Dandona, L.; et al. Global, Regional, and National Cancer Incidence, Mortality, Years of Life Lost, Years Lived With Disability, and Disability-Adjusted Life-years for 32 Cancer Groups, 1990 to 2015: A Systematic Analysis for the Global Burden of Disease Study. *JAMA Oncol.* **2017**, *3*, 524–548. [PubMed]

2. DeBerardinis, R.J.; Lum, J.J.; Hatzivassiliou, G.; Thompson, C.B. The biology of cancer: Metabolic reprogramming fuels cell growth and proliferation. *Cell Metab.* **2008**, *7*, 11–20. [CrossRef] [PubMed]

3. Kaelin, W.G.; Thompson, C.B. Q&A: Cancer: Clues from cell metabolism. *Nature* **2010**, *465*, 562–564. [PubMed]

4. Jiang, L.; Xiao, L.; Sugiura, H.; Huang, X.; Ali, A.; Kuro-o, M.; Deberardinis, R.J.; Boothman, D.A. Metabolic reprogramming during TGFβ1-induced epithelial-to-mesenchymal transition. *Oncogene* **2015**, *34*, 3908–3916. [CrossRef] [PubMed]

5. Fisher, K.E.; Pop, A.; Koh, W.; Anthis, N.J.; Saunders, W.B.; Davis, G.E. Tumor cell invasion of collagen matrices requires coordinate lipid agonist-induced G-protein and membrane-type matrix metalloproteinase-1-dependent signaling. *Mol. Cancer* **2006**. [CrossRef] [PubMed]

6. Sánchez-Martínez, R.; Cruz-Gil, S.; Gómez de Cedrón, M.; Álvarez-Fernández, M.; Vargas, T.; Molina, S.; García, B.; Herranz, J.; Moreno-Rubio, J.; Reglero, G.; et al. A link between lipid metabolism and epithelial-mesenchymal transition provides a target for colon cancer therapy. *Oncotarget* **2015**, *6*, 38719–38736. [CrossRef] [PubMed]

7. English, D.; Brindley, D.N.; Spiegel, S.; Garcia, J.G.N. Lipid mediators of angiogenesis and the signalling pathways they initiate. *Biochim. Biophys. Acta* **2002**, *1582*, 228–239. [CrossRef]

8. Wong, B.W.; Wang, X.; Zecchin, A.; Thienpont, B.; Cornelissen, I.; Kalucka, J.; García-Caballero, M.; Missiaen, R.; Huang, H.; Brüning, U.; et al. The role of fatty acid β-oxidation in lymphangiogenesis. *Nature* **2017**, *542*, 49–54. [CrossRef] [PubMed]

9. Luo, X.; Cheng, C.; Tan, Z.; Li, N.; Tang, M.; Yang, L.; Cao, Y. Emerging roles of lipid metabolism in cancer metastasis. *Mol. Cancer* **2017**. [CrossRef] [PubMed]

10. Vargas, T.; Moreno-Rubio, J.; Herranz, J.; Cejas, P.; Molina, S.; González-Vallinas, M.; Mendiola, M.; Burgos, E.; Aguayo, C.; Custodio, A.B.; et al. ColoLipidGene: Signature of lipid metabolism-related genes to predict prognosis in stage-II colon cancer patients. *Oncotarget* **2015**, *6*, 7348–7363. [CrossRef] [PubMed]

11. Vargas, T.; Moreno-Rubio, J.; Herranz, J.; Cejas, P.; Molina, S.; Mendiola, M.; Burgos, E.; Custodio, A.B.; De Miguel, M.; Martín-Hernández, R.; et al. 3′UTR Polymorphism in ACSL1 Gene Correlates with Expression Levels and Poor Clinical Outcome in Colon Cancer Patients. *PLoS ONE* **2016**, *11*, e0168423. [CrossRef] [PubMed]

12. Guinney, J.; Dienstmann, R.; Wang, X.; de Reyniès, A.; Schlicker, A.; Soneson, C.; Marisa, L.; Roepman, P.; Nyamundanda, G.; Angelino, P.; et al. The consensus molecular subtypes of colorectal cancer. *Nat. Med.* **2015**, *21*, 1350–1356. [CrossRef] [PubMed]

13. Blatter, S.; Rottenberg, S. Minimal residual disease in cancer therapy—Small things make all the difference. *Drug Resist. Updat. Rev. Comment. Antimicrob. Anticancer Chemother.* **2015**, *21–22*, 1–10. [CrossRef] [PubMed]

14. Simonds, N.I.; Ghazarian, A.A.; Pimentel, C.B.; Schully, S.D.; Ellison, G.L.; Gillanders, E.M.; Mechanic, L.E. Review of the Gene-Environment Interaction Literature in Cancer: What Do We Know? *Genet. Epidemiol.* **2016**, *40*, 356–365. [CrossRef] [PubMed]

15. Thomas, D. Gene—Environment-wide association studies: Emerging approaches. *Nat. Rev. Genet.* **2010**, *11*, 259–272. [CrossRef] [PubMed]

16. Sharma, S.V.; Lee, D.Y.; Li, B.; Quinlan, M.P.; Takahashi, F.; Maheswaran, S.; McDermott, U.; Azizian, N.; Zou, L.; Fischbach, M.A.; et al. A chromatin-mediated reversible drug-tolerant state in cancer cell subpopulations. *Cell* **2010**, *141*, 69–80. [CrossRef] [PubMed]

17. Biro, F.M.; Wien, M. Childhood obesity and adult morbidities. *Am. J. Clin. Nutr.* **2010**, *91*, 1499S–1505S. [CrossRef] [PubMed]

18. Marusyk, A.; Almendro, V.; Polyak, K. Intra-tumour heterogeneity: A looking glass for cancer? *Nat. Rev. Cancer* **2012**, *12*, 323–334. [CrossRef] [PubMed]

19. Junttila, M.R.; de Sauvage, F.J. Influence of tumour micro-environment heterogeneity on therapeutic response. *Nature* **2013**, *501*, 346–354. [CrossRef] [PubMed]
20. Armstrong, B.; Doll, R. Environmental factors and cancer incidence and mortality in different countries, with special reference to dietary practices. *Int. J. Cancer* **1975**, *15*, 617–631. [CrossRef] [PubMed]
21. Burkitt, D.P. Epidemiology of cancer of the colon and rectum. *Cancer* **1971**, *28*, 3–13. [CrossRef]
22. Moghaddam, A.A.; Woodward, M.; Huxley, R. Obesity and Risk of Colorectal Cancer: A Meta-analysis of 31 Studies with 70,000 Events. *Cancer Epidemiol. Prev. Biomark.* **2007**, *16*, 2533–2547. [CrossRef] [PubMed]
23. Ferguson, L.R.; De Caterina, R.; Görman, U.; Allayee, H.; Kohlmeier, M.; Prasad, C.; Choi, M.S.; Curi, R.; de Luis, D.A.; Gil, Á.; et al. Guide and Position of the International Society of Nutrigenetics/Nutrigenomics on Personalised Nutrition: Part 1—Fields of Precision Nutrition. *J. Nutr. Nutr.* **2016**, *9*, 12–27. [CrossRef] [PubMed]
24. Thorisson, G.A.; Stein, L.D. The SNP Consortium website: Past, present and future. *Nucleic Acids Res.* **2003**, *31*, 124–127. [CrossRef] [PubMed]
25. Hesketh, J. Personalised nutrition: How far has nutrigenomics progressed? *Eur. J. Clin. Nutr.* **2013**, *67*, 430–435. [CrossRef] [PubMed]
26. Hanahan, D.; Weinberg, R.A. Hallmarks of Cancer: The Next Generation. *Cell* **2011**, *144*, 646–674. [CrossRef] [PubMed]
27. Schug, Z.T.; Gottlieb, E. Cardiolipin acts as a mitochondrial signalling platform to launch apoptosis. *Biochim. Biophys. Acta* **2009**, *1788*, 2022–2031. [CrossRef] [PubMed]
28. Zhao, W.; Prijic, S.; Urban, B.C.; Tisza, M.J.; Zuo, Y.; Li, L.; Tan, Z.; Chen, X.; Mani, S.A.; Chang, J.T. Candidate Antimetastasis Drugs Suppress the Metastatic Capacity of Breast Cancer Cells by Reducing Membrane Fluidity. *Cancer Res.* **2016**, *76*, 2037–2049. [CrossRef] [PubMed]
29. Carracedo, A.; Cantley, L.C.; Pandolfi, P.P. Cancer metabolism: Fatty acid oxidation in the limelight. *Nat. Rev. Cancer* **2013**, *13*, 227–232. [CrossRef] [PubMed]
30. Röhrig, F.; Schulze, A. The multifaceted roles of fatty acid synthesis in cancer. *Nat. Rev. Cancer* **2016**, *16*, 732–749. [CrossRef] [PubMed]
31. Carito, V.; Bonuccelli, G.; Martinez-Outschoorn, U.E.; Whitaker-Menezes, D.; Caroleo, M.C.; Cione, E.; Howell, A.; Pestell, R.G.; Lisanti, M.P.; Sotgia, F. Metabolic remodeling of the tumor microenvironment: Migration stimulating factor (MSF) reprograms myofibroblasts toward lactate production, fueling anabolic tumor growth. *Cell Cycle Georget. Tex* **2012**, *11*, 3403–3414. [CrossRef] [PubMed]
32. Guaita-Esteruelas, S.; Gumà, J.; Masana, L.; Borràs, J. The peritumoural adipose tissue microenvironment and cancer. The roles of fatty acid binding protein 4 and fatty acid binding protein 5. *Mol. Cell. Endocrinol.* **2017**. [CrossRef] [PubMed]
33. Gupta, S.; Roy, A.; Dwarakanath, B.S. Metabolic Cooperation and Competition in the Tumor Microenvironment: Implications for Therapy. *Front. Oncol.* **2017**. [CrossRef] [PubMed]
34. Ventura, R.; Mordec, K.; Waszczuk, J.; Wang, Z.; Lai, J.; Fridlib, M.; Buckley, D.; Kemble, G.; Heuer, T.S. Inhibition of de novo Palmitate Synthesis by Fatty Acid Synthase Induces Apoptosis in Tumor Cells by Remodeling Cell Membranes, Inhibiting Signaling Pathways, and Reprogramming Gene Expression. *EBioMedicine* **2015**, *2*, 808–824. [CrossRef] [PubMed]
35. Wang, D.; Dubois, R.N. Eicosanoids and cancer. *Nat. Rev. Cancer* **2010**, *10*, 181–193. [CrossRef] [PubMed]
36. Tiper, I.V.; East, J.E.; Subrahmanyam, P.B.; Webb, T.J. Sphingosine 1-phosphate signaling impacts lymphocyte migration, inflammation and infection. *Pathog. Dis.* **2016**, *74*. [CrossRef] [PubMed]
37. Baró, L.; Hermoso, J.C.; Núñez, M.C.; Jiménez-Rios, J.A.; Gil, A. Abnormalities in plasma and red blood cell fatty acid profiles of patients with colorectal cancer. *Br. J. Cancer* **1998**, *77*, 1978–1983. [CrossRef] [PubMed]
38. Cao, W.; Ma, Z.; Rasenick, M.M.; Yeh, S.; Yu, J. N-3 poly-unsaturated fatty acids shift estrogen signaling to inhibit human breast cancer cell growth. *PLoS ONE* **2012**, *7*, e52838. [CrossRef] [PubMed]
39. Lim, K.; Han, C.; Dai, Y.; Shen, M.; Wu, T. Omega-3 polyunsaturated fatty acids inhibit hepatocellular carcinoma cell growth through blocking beta-catenin and cyclooxygenase-2. *Mol. Cancer Ther.* **2009**, *8*, 3046–3055. [CrossRef] [PubMed]
40. Ma, C.-J.; Wu, J.-M.; Tsai, H.-L.; Huang, C.-W.; Lu, C.-Y.; Sun, L.-C.; Shih, Y.-L.; Chen, C.-W.; Chuang, J.-F.; Wu, M.-H.; et al. Prospective double-blind randomized study on the efficacy and safety of an n-3 fatty acid enriched intravenous fat emulsion in postsurgical gastric and colorectal cancer patients. *Nutr. J.* **2015**, *14*, 9. [CrossRef] [PubMed]

41. Whelan, J.; McEntee, M.F. Dietary (n-6) PUFA and intestinal tumorigenesis. *J. Nutr.* **2004**, *134*, 3421S–3426S. [PubMed]

42. Kim, E.K.; Ha, J.M.; Kim, Y.W.; Jin, S.Y.; Ha, H.K.; Bae, S.S. Inhibitory role of polyunsaturated fatty acids on lysophosphatidic acid-induced cancer cell migration and adhesion. *FEBS Lett.* **2014**, *588*, 2971–2977. [CrossRef] [PubMed]

43. Xia, H.; Ma, S.; Wang, S.; Sun, G. Meta-Analysis of Saturated Fatty Acid Intake and Breast Cancer Risk. *Medicine* **2015**, *94*, e2391. [CrossRef] [PubMed]

44. Bayerdörffer, E.; Mannes, G.A.; Richter, W.O.; Ochsenkühn, T.; Seeholzer, G.; Köpcke, W.; Wiebecke, B.; Paumgartner, G. Decreased high-density lipoprotein cholesterol and increased low-density cholesterol levels in patients with colorectal adenomas. *Ann. Intern. Med.* **1993**, *118*, 481–487. [CrossRef] [PubMed]

45. Morad, S.A.F.; Madigan, J.P.; Levin, J.C.; Abdelmageed, N.; Karimi, R.; Rosenberg, D.W.; Kester, M.; Shanmugavelandy, S.S.; Cabot, M.C. Tamoxifen magnifies therapeutic impact of ceramide in human colorectal cancer cells independent of p53. *Biochem. Pharmacol.* **2013**, *85*, 1057–1065. [CrossRef] [PubMed]

46. Tsukahara, T.; Tsukahara, R.; Fujiwara, Y.; Yue, J.; Cheng, Y.; Guo, H.; Bolen, A.; Zhang, C.; Balazs, L.; Re, F.; et al. Phospholipase D2-dependent inhibition of the nuclear hormone receptor PPARgamma by cyclic phosphatidic acid. *Mol. Cell* **2010**, *39*, 421–432. [CrossRef] [PubMed]

47. Kurabe, N.; Hayasaka, T.; Ogawa, M.; Masaki, N.; Ide, Y.; Waki, M.; Nakamura, T.; Kurachi, K.; Kahyo, T.; Shinmura, K.; et al. Accumulated phosphatidylcholine (16:0/16:1) in human colorectal cancer; possible involvement of LPCAT4. *Cancer Sci.* **2013**, *104*, 1295–1302. [CrossRef] [PubMed]

48. Mjabri, B.; Boucrot, P.; Aubry, J. The 1-*O*-octadecyl-2-*O*-methyl-sn-glycero-3-phosphocholine causes a differential incorporation of hexadecanol into neutral ether ester glycerolipids of 2 variant cell lines of rat colon carcinoma. *Arch. Int. Physiol. Biochim. Biophys.* **1992**, *100*, 237–240. [CrossRef] [PubMed]

49. Mayne, S.T.; Playdon, M.C.; Rock, C.L. Diet, nutrition, and cancer: Past, present and future. *Nat. Rev. Clin. Oncol.* **2016**, *13*, 504–515. [CrossRef] [PubMed]

50. Martín-Timón, I.; Sevillano-Collantes, C.; Segura-Galindo, A.; del Cañizo-Gómez, F.J. Type 2 diabetes and cardiovascular disease: Have all risk factors the same strength? *World J. Diabetes* **2014**, *5*, 444–470. [CrossRef] [PubMed]

51. Dobbins, M.; Decorby, K.; Choi, B.C.K. The Association between Obesity and Cancer Risk: A Meta-Analysis of Observational Studies from 1985 to 2011. *Int. Sch. Res. Not.* **2013**, *2013*, e680536. [CrossRef] [PubMed]

52. Calle, E.E.; Rodriguez, C.; Walker-Thurmond, K.; Thun, M.J. Overweight, obesity, and mortality from cancer in a prospectively studied cohort of U.S. adults. *N. Engl. J. Med.* **2003**, *348*, 1625–1638. [CrossRef] [PubMed]

53. Nieman, K.M.; Romero, I.L.; Van Houten, B.; Lengyel, E. Adipose tissue and adipocytes support tumorigenesis and metastasis. *Biochim. Biophys. Acta* **2013**, *1831*, 1533–1541. [CrossRef] [PubMed]

54. Zhang, X.; Zhou, G.; Sun, B.; Zhao, G.; Liu, D.; Sun, J.; Liu, C.; Guo, H. Impact of obesity upon prostate cancer-associated mortality: A meta-analysis of 17 cohort studies. *Oncol. Lett.* **2015**, *9*, 1307–1312. [CrossRef] [PubMed]

55. Zhang, Y.; Liu, H.; Yang, S.; Zhang, J.; Qian, L.; Chen, X. Overweight, obesity and endometrial cancer risk: Results from a systematic review and meta-analysis. *Int. J. Biol. Markers* **2014**, *29*, e21–29. [CrossRef] [PubMed]

56. Liu, Z.; Zhang, T.-T.; Zhao, J.-J.; Qi, S.-F.; Du, P.; Liu, D.-W.; Tian, Q.-B. The association between overweight, obesity and ovarian cancer: A meta-analysis. *Jpn. J. Clin. Oncol.* **2015**, *45*, 1107–1115. [CrossRef] [PubMed]

57. Qin, Q.; Xu, X.; Wang, X.; Zheng, X.-Y. Obesity and risk of bladder cancer: A meta-analysis of cohort studies. *Asian Pac. J. Cancer Prev.* **2013**, *14*, 3117–3121. [CrossRef] [PubMed]

58. Chen, Y.; Wang, X.; Wang, J.; Yan, Z.; Luo, J. Excess body weight and the risk of primary liver cancer: An updated meta-analysis of prospective studies. *Eur. J. Cancer* **2012**, *48*, 2137–2145. [CrossRef] [PubMed]

59. Turati, F.; Tramacere, I.; La Vecchia, C.; Negri, E. A meta-analysis of body mass index and esophageal and gastric cardia adenocarcinoma. *Ann. Oncol.* **2013**, *24*, 609–617. [CrossRef] [PubMed]

60. Larsson, S.C.; Wolk, A. Overweight, obesity and risk of liver cancer: A meta-analysis of cohort studies. *Br. J. Cancer* **2007**, *97*, 1005–1008. [CrossRef] [PubMed]

61. Wang, F.; Xu, Y. Body mass index and risk of renal cell cancer: A dose-response meta-analysis of published cohort studies. *Int. J. Cancer* **2014**, *135*, 1673–1686. [CrossRef] [PubMed]

62. Ma, J.; Huang, M.; Wang, L.; Ye, W.; Tong, Y.; Wang, H. Obesity and Risk of Thyroid Cancer: Evidence from a Meta-Analysis of 21 Observational Studies. *Med. Sci. Monit. Int. Med. J. Exp. Clin. Res.* **2015**, *21*, 283–291.

63. Heianza, Y.; Qi, L. Gene-Diet Interaction and Precision Nutrition in Obesity. *Int. J. Mol. Sci.* **2017**, *18*. [CrossRef] [PubMed]

64. Oh, T.-H.; Byeon, J.-S.; Myung, S.-J.; Yang, S.-K.; Choi, K.-S.; Chung, J.-W.; Kim, B.; Lee, D.; Byun, J.H.; Jang, S.J.; et al. Visceral obesity as a risk factor for colorectal neoplasm. *J. Gastroenterol. Hepatol.* **2008**, *23*, 411–417. [CrossRef] [PubMed]

65. Clayton, P.E.; Banerjee, I.; Murray, P.G.; Renehan, A.G. Growth hormone, the insulin-like growth factor axis, insulin and cancer risk. *Nat. Rev. Endocrinol.* **2011**, *7*, 11–24. [CrossRef] [PubMed]

66. Khandekar, M.J.; Cohen, P.; Spiegelman, B.M. Molecular mechanisms of cancer development in obesity. *Nat. Rev. Cancer* **2011**, *11*, 886–895. [CrossRef] [PubMed]

67. Pollak, M. The insulin and insulin-like growth factor receptor family in neoplasia: An update. *Nat. Rev. Cancer* **2012**, *12*, 159–169. [CrossRef] [PubMed]

68. Teoh, S.L.; Das, S. Tumour biology of obesity-related cancers: Understanding the molecular concept for better diagnosis and treatment. *Tumour Biol. J. Int. Soc. Oncodevelopmental Biol. Med.* **2016**, *37*, 14363–14380. [CrossRef] [PubMed]

69. DeGruttola, A.K.; Low, D.; Mizoguchi, A.; Mizoguchi, E. Current understanding of dysbiosis in disease in human and animal models. *Inflamm. Bowel Dis.* **2016**, *22*, 1137–1150. [CrossRef] [PubMed]

70. Font-Burgada, J.; Sun, B.; Karin, M. Obesity and Cancer: The Oil that Feeds the Flame. *Cell Metab.* **2016**, *23*, 48–62. [CrossRef] [PubMed]

71. Sheflin, A.M.; Whitney, A.K.; Weir, T.L. Cancer-Promoting Effects of Microbial Dysbiosis. *Curr. Oncol. Rep.* **2014**, *16*, 406. [CrossRef] [PubMed]

72. Louis, P.; Hold, G.L.; Flint, H.J. The gut microbiota, bacterial metabolites and colorectal cancer. *Nat. Rev. Microbiol.* **2014**, *12*, 661–672. [CrossRef] [PubMed]

73. Ou, J.; Carbonero, F.; Zoetendal, E.G.; DeLany, J.P.; Wang, M.; Newton, K.; Gaskins, H.R.; O'Keefe, S.J.D. Diet, microbiota, and microbial metabolites in colon cancer risk in rural Africans and African Americans. *Am. J. Clin. Nutr.* **2013**, *98*, 111–120. [CrossRef] [PubMed]

74. Raman, M.; Ambalam, P.; Kondepudi, K.K.; Pithva, S.; Kothari, C.; Patel, A.T.; Purama, R.K.; Dave, J.M.; Vyas, B.R.M. Potential of probiotics, prebiotics and synbiotics for management of colorectal cancer. *Gut Microbes* **2013**, *4*, 181–192. [CrossRef] [PubMed]

75. Dimitrov, D.V. The human gutome: Nutrigenomics of the host-microbiome interactions. *Omics J. Integr. Biol.* **2011**, *15*, 419–430. [CrossRef] [PubMed]

76. Gagnière, J.; Raisch, J.; Veziant, J.; Barnich, N.; Bonnet, R.; Buc, E.; Bringer, M.-A.; Pezet, D.; Bonnet, M. Gut microbiota imbalance and colorectal cancer. *World J. Gastroenterol.* **2016**, *22*, 501–518. [CrossRef] [PubMed]

77. Kich, D.M.; Vincenzi, A.; Majolo, F.; Volken de Souza, C.F.; Goettert, M.I. Probiotic: Effectiveness nutrition in cancer treatment and prevention. *Nutr. Hosp.* **2016**, *33*, 1430–1437. [CrossRef] [PubMed]

78. Steeg, P.S. Targeting metastasis. *Nat. Rev. Cancer* **2016**, *16*, 201–218. [CrossRef] [PubMed]

79. Cremolini, C.; Schirripa, M.; Antoniotti, C.; Moretto, R.; Salvatore, L.; Masi, G.; Falcone, A.; Loupakis, F. First-line chemotherapy for mCRC—A review and evidence-based algorithm. *Nat. Rev. Clin. Oncol.* **2015**, *12*, 607–619. [CrossRef] [PubMed]

80. Dienstmann, R.; Vermeulen, L.; Guinney, J.; Kopetz, S.; Tejpar, S.; Tabernero, J. Consensus molecular subtypes and the evolution of precision medicine in colorectal cancer. *Nat. Rev. Cancer* **2017**, *17*, 79–92. [CrossRef] [PubMed]

81. Rattray, N.J.W.; Charkoftaki, G.; Rattray, Z.; Hansen, J.E.; Vasiliou, V.; Johnson, C.H. Environmental influences in the etiology of colorectal cancer: The premise of metabolomics. *Curr. Pharmacol. Rep.* **2017**, *3*, 114–125. [CrossRef] [PubMed]

82. Meyer, J.E.; Narang, T.; Schnoll-Sussman, F.H.; Pochapin, M.B.; Christos, P.J.; Sherr, D.L. Increasing incidence of rectal cancer in patients aged younger than 40 years: An analysis of the surveillance, epidemiology, and end results database. *Cancer* **2010**, *116*, 4354–4359. [CrossRef] [PubMed]

83. Lee, D.H.; Keum, N.; Giovannucci, E.L. Colorectal Cancer Epidemiology in the Nurses' Health Study. *Am. J. Public Health* **2016**, *106*, 1599–1607. [CrossRef] [PubMed]

84. Raay, T.V.; Allen-Vercoe, E. Microbial Interactions and Interventions in Colorectal Cancer. *Microbiol. Spectr.* **2017**, *5*. [CrossRef]

85. Domingo, J.L.; Nadal, M. Carcinogenicity of consumption of red meat and processed meat: A review of scientific news since the IARC decision. *Food Chem. Toxicol. Int. J. Publ. Br. Ind. Biol. Res. Assoc.* **2017**, *105*, 256–261. [CrossRef] [PubMed]

86. Jeyakumar, A.; Dissabandara, L.; Gopalan, V. A critical overview on the biological and molecular features of red and processed meat in colorectal carcinogenesis. *J. Gastroenterol.* **2017**, *52*, 407–418. [CrossRef] [PubMed]

87. Bouvard, V.; Loomis, D.; Guyton, K.Z.; Grosse, Y.; Ghissassi, F.E.; Benbrahim-Tallaa, L.; Guha, N.; Mattock, H.; Straif, K.; International Agency for Research on Cancer Monograph Working Group. Carcinogenicity of consumption of red and processed meat. *Lancet Oncol.* **2015**, *16*, 1599–1600. [CrossRef]

88. Carr, P.R.; Walter, V.; Brenner, H.; Hoffmeister, M. Meat subtypes and their association with colorectal cancer: Systematic review and meta-analysis. *Int. J. Cancer* **2016**, *138*, 293–302. [CrossRef] [PubMed]

89. Carr, P.R.; Jansen, L.; Walter, V.; Kloor, M.; Roth, W.; Bläker, H.; Chang-Claude, J.; Brenner, H.; Hoffmeister, M. Associations of red and processed meat with survival after colorectal cancer and differences according to timing of dietary assessment. *Am. J. Clin. Nutr.* **2016**, *103*, 192–200. [CrossRef] [PubMed]

90. Ward, H.A.; Norat, T.; Overvad, K.; Dahm, C.C.; Bueno-de-Mesquita, H.B.; Jenab, M.; Fedirko, V.; van Duijnhoven, F.J.B.; Skeie, G.; Romaguera-Bosch, D.; et al. Pre-diagnostic meat and fibre intakes in relation to colorectal cancer survival in the European Prospective Investigation into Cancer and Nutrition. *Br. J. Nutr.* **2016**, *116*, 316–325. [CrossRef] [PubMed]

91. Helmus, D.S.; Thompson, C.L.; Zelenskiy, S.; Tucker, T.C.; Li, L. Red meat-derived heterocyclic amines increase risk of colon cancer: A population-based case-control study. *Nutr. Cancer* **2013**, *65*, 1141–1150. [CrossRef] [PubMed]

92. Park, Y.; Hunter, D.J.; Spiegelman, D.; Bergkvist, L.; Berrino, F.; van den Brandt, P.A.; Buring, J.E.; Colditz, G.A.; Freudenheim, J.L.; Fuchs, C.S.; et al. Dietary fiber intake and risk of colorectal cancer: A pooled analysis of prospective cohort studies. *JAMA* **2005**, *294*, 2849–2857. [CrossRef] [PubMed]

93. Giovannucci, E.; Stampfer, M.J.; Colditz, G.A.; Hunter, D.J.; Fuchs, C.; Rosner, B.A.; Speizer, F.E.; Willett, W.C. Multivitamin use, folate, and colon cancer in women in the Nurses' Health Study. *Ann. Intern. Med.* **1998**, *129*, 517–524. [CrossRef] [PubMed]

94. Mason, J.B.; Tang, S.Y. Folate status and colorectal cancer risk: A 2016 update. *Mol. Aspects Med.* **2017**, *53*, 73–79. [CrossRef] [PubMed]

95. Bariol, C.; Suter, C.; Cheong, K.; Ku, S.-L.; Meagher, A.; Hawkins, N.; Ward, R. The Relationship between Hypomethylation and CpG Island Methylation in Colorectal Neoplasia. *Am. J. Pathol.* **2003**, *162*, 1361–1371. [CrossRef]

96. Gibson, T.M.; Weinstein, S.J.; Pfeiffer, R.M.; Hollenbeck, A.R.; Subar, A.F.; Schatzkin, A.; Mayne, S.T.; Stolzenberg-Solomon, R. Pre- and postfortification intake of folate and risk of colorectal cancer in a large prospective cohort study in the United States123. *Am. J. Clin. Nutr.* **2011**, *94*, 1053–1062. [CrossRef] [PubMed]

97. Cho, E.; Smith-Warner, S.A.; Spiegelman, D.; Beeson, W.L.; van den Brandt, P.A.; Colditz, G.A.; Folsom, A.R.; Fraser, G.E.; Freudenheim, J.L.; Giovannucci, E.; et al. Dairy foods, calcium, and colorectal cancer: A pooled analysis of 10 cohort studies. *J. Natl. Cancer Inst.* **2004**, *96*, 1015–1022. [CrossRef] [PubMed]

98. Huncharek, M.; Muscat, J.; Kupelnick, B. Colorectal Cancer Risk and Dietary Intake of Calcium, Vitamin D, and Dairy Products: A Meta-Analysis of 26,335 Cases from 60 Observational Studies. *Nutr. Cancer* **2008**, *61*, 47–69. [CrossRef] [PubMed]

99. Park, J.; Morley, T.S.; Kim, M.; Clegg, D.J.; Scherer, P.E. Obesity and cancer—mechanisms underlying tumour progression and recurrence. *Nat. Rev. Endocrinol.* **2014**, *10*, 455–465. [CrossRef] [PubMed]

100. Eussen, S.J.P.M.; Vollset, S.E.; Igland, J.; Meyer, K.; Fredriksen, A.; Ueland, P.M.; Jenab, M.; Slimani, N.; Boffetta, P.; Overvad, K.; et al. Plasma folate, related genetic variants, and colorectal cancer risk in EPIC. *Cancer Epidemiol. Biomark. Prev. Publ. Am. Assoc. Cancer Res. Cosponsored Am. Soc. Prev. Oncol.* **2010**, *19*, 1328–1340. [CrossRef] [PubMed]

101. Ulrich, C.M.; Kampman, E.; Bigler, J.; Schwartz, S.M.; Chen, C.; Bostick, R.; Fosdick, L.; Beresford, S.A.; Yasui, Y.; Potter, J.D. Colorectal adenomas and the C677T MTHFR polymorphism: Evidence for gene-environment interaction? *Cancer Epidemiol. Biomark. Prev. Publ. Am. Assoc. Cancer Res. Cosponsored Am. Soc. Prev. Oncol.* **1999**, *8*, 659–668.

102. Kennedy, D.A.; Stern, S.J.; Matok, I.; Moretti, M.E.; Sarkar, M.; Adams-Webber, T.; Koren, G. Folate Intake, MTHFR Polymorphisms, and the Risk of Colorectal Cancer: A Systematic Review and Meta-Analysis. *J. Cancer Epidemiol.* **2012**, *2012*. [CrossRef] [PubMed]

103. Economopoulos, K.P.; Sergentanis, T.N. GSTM1, GSTT1, GSTP1, GSTA1 and colorectal cancer risk: A comprehensive meta-analysis. *Eur. J. Cancer Oxf. Engl. 1990* **2010**, *46*, 1617–1631. [CrossRef] [PubMed]

104. Qin, X.; Zhou, Y.; Chen, Y.; Li, N.; Chen, B.; Yang, P.; Wu, X. Glutathione S-transferase T1 gene polymorphism and colorectal cancer risk: An updated analysis. *Clin. Res. Hepatol. Gastroenterol.* **2013**, *37*, 626–635. [CrossRef] [PubMed]

105. Riscuta, G.; Dumitrescu, R.G. Nutrigenomics: Implications for breast and colon cancer prevention. *Methods Mol. Biol. Clifton NJ* **2012**, *863*, 343–358.

106. Murtaugh, M.A.; Sweeney, C.; Ma, K.-N.; Potter, J.D.; Caan, B.J.; Wolff, R.K.; Slattery, M.L. Vitamin D receptor gene polymorphisms, dietary promotion of insulin resistance, and colon and rectal cancer. *Nutr. Cancer* **2006**, *55*, 35–43. [CrossRef] [PubMed]

107. Ross, S.A. Nutritional genomic approaches to cancer prevention research. *Exp. Oncol.* **2007**, *29*, 250–256. [PubMed]

108. Park, Y.; Kim, J. Association of Dietary Vitamin D and Calcium with Genetic Polymorphisms in Colorectal Neoplasia. *J. Cancer Prev.* **2015**, *20*, 97–105. [CrossRef] [PubMed]

109. Sheng, S.; Chen, Y.; Shen, Z. Correlation between polymorphism of vitamin D receptor TaqI and susceptibility to colorectal cancer. *Medicine (Baltimore)* **2017**, *96*. [CrossRef] [PubMed]

110. Dai, Q.; Shrubsole, M.J.; Ness, R.M.; Schlundt, D.; Cai, Q.; Smalley, W.E.; Li, M.; Shyr, Y.; Zheng, W. The relation of magnesium and calcium intakes and a genetic polymorphism in the magnesium transporter to colorectal neoplasia risk. *Am. J. Clin. Nutr.* **2007**, *86*, 743–751. [PubMed]

111. Brevik, A.; Joshi, A.D.; Corral, R.; Onland-Moret, N.C.; Siegmund, K.D.; Le Marchand, L.; Baron, J.A.; Martinez, M.E.; Haile, R.W.; Ahnen, D.J.; et al. Polymorphisms in base excision repair genes as colorectal cancer risk factors and modifiers of the effect of diets high in red meat. *Cancer Epidemiol. Biomark. Prev. Publ. Am. Assoc. Cancer Res. Cosponsored Am. Soc. Prev. Oncol.* **2010**, *19*, 3167–3173. [CrossRef] [PubMed]

112. Sharafeldin, N.; Slattery, M.L.; Liu, Q.; Franco-Villalobos, C.; Caan, B.J.; Potter, J.D.; Yasui, Y. A Candidate-Pathway Approach to Identify Gene-Environment Interactions: Analyses of Colon Cancer Risk and Survival. *J. Natl. Cancer Inst.* **2015**, *107*. [CrossRef] [PubMed]

113. Fenech, M.F. Nutriomes and nutrient arrays—The key to personalised nutrition for DNA damage prevention and cancer growth control. *Genome Integr.* **2010**, *1*, 11. [CrossRef] [PubMed]

114. Ordovas, J.M. Nutrigenetics, plasma lipids, and cardiovascular risk. *J. Am. Diet. Assoc.* **2006**, *106*, 1074–1081. [CrossRef] [PubMed]

115. Yeh, J.C.; Ong, E.; Fukuda, M. Molecular cloning and expression of a novel beta-1, 6-*N*-acetylglucosaminyltransferase that forms core 2, core 4, and I branches. *J. Biol. Chem.* **1999**, *274*, 3215–3221. [CrossRef] [PubMed]

116. González-Vallinas, M.; Vargas, T.; Moreno-Rubio, J.; Molina, S.; Herranz, J.; Cejas, P.; Burgos, E.; Aguayo, C.; Custodio, A.; Reglero, G.; et al. Clinical relevance of the differential expression of the glycosyltransferase gene GCNT3 in colon cancer. *Eur. J. Cancer Oxf. Engl. 1990* **2015**, *51*, 1–8. [CrossRef] [PubMed]

117. Huang, M.-C.; Chen, H.-Y.; Huang, H.-C.; Huang, J.; Liang, J.-T.; Shen, T.-L.; Lin, N.-Y.; Ho, C.-C.; Cho, I.-M.; Hsu, S.-M. C2GnT-M is downregulated in colorectal cancer and its re-expression causes growth inhibition of colon cancer cells. *Oncogene* **2006**, *25*, 3267–3276. [CrossRef] [PubMed]

118. Liu, T.; Zhang, S.; Chen, J.; Jiang, K.; Zhang, Q.; Guo, K.; Liu, Y. The transcriptional profiling of glycogenes associated with hepatocellular carcinoma metastasis. *PLoS ONE* **2014**, *9*, e107941. [CrossRef] [PubMed]

119. Rao, C.V.; Janakiram, N.B.; Madka, V.; Kumar, G.; Scott, E.J.; Pathuri, G.; Bryant, T.; Kutche, H.; Zhang, Y.; Biddick, L.; et al. Small-Molecule Inhibition of GCNT3 Disrupts Mucin Biosynthesis and Malignant Cellular Behaviors in Pancreatic Cancer. *Cancer Res.* **2016**, *76*, 1965–1974. [CrossRef] [PubMed]

120. Ulbricht, C.; Abrams, T.R.; Brigham, A.; Ceurvels, J.; Clubb, J.; Curtiss, W.; Kirkwood, C.D.; Giese, N.; Hoehn, K.; Iovin, R.; et al. An evidence-based systematic review of rosemary (Rosmarinus officinalis) by the Natural Standard Research Collaboration. *J. Diet. Suppl.* **2010**, *7*, 351–413. [CrossRef] [PubMed]

121. González-Vallinas, M.; Reglero, G.; Molina, A.R. de Rosemary (Rosmarinus officinalis L.) Extract as a Potential Complementary Agent in Anticancer Therapy. *Nutr. Cancer* **2015**, *67*, 1223–1231. [CrossRef] [PubMed]

122. González-Vallinas, M.; Molina, S.; Vicente, G.; Zarza, V.; Martín-Hernández, R.; García-Risco, M.R.; Fornari, T.; Reglero, G.; Ramírez de Molina, A. Expression of microRNA-15b and the glycosyltransferase GCNT3

correlates with antitumor efficacy of Rosemary diterpenes in colon and pancreatic cancer. *PLoS ONE* **2014**, *9*, e98556. [CrossRef] [PubMed]

123. Giráldez, M.D.; Lozano, J.J.; Ramírez, G.; Hijona, E.; Bujanda, L.; Castells, A.; Gironella, M. Circulating microRNAs as biomarkers of colorectal cancer: Results from a genome-wide profiling and validation study. *Clin. Gastroenterol. Hepatol.* **2013**, *11*, 681–688. [CrossRef] [PubMed]

124. Gonsalves, W.I.; Mahoney, M.R.; Sargent, D.J.; Nelson, G.D.; Alberts, S.R.; Sinicrope, F.A.; Goldberg, R.M.; Limburg, P.J.; Thibodeau, S.N.; Grothey, A.; et al. Patient and Tumor Characteristics and BRAF and KRAS Mutations in Colon Cancer, NCCTG/Alliance N0147. *JNCI J. Natl. Cancer Inst.* **2014**, *106*. [CrossRef] [PubMed]

125. Chen, K.; Xia, G.; Zhang, C.; Sun, Y. Correlation between smoking history and molecular pathways in sporadic colorectal cancer: A meta-analysis. *Int. J. Clin. Exp. Med.* **2015**, *8*, 3241–3257. [PubMed]

126. Porta, M.; Crous-Bou, M.; Wark, P.A.; Vineis, P.; Real, F.X.; Malats, N.; Kampman, E. Cigarette smoking and K-ras mutations in pancreas, lung and colorectal adenocarcinomas: Etiopathogenic similarities, differences and paradoxes. *Mutat. Res.* **2009**, *682*, 83–93. [CrossRef] [PubMed]

127. Jayasekara, H.; MacInnis, R.J.; Williamson, E.J.; Hodge, A.M.; Clendenning, M.; Rosty, C.; Walters, R.; Room, R.; Southey, M.C.; Jenkins, M.A.; et al. Lifetime alcohol intake is associated with an increased risk of KRAS+ and BRAF-/KRAS- but not BRAF+ colorectal cancer. *Int. J. Cancer* **2017**, *140*, 1485–1493. [CrossRef] [PubMed]

128. Gilsing, A.M.J.; Fransen, F.; de Kok, T.M.; Goldbohm, A.R.; Schouten, L.J.; de Bruïne, A.P.; van Engeland, M.; van den Brandt, P.A.; de Goeij, A.F.P.M.; Weijenberg, M.P. Dietary heme iron and the risk of colorectal cancer with specific mutations in KRAS and APC. *Carcinogenesis* **2013**, *34*, 2757–2766. [CrossRef] [PubMed]

129. Beloribi-Djefaflia, S.; Vasseur, S.; Guillaumond, F. Lipid metabolic reprogramming in cancer cells. *Oncogenesis* **2016**, *5*, e189. [CrossRef] [PubMed]

130. Hoeft, B.; Linseisen, J.; Beckmann, L.; Müller-Decker, K.; Canzian, F.; Hüsing, A.; Kaaks, R.; Vogel, U.; Jakobsen, M.U.; Overvad, K.; et al. Polymorphisms in fatty acid metabolism-related genes are associated with colorectal cancer risk. *Carcinogenesis* **2010**, *31*, 466–472. [CrossRef] [PubMed]

131. Crous-Bou, M.; Rennert, G.; Salazar, R.; Rodriguez-Moranta, F.; Rennert, H.S.; Lejbkowicz, F.; Kopelovich, L.; Lipkin, S.M.; Gruber, S.B.; Moreno, V. Genetic polymorphisms in fatty acid metabolism genes and colorectal cancer. *Mutagenesis* **2012**, *27*, 169–176. [CrossRef] [PubMed]

132. Huang, J.; Frohlich, J.; Ignaszewski, A.P. The impact of dietary changes and dietary supplements on lipid profile. *Can. J. Cardiol.* **2011**, *27*, 488–505. [CrossRef] [PubMed]

133. Daimiel, L.; Vargas, T.; Ramírez de Molina, A. Nutritional genomics for the characterization of the effect of bioactive molecules in lipid metabolism and related pathways. *Electrophoresis* **2012**, *33*, 2266–2289. [CrossRef] [PubMed]

134. Hori, S.; Butler, E.; McLoughlin, J. Prostate cancer and diet: Food for thought? *BJU Int.* **2011**, *107*, 1348–1359. [CrossRef] [PubMed]

135. Huang, W.-Y.; Cai, Y.-Z.; Zhang, Y. Natural phenolic compounds from medicinal herbs and dietary plants: Potential use for cancer prevention. *Nutr. Cancer* **2010**, *62*, 1–20. [CrossRef] [PubMed]

136. Nishiumi, S.; Miyamoto, S.; Kawabata, K.; Ohnishi, K.; Mukai, R.; Murakami, A.; Ashida, H.; Terao, J. Dietary flavonoids as cancer-preventive and therapeutic biofactors. *Front. Biosci. Sch. Ed.* **2011**, *3*, 1332–1362. [CrossRef]

137. Gillies, P.J.; Bhatia, S.K.; Belcher, L.A.; Hannon, D.B.; Thompson, J.T.; Heuvel, J.P.V. Regulation of inflammatory and lipid metabolism genes by eicosapentaenoic acid-rich oil. *J. Lipid Res.* **2012**, *53*, 1679–1689. [CrossRef] [PubMed]

138. Biswas, S.K.; McClure, D.; Jimenez, L.A.; Megson, I.L.; Rahman, I. Curcumin induces glutathione biosynthesis and inhibits NF-kappaB activation and interleukin-8 release in alveolar epithelial cells: Mechanism of free radical scavenging activity. *Antioxid. Redox Signal.* **2005**, *7*, 32–41. [CrossRef] [PubMed]

139. Iio, A.; Ohguchi, K.; Iinuma, M.; Nozawa, Y.; Ito, M. Hesperetin upregulates ABCA1 expression and promotes cholesterol efflux from THP-1 macrophages. *J. Nat. Prod.* **2012**, *75*, 563–566. [CrossRef] [PubMed]

140. Wang, L.; Wesemann, S.; Krenn, L.; Ladurner, A.; Heiss, E.H.; Dirsch, V.M.; Atanasov, A.G. Erythrodiol, an Olive Oil Constituent, Increases the Half-Life of ABCA1 and Enhances Cholesterol Efflux from THP-1-Derived Macrophages. *Front. Pharmacol.* **2017**, *8*, 375. [CrossRef] [PubMed]

141. Jun, H.; Hoang, M.-H.; Yeo, S.-K.; Jia, Y.; Lee, S.-J. Induction of ABCA1 and ABCG1 expression by the liver X receptor modulator cineole in macrophages. *Bioorg. Med. Chem. Lett.* **2013**, *23*, 579–583. [CrossRef] [PubMed]

142. Wang, L.; Palme, V.; Rotter, S.; Schilcher, N.; Cukaj, M.; Wang, D.; Ladurner, A.; Heiss, E.H.; Stangl, H.; Dirsch, V.M.; Atanasov, A.G. Piperine inhibits ABCA1 degradation and promotes cholesterol efflux from THP-1-derived macrophages. *Mol. Nutr. Food Res.* **2017**, *61*. [CrossRef] [PubMed]

143. Wang, L.; Rotter, S.; Ladurner, A.; Heiss, E.H.; Oberlies, N.H.; Dirsch, V.M.; Atanasov, A.G. Silymarin Constituents Enhance ABCA1 Expression in THP-1 Macrophages. *Mol. Basel Switz.* **2015**, *21*. [CrossRef] [PubMed]

144. Madden, A.J.; Krehbiel, M.D.; Clarke, S.L. Garlic-derived Compounds Increase Expression of ABCA1 mRNA in RAW 264.7 Murine Macrophages. *FASEB J.* **2017**, *31*, 973.1.

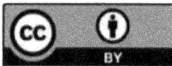

![nutrients logo] *nutrients*

MDPI

Review

Fatty Acids Consumption: The Role Metabolic Aspects Involved in Obesity and Its Associated Disorders

Priscila Silva Figueiredo [1,*], Aline Carla Inada [1], Gabriela Marcelino [1],
Carla Maiara Lopes Cardozo [1], Karine de Cássia Freitas [1], Rita de Cássia Avellaneda Guimarães [1],
Alinne Pereira de Castro [2], Valter Aragão do Nascimento [1] and Priscila Aiko Hiane [1]

[1] Post Graduate Program in Health and Development in the Central-West Region of Brazil, Federal University of Mato Grosso do Sul-UFMS, Campo Grande, MS 79079-900, Brazil; inada.aline@gmail.com (A.C.I.); gabi19ac@gmail.com (G.M.); carlinhalopescardozo@hotmail.com (C.M.L.C.); kcfreitas@gmail.com (K.d.C.F.); rita.guimares@ufms.br (R.d.C.A.G); aragao60@hotmail.com (V.A.d.N); priscila.hiane@ufms.br (P.A.H.)

[2] Post-Graduate Program in Biotechnology, Catholic University Dom Bosco, Campo Grande, MS 79117-900, Brazil; alinne_castro@ucdb.br

* Correspondence: priscilas.figueiredo@hotmail.com; Tel.: +55-67-3345-7445

Received: 1 September 2017; Accepted: 9 October 2017; Published: 22 October 2017

Abstract: Obesity and its associated disorders, such as insulin resistance, dyslipidemia, metabolic inflammation, dysbiosis, and non-alcoholic hepatic steatosis, are involved in several molecular and inflammatory mechanisms that alter the metabolism. Food habit changes, such as the quality of fatty acids in the diet, are proposed to treat and prevent these disorders. Some studies demonstrated that saturated fatty acids (SFA) are considered detrimental for treating these disorders. A high fat diet rich in palmitic acid, a SFA, is associated with lower insulin sensitivity and it may also increase atherosclerosis parameters. On the other hand, a high intake of eicosapentaenoic (EPA) and docosahexaenoic (DHA) fatty acids may promote positive effects, especially on triglyceride levels and increased high-density lipoprotein (HDL) levels. Moreover, polyunsaturated fatty acids (PUFAs) and monounsaturated fatty acids (MUFAs) are effective at limiting the hepatic steatosis process through a series of biochemical events, such as reducing the markers of non-alcoholic hepatic steatosis, increasing the gene expression of lipid metabolism, decreasing lipogenic activity, and releasing adiponectin. This current review shows that the consumption of unsaturated fatty acids, MUFA, and PUFA, and especially EPA and DHA, which can be applied as food supplements, may promote effects on glucose and lipid metabolism, as well as on metabolic inflammation, gut microbiota, and hepatic metabolism.

Keywords: fatty acids; obesity; obesity-related metabolic dysfunction; chronic diseases

---

1. Introduction

Obesity acts as a stressing agent both in adipose metabolism and in metabolic organs, including the liver, muscle, and pancreas, resulting in insulin resistance and type II diabetes mellitus DM II [1]. With the presence of obesity and the progressive expansion of adipocytes, the blood supply to the adipocytes decreases with ensuing hypoxia [2]. This expansion of adipocytes and hypoxia has been related to the onset of macrophage necrosis and infiltration into adipose tissue, leading to an overproduction of active metabolites called adipocytokines, such as glycerol, plasminogen activator inhibitor-1 (PAI-1), C-reactive protein (PCR), and proinflammatory mediators, including tumor necrosis factor alpha and interleukin-6 (TNFα and IL-6), and free fatty acids [3]. These changes initially result in an inflammatory process located in the adipose tissue, which expands to systemic inflammation associated with the development of obesity-related comorbidities [4].

The increased body fat observed in obesity is an increase in the number and/or size of adipocytes that are linked to metabolic and hemodynamic processes in the production of adipokines, which are responsible for causing insulin resistance and atherosclerosis, which are mediated by inflammatory cytokines [5]. Obese, but metabolically healthy individuals, have smaller adipocytes when compared to metabolically abnormal obese individuals, suggesting that hypertrophy of adipocytes is associated with the development of metabolic disorders [5].

With obesity, immune cells display phenotypic changes according to the type of dietary fatty acids, causing a change in the M2 macrophage, which has anti-inflammatory properties on M1 macrophages, which have pro-inflammatory properties. The consumption of saturated fatty acids (SFA) activate M1 genes that stimulate -α and IL-6 TNF production, whereas monounsaturated fatty acids (MUFA) activate the M2 genes related to the expression of Arginase-1 and interleukin-10, which are cytokines with anti-inflammatory action [6], as illustrated in Figure 1.

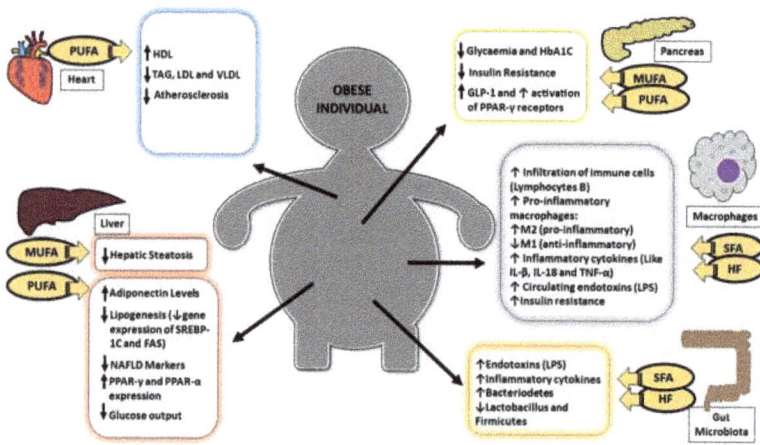

Figure 1. Different metabolic changes involved after consumption of different types of fatty acids: saturated (SFA), monounsaturated (MUFA), and polyunsaturated (PUFA) fatty acids. Different types of fatty acids have different effects on the major metabolic organs of the body. Diets with high levels of SFA, especially high fat (HF), modulate the inflammatory process with the infiltration of macrophages and other immunological cells, promoting higher production of type M2 macrophages, considered pro-inflammatory, with a reduction in type M1 macrophages, which are anti-inflammatory, in addition to the expression of inflammatory cytokines and circulating endotoxins, which promote insulin resistance. This inflammatory process is related to the microbiota, which also has a greater expression of inflammatory endotoxins and cytokines, as well as transitions in intestinal colonization, with increase of strains of the genus Firmicutes, and decrease of Bacteroidetes and Lactobacillus genus after consumption of HF diets rich in SFA. On the other hand, the consumption of MUFA and PUFA has positive effects on glucose metabolism, with a reduction in some parameters related to type II diabetes mellitus (DM II), such as hemoglobin A1c (HbA1c) and glycaemia, and a reduction of hepatic steatosis and related parameters. Intake of PUFA is linked to increased expression of adiponectin, an anti-inflammatory cytokine, which promotes hepatic metabolic enhancement, and reduces the risk of atherosclerosis, such as increased high density lipoprotein (HDL) and decreased triacyclglycerols (TAG). LDL; very low density lipoprotein (VLDL); glucagon-like peptide-1 (GLP-1) receptor; peroxisome proliferator-activated receptor-γ (PPAR-γ); free fatty acids (FFA); sterol regulatory element-binding protein -1C (SREBP-1C); Non-alcoholic fatty liver disease (NAFLD); interleukin (IL); tumor necrosis factor (TNF); lipopolyssacharide (LPS); high fat (HF).

At the end of the 1950s, the different types of fatty acids ingested in the diet were thought to influence glucose homeostasis. Many decades later, new in vitro and in vivo studies maintained this hypothesis, pointing to different influences according to chain length and the number of double bonds in fatty acids, altering sensitivity, pro- or anti-lipotoxic action, and insulinotropic influence [7,8].

In order to control this inflammatory process and the obesity comorbidities, some strategies are used, such as changes in diet, which include the reduction of SFA sources and an increase in the consumption of MUFA and polyunsaturated fatty acids (PUFA), which are associated with cardiovascular protection, acting on atherosclerosis [9–11].

Mammals are able to desaturate fatty acids at positions Δ5, Δ6, and Δ9 [12]. The latter desaturase is called stearoyl-CoA desaturase (SCD-1) and it converts SFAs, such as stearic acid (18:0), into oleic acid, a MUFA; while Δ5 and Δ6 desaturases are required for long-chain PUFA desaturation. These kind of PUFAs are classified as omega-3 (ω-3) and omega-6 (ω-6) [13]. Araquidonic acid (AA) is the principal ω-6 fatty acid, whereas eicosapentaenoic (EPA) and docosahexaenoic (DHA) fatty acids are the main ω-3 FAs [14]. These FAs are defined as essential fatty acids because they cannot be synthesized in human cells, and therefore must be obtained from dietary linoleic acid (C18:2 n-6) and α-linolenic acid (C18:3 n-3) [15].

Considering the importance and the effects of fatty acid intake, the global problem of obesity, and the risk factors associated with obesity and chronic diseases, FAs are usually a component of nutrition educational programs and those individuals receive guidance for lifestyle changes. For many years, highlighting the consumption pattern of lipid content and quality in the diet, aiming at a reduction in the consumption of saturated fatty acids, was a key component of an obesity-targeted diet [16,17]. Because some lipid sources of saturated fatty acids have shown positive results, as in the case of coconut oil, extensive discussion has been generated about the quality of lipids that should be used in the diet. In addition, other measures related to lipid ingestion, proposed in the treatment of chronic diseases, should be considered, and deserves further elucidation to avoid such controversies [18].

The objective of this review is to determine the metabolic effect related to the mechanism of actions of the different types of fatty acids, including saturated, monounsaturated, and polyunsaturated acids, in obesity and its related disorders, (i.e., insulin resistance, dyslipidemia, inflammation, non-alcoholic fatty liver, and intestinal microbiota) through the compilation of several scientific papers published in the last five years.

2. Insulin Resistance and Associated Comorbidities

The main factors responsible for the development of type 2 diabetes mellitus (DM II) are the high production of hepatic glucose, impaired insulin secretion, and insulin resistance, which is common in obesity [19]. During DM II evolution, adipocytes become resistant to the anti-lipolytic activity of insulin, which leads to increased concentrations of free fatty acids in both the fed and postprandial states. This situation worsens considerably as the function of beta cells is impaired and insulin secretion decreases [20].

Dietary fatty acids play an important role in cell membranes and insulin sensitivity, interfering with the metabolic control of diabetes. Observational studies show a strong association between diets with a high amount of SFAs, being mainly palmitic acid, and a small amount of PUFA, with insulin resistance (Figure 1) [21]. Hypercaloric diets, especially hyperlipidic ones, are related to the induction of insulin resistance [22].

An excess of nutrient intake also directly regulates tumor cell growth, and saturated fatty acids are more associated with this inducement of proliferation than unsaturated fatty acids, which promote apoptosis [23]. A diet low in saturated fatty acids is recommended for the treatment of DM II. Among the SFAs, palmitic acid (16:0) is believed to be responsible for the damage caused to β-pancreatic cell function and to insulin resistance [24].

In a recent study [22], a hypercaloric and hyperlipidic diet in the induction of insulin resistance in humans was developed and tested. The effects of a diet rich in saturated fatty acids after 24 h included increases in glycaemia, insulin, and HDL-cholesterol levels when compared to a normocaloric and normolipid diet, whose lipid composition corresponded to 25% of the total calories, being 12% MUFA, 8% PUFA, and 5% SFA (Table 1). The negative effect of the SFAs was suggested to be greater when associated with a hypercaloric diet (>27 kcal/kg), since the SFAs probably enter the cell membranes by altering the insulin receptors and their secretion, resulting in insulin resistance [25].

Table 1. Effects of different types of fatty acids on insulin resistance and associated comorbidities during human studies.

Host	Fatty Acid Composition	Glycaemia-Related Effects in Obesity	References
Humans	Diets with 63% SFA (42% palmitic, 29% MUFA, 4% PUFA)	Increased glycaemia (3.70%) Increased insulin (25%)	[22]
Hypertensive women with DM II	(1) 1.5 g fish oil (21.9% EPA, 14.1% DHA) (2) 2.5 g fish oil (21.9% EPA, 14.1% DHA) (3) Control group.	Glucose, mg/dL; glycated hemoglobin, %; insulin, μU/mL and HOMA-IR without changes.	[26]
Diabetics and nondiabetics individuals	(1) 300 g of vegetables and 25 mL of PUFA-rich plants (61.8% linoleic, 11.5% linolenic, and 16.4% of oleic fatty acid) per day	Reduction of HbA1c (hemoglobin A1c) (%) after 4 and 8 weeks	[27]
Subjects with early-stage DM II or metabolic syndrome	Individuals received corn oil (CO); a combination of borage [*Borago officinalis* L.] and echium oil [*Echium plantagineum* L.] (BO) or fish oil (FO): 9 CO capsules, 10 BO capsules (3 borage and 7 echium), or 9 FO capsules	Statistically significant increase in insulin and reduction in HbA1c of FO group.	[28]
DM II subjects	Supplementation of 3 g/day of ALA or placebo for 60 days	ALA group improved IS corrected for FFM (M/FFM)—Insulin sensitivity corrected for fat-free mass.	[29]
DM II subjects	(1) High-carbohydrate/high-fiber/low-glycemic index diet (CHO/fiber group) (2) High-MUFA diet (MUFA group) (3) High-carbohydrate/high-fiber/low-glycemic index diet plus physical activity program (CHO/fiber + Exercise group) (4) High-MUFA diet plus physical activity program (MUFA + Ex group).	Reduction of HbA1c levels in the MUFA group.	[30]
Human clinical trials: obese children	Supplementation of CLA (3 g/day) with 50:50 isomers c9, t11, and t10, c12 or placebo (1 g/day) 3 times per day for 16 weeks	Significant improvement in insulin, fasting insulinemia, and HOMA-IR in CLA group.	[31]

Abbreviations: Saturated fatty acids (SFA); monounsaturated fatty acids (MUFA); polyunsaturated fatty acids (PUFA); type II diabetes mellitus (DM II); docosahexaenoic (DHA) fatty acids; alfa-linolenic fatty acid (ALA); homeostasis model assessment-estimated insulin resistance (HOMA-IR); hemoglobin A1c (HbA1c); insulin sensitivity corrected for fat-free mass (FFM); carbohydrate (CHO); conjugated linoleic acid (CLA).

In a study by Crochemore et al. [26] (Table 1), women with DM II and hypertension had no statistically significant difference among the groups that received supplementation of 1.5 g and 2.5 g fish oil, with 21.9% EPA and 14.1% DHA, respectively, and a control group, for glucose, glycated hemoglobin, insulin, or homeostasis model assessment-estimated insulin resistance (HOMA-IR), regardless of the dosage. The doses of fish oil and the duration of the study, at only 30 days, were potentially inadequate to note a significant difference in this population, which also had a hypertension frame. Additionally, despite the absence of a statistical difference, the groups supplemented with fish oil presented a trend in HOMA-IR improvement, which decreased 21.4% and 35.7%, respectively, in both the supplemented groups when compared to the baseline.

Another parameter used is Hemoglobin A1c, which reflects the cumulative changes that occur over several weeks to months, so the duration of treatment may be particularly important for this biomarker. Glycation refers to the non-enzymatic reaction of reducing sugars with primary amino groups' Schiff bases that undergo an Amadori rearrangement, which is well-studied for proteins and peptides. Glycation sites derived from glucose have been reported and characterized by many proteins in the last decades, with the glycated N-terminal hemoglobin A (HbA1c) being a well-established biomarker to diagnose and control diabetes [32]. Müllner et al. [27] showed a decrease in this parameter after implementing a diet including 300 g of vegetables and 25 mL of PUFA-rich plant oil daily. Additionally, a significant decrease in hemoglobin A1c occurred during the eight-week test with the fish oil group, where each capsule had 3.58 g of EPA and 2.44 g of DHA [28], demonstrating the positive effects on glycated hemoglobin after the intake of polyunsaturated sources, whether of vegetable or marine origin.

Another study with DM II subjects did not show significant improvements in a large part of the glucose homeostasis parameters. The ALA group had improved insulin sensitivity, which may be associated with the greater increase in adiponectin levels also evaluated in this study, which has an inverse correlation with HOMA-IR, reinforcing the positive effect of ALA supplementation on IR [29]. Patients with DM II exhibit lower postprandial glucagon-like peptide-1 (GLP-1) responses as compared to healthy individuals [33]. GLP-1 is secreted from intestinal endocrine cells in response to nutrient intake and plays several different roles in metabolic homeostasis after its absorption [33].

The supplementation of Conjugated Linoleic Acid (CLA) resulted in improvements in obese children after four months of intervention, combined with lifestyle changes for both the children and their parents. Garibay-Nieto et al. [31] implemented a program consisting of monthly visits that included a one-hour structured physical activity session, followed by a psychoeducational group session, with consultations with nutritionists, and supplementation of CLA (3 g/day) or placebo (1 g/day) for obese children three times a day for 16 weeks, which resulted in insulin reductions (μU/mL), fasting insulinemia, and HOMA-IR in the CLA group.

CLA represents a group of positional and geometric isomers of linoleic acid (18:2n-6), whose predominant form is cis-9, trans-11 isomers, and due to its high composition of PUFA, promotes benefits in the membrane phospholipid composition, thus improving its fluidity. Another possible mechanism for the antidiabetic effects of CLA supplementation is the activation of peroxisome proliferator-activated receptor-γ (PPAR-γ) receptors [34], which participate in lipid homeostasis and are predominantly expressed in adipose tissue. With the activation of PPAR-γ, CLA also increases the gene expression of adiponectin and thus may affect glucose metabolism and insulin sensitivity [35].

Furthermore, some in vivo and in vitro studies presented positive results after the use of unsaturated sources, especially the n-3 series, and with MUFA, basically oleic fatty acid, which are demonstrated in Table 2. An in vitro study [36] demonstrated that oleate did not induce insulin resistance in cardiovascular cells, such as cardiomyocyte, vascular smooth muscle cells, or endothelial cells, which are otherwise palmitate induced, showing the beneficial cardiovascular effects in relation to insulin signaling with oleate. Previous studies showed this induction of resistance insulin with palmitate also being observed in other tissues, such as adipocytes and skeletal muscle [37,38]. Oleate was able to prevent insulin resistance in the myotubes through the activation of PI3K and a mechanism dependent on amp-activated protein kinase (AMPK) [36].

Malinska et al. [39] found an increase in insulin sensitivity in hypertriglyceridemia-induced dyslipidemia rats fed a high sucrose diet, supplemented with either sunflower oil or Conjugated Linoleic Acid (CLA) (2 g/100 g diet), for eight weeks. CLA possibly present anti-diabetic effects related to the activation of PPAR-γ receptors [34].

The MUFA intake also showed positive results on the glucose parameters, with a statistically significant reduction in the HbA1c levels [30]. A high-MUFA diet also showed an improvement in insulin resistance when compared to a high-SFA diet in mice, with significantly lower fasting glucose and insulin concentrations and attenuated insulin secretion, in response to glucose challenge. These challenges included intraperitoneal glucose, insulin tolerance testing, and insulin secretion response in overnight fasted mice after intraperitoneal injection with 1.5 g/kg glucose [40]. Carbohydrates and fatty acid components of a meal can directly influence postprandial GLP-1 responses [33]. MUFAs seem to be powerful stimulators of GLP-1 secretion, both in the enterocytes cultured from mice in vivo fand in Zucker rats that were genetically obese [41,42].

Table 2. Effects of different types of fatty acids on insulin resistance and associated comorbidities during in vivo and in vitro studies.

Host	Fatty Acid Composition	Glycaemia-Related Effects in Obesity	References
In vitro insulin resistance at cellular level from thoracic aorta arteries of three 8-week-old wild-type male mice	Cell lines were cultured with high glucose and were serum-starved for insulin signaling and relatives free fatty acids (palmitate or oleate)	Oleate treatment for 2 h did not produce insulin resistance. Palmitate significantly induced insulin resistance for 18 h.	[36]
C57BL/6 male mice	SFA High Fat Diet (HFD) with 45% palmitic acid; MUFA-HFD (45% oleic acid), and a standard chow as a control group (5.2% fat: 0.9% SFA, 1.3% MUFA, and 3.4% PUFA)	Lower fast glucose, insulin concentrations and insulin secretion in MUFA-HFD group compared to the SFA-HFD group.	[40]
Hypertriglyceridemia-induced dyslipidemia rats	High sucrose diet supplemented with either sunflower oil or Conjugated Linoleic Acid (CLA) (2 g/100 g diet)	Decrease in glucose and insulin (mmol/L) in CLA supplemented group.	[39]
Diet-induced IR rat model	Supplementation of fish oil (n-3 PUFA), sunflower oil (n-6 PUFA), and high oleic sunflower oil (n-9 MUFA)	Reduction of HOMA-IR in n-3 PUFA.	[43]

Abbreviations: Saturated fatty acids (SFA); monounsaturated fatty acids (MUFA); polyunsaturated fatty acids (PUFA); homeostasis model assessment-estimated insulin resistance (HOMA-IR); conjugated linoleic acid (CLA); high fat diet (HFD).

The liver plays a unique role in regulating glucose homeostasis by maintaining blood glucose concentration within a normal range. However, impaired insulin action in the liver leads to insulin resistance, characterized by an impaired insulin capacity to inhibit glucose production. Thus, insulin resistance in the liver, which is the reduced sensitivity to insulin in the liver, causes gluconeogenesis and hyperglycemia. As a result of insulin resistance, adipocytes increase the release of free fatty acids (FFA) in the circulatory system [44].

A study with a diet-induced IR rat model [43] showed a significant reduction in HOMA-IR after supplementation of 12 g per 100 g for 12 weeks with fish oil, when compared to the n-6 PUFA and MUFA groups (Table 2). The evidence indicates positive effects on insulin resistance and glycemic metabolism with consumption of ω-3 PUFA, which can be explained by the alteration in serum fatty acid composition, which influences the membrane fluidity with the ingestion of these polyunsaturated sources, allowing for greater insulin binding. Subsequent events, such as aggregation, internalization of the insulin-receptor complex, and the movement of the glucose transporter to the cell membrane, could be facilitated by changes in membrane fluidity [45].

The evidence indicates that the composition of dietary fatty acid intake can change the fatty acid composition of the cell membrane, thereby affecting insulin sensitivity [46]. A diet rich in unsaturated fatty acids, present in oilseeds, plays an important role in the prevention of insulin resistance, increasing insulin affinity for the receptors [47]. Furthermore, the composition of oilseeds with high magnesium [48,49], high fiber content [50,51], and low glycemic index [52,53] have also been linked to a lower risk of diabetes.

In addition to the previously mentioned factors associated with glucose metabolism and insulin resistance, the metabolism of this comorbidity is known to be complex, being associated with cardiovascular diseases (CVD). CVD mortality has been strongly linked to the prevalence of diabetes, in which CVD is considered an important risk factor for DM and vice versa. The metabolism involved in the CVD should be addressed with the consumption of different lipid sources, accessing the different influences in the comorbidities linked to obesity [54].

3. Dyslipidemias

Dyslipidemia is characterized by the change in lipid concentrations in the bloodstream with the accumulation of one or more classes of lipoproteins [55]. In this case, this process is called hypercholesterolemia, which is the accumulation of low density lipoprotein (LDL) in the plasma by alterations in the genes of the LDL receptor (LDLR), or apolipoprotein B-100, which is considered as one of the most important components of atherogenic lipoproteins [55]. Hypertriglyceridemia is the result of chylomicron condensation of very low density lipoprotein (VLDL), or both lipoproteins in the plasma, with a decrease in high density lipoprotein (HDL) [56]. These condensations are as a result of lipoprotein lipase (LPL), which is responsible for promoting triglyceride breakdown with apolipoprotein A5 (APOA5) mutations, and the inhibition of LPL and hepatic lipase by apolipoprotein C-III (APOC3), contributing to the triglycerides concentration increase [57].

The atherogenic process occurs when Lymphocytes T migrates to the intima layer of the arteries by proinflammatory cytokines, producing macrophages by monocytes and increasing the LDL levels, resulting in atherosclerotic plaques [58]. These plaques originate in the intima and media layers of medium and large arteries, and are thus the principal factor related to CVD [59].

Some types of treatment and prevention methods are available to address dyslipidemia and atherosclerosis, such as specific medicines, as well as the adoption of a healthy lifestyle, which includes an improvement in eating habits [60]. One of the reasons for changing these habits is to improve the quality of lipids consumed in the diet, involving recommendations to reduce SFAs, which are associated with the dyslidemia process because they cause an increase in LDL, which is due to a reduction in the production and activity of the LDLR gene, related to alter the hepatic metabolic processes and fatty acid biosynthesis [61].

Besides that, recommendations are proposed to increase the ingestion of PUFA sources in detrimental of SFA reduce. The n-3 PUFA consumption operates on the reduction of plasma triacyclglycerols (TAG), VLDL, and apolipoprotein B-100 (APOB-100) [62,63]. A multinacional study (Table 3) with individuals at least 18 years of age with average serum TG concentrations >500 mg/dL but <2000 mg/dL at screening (1 and 2 weeks before random assignment) who were either untreated for dyslipidemia or were using a stable (for at least 6 weeks before the first qualifying lipid measurement) dosage of a statin, CAI, or their combination. The individuals were divided into four groups, which one of them was a control group with 4g/day of olive oil supplemented. There were three groups that receive the supplementation of fish oil (EPA + DHA) in capsules of 2, 3, and 4 g/day. All of the groups that receive the fish oil presented decreasing values for TG, non-HDL, LDL, VLDL and ApoB-100 from baseline [63]. n-3 PUFA acts on ApoB-100 by inhibiting its synthesis and, consequently, decreasing the plasma concentration of all lipoproteins composed with Apo-B, especially VLDL and LDL [64]. DHA also presents an important mechanism in the signaling pathway, inhibiting the delta-6 desaturase, an indispensable enzyme that produces gamma linolenic and dihomo-gamma-linolenic acids from linolenic acid, to the detriment of the production of araquidonic acid (AA). In addition, DHA acts to improve cellular membrane fluids, which enables the flexibility of the arteries, aiding in the removal of lipids, as well as possible inflammatory agents, that are deposited in the membrane [63].

Table 3. Effects of consuming different types of fatty acids during human studies on dyslipidemia.

Host	Fatty Acid Composition	Effects	References
Humans with hypertriglyceridemia	n-3 PUFA (2,3 and 4 g of fish oil)	Reduction in VLDL, TG, non-HDL, LDL and Apo-B	[62]
Humans: Hemodialysis Patients	2 capsules of EPA and 1.28 g DHA/day	TG, TC, and LDL (no differences) EPA/DHA and placebo. Increase in HDL.	[65]
Humans	2 capsules of 900 mg/day containing EPA and DHA	Increase in HDL, reduction in LDL and TG. Improvement Protein C reactive levels.	[66]
Humans	4 capsules of 1 g/day containing EPA and DHA for 6 months	Reduction in TG, increase in HDL. No difference in TC and LDL.	[67]
Humans	4 different foods enriched with 3 rich-n-3-PUFA oils	Increase in HDL. LDL—no differences.	[68]

Abbreviations: Polyunsaturated fatty acids (PUFA); very low density lipoprotein (VLDL); triacylglycerol (TG); unlike LDL-C (non-HDL); low density lipoprotein (LDL); apolipoprotein-B (Apo-B); total cholesterol (TC); eicosapentaenoic (EPA); docosahexaenoic (DHA); high density lipoprotein (HDL).

Mattos et al. [65] performed a randomized study with administration of two fish oil capsules per day in hemodialysis patients for 12 weeks. The results did not demonstrate differences between the groups that received n-3-PUFA and the control group that received a placebo. This may have occurred because hemodialysis patients are have a higher propensity of developing CVD.

In another study [68], after the use of flaxseed oil, Echium seed oil, and microalgae oil, which is another source of n-3-PUFA with high DHA, changes in LDL levels were not seen, however, they observed an increase in HDL levels. This result corroborates with a study by Wang et al. [67], who observed that individuals that consumed four capsules of fish oil, containing EPA and DHA, for six weeks showed no differences in total cholesterol (TC) and LDL, whereas TAG levels were reduced.

The following molecular mechanisms responsible for the reduction of serum TAGs, after EPA and DHA ingestion, have been proposed to create this beneficial effect: the decreased expression of sterol regulatory element-binding protein-1c (SREBP-1c) may be one of the factors responsible for the reduced secretion of VLDL-TAG, or the increased mitochondrial oxidation rates, or peroxisome that reduces the substrate for TAG synthesis [69].

The expression of decreased SREBP-1c can be mediated by the inhibition of liver X-receptor binding (LXR) to the LXR/retinoid X receptor. The increase in peroxisomal oxidation rates may result in the increase of peroxisome proliferator-activated receptor-α (PPAR-α) on the expression of the acyl-coenzyme A oxidase gene. In addition, the reduction in the activity of the enzymes that perform TAG synthesis decreases the distribution of non-esterified fatty acids from adipose tissue and decreases the availability of apoprotein B, which potentially results in a lower release of VLDL-TAG. On the periphery, increased lipoprotein lipase activity may lead to increased clearance of VLDL-TAG, possibly due to increased PPAR-γ and/or PPAR-α gene expression [69]. Additionally, EPA and DHA fatty acids are capable of preventing the synthesis and the secretion of hepatic VLDL and TAG, increasing the TAG clearance by chylomicrons and VLDL particles. Furthermore, both EPA and DHA are preferably diverted for phospholipid synthesis paths, whereas other fatty acids, such as oleic acid, are generally incorporated into TAG [70].

Furthermore, n-3 PUFAs promoted an increase in HDL in the studies that used EPA and DHA. This mechanism may improve the atherosclerosis protection due to the fact that n-3-PUFAs act in reverse cholesterol trafficking [71]. This involves of the transportation of cholesterol molecules present in high concentration in the tissue, back to the liver to be eliminated by bile in feces, improving the endothelial dysfunction and promoting antioxidants and anti-inflammatory effects [71].

Considering that animal models are extremely important for elucidating the etiology of diseases in humans, having an integrated view of disorders mechanisms [72], there are some in vivo studies in Table 4 on dyslipidemia. A treatment with rats demonstrated that a high amount of SFAs in the diet during a 30-day study resulted in increased levels of total cholesterol (TC), TGA, LDL, and VLDL in the bloodstream, as shown in Table 4 [73]. On the other hand, after 180 days of diet, TC, HDL, and LDL serum levels increased, while VLDL and TGA levels diminished. The data showed that a diet rich in SFA exerted a hyperlipidemic effect only on the 30th day, but a long-term diet displayed beneficial effects on hyperlipidemia (Table 4) [73], which could be a consequence of the decrease in apolipoprotein synthesis and the formation of VLDL in the liver [74,75].

SFA and n-6 PUFA showed a negative effect on TC, HDL, and TAG levels, which increased in relation to the groups that received flaxseed oil, including alfa-linolenic fatty acid (ALA) and SFO (a combination of sesame and flaxseed oil; n-3 and n-6 PUFA), in wistar rats after 65 days of treatment with a standard diet poor in lipid sources, at 7% fat [76]. The SFO groups also demonstrated an improvement in non-HDL and LDL levels when compared to others (Table 4). This could be explained by the proportion of n-6 to n-3 PUFA in this diet, which was 1:1, which is considered the best proportion of essential fatty acids associated with cardioprotective effects [77]. According to another study with pigs, a diet with the proportions of n-6:n-3 from 1:1 up to 5:1 better assisted in the use and absorption of fatty acids, also promoting an anti-inflammatory action [78].

Table 4. Effects of consuming different types of fatty acids during in vivo studies on dyslipidemia.

Host	Fatty Acid Composition	Effects	References
Wistar rats	Three diets and a control group (7% fat): CG (Saturated fatty acid); SO (Sesame oil—oleic and linoleic fatty acid); FO (Flaxseed oil—alfa-linolenic fatty acid), and SFO (flaxseed and sesame oil)	Increased levels of total cholesterol, HDL, VLDL, and TAG in CG and SO groups. Reduction in levels in non-HDL and LDL for SFO group.	[76]
Wistar rats	6 groups: control (AIN-93G—7% soy oil); extra virgin oil (OO-C) (7% soy oil and 13% extra virgin); sunflower oil (HOSO) (7% soy oil and 13% sunflower oil); Atherogenic diet (AT), (rich-SFAs (12.3 g %) and cholesterol (4 g %); Experimental diets were: OO and HOSO (11.82% and 12.9 % MUFA and 4% cholesterol).	HOSO: Increase in TC and non-HDL, HDL diminished and decrease in TG in comparison to AT. OO: Reduced TC and non-HDL.	[79]
Wistar rats	4 groups over 5 weeks: Extra virgin olive oil group (OO) (SFA 12.0%, MUFA 81.9%, PUFA 6.10%), sunflower group (HOSO) (SFA 7.82%, MUFA 87.11%, PUFA 4.75%), sunflower oil and phytosterols group (HOSO-F) (1% phytosterols); sunflower oil and n-3-PUFA (HOSO-P) (6.5% fish oil).	HOSO: Increase in TC and non-HDL and reduction in HDL; HOSO-P and HOSO-F: Decrease in TC, non-HDL and TAG and increase in HDL in comparison to the OO group.	[80]
Wistar rats	High fat (HF) diets enriched in saturated fatty acids (SFAs); MUFA (oleic acid); PUFA n-6 and PUFA n-3.	TG decreased in MUFA and PUFA n-6 just at first day; Reduction in TG levels with a longer time feeding (21 days)	[81]

Abbreviations: Polyunsaturated fatty acids (PUFA); very low density lipoprotein (VLDL); triacylglycerol (TG); unlike LDL-C (non-HDL); low density lipoprotein (LDL); total cholesterol (TC); high density lipoprotein (HDL); American Institute of Nutrition Rodent Diets for growth (AIN-93G); sunflower group (HOSO); Extra virgin olive oil group (OO);

For MUFA, Macri et al. [79] showed that sunflower oil consumption resulted in an increase in visceral fat depots and liver weight, due to cholesterol esters that are supplied by oleic acid from the diet, contributing to cholesterol oleate synthesis in the liver and to the secretion of lipoproteins that possess ApoB, like LDL. On the other hand, olive oil led to a reduction in TC and LDL, which contributes to the anti-atherogenic effect.

In a similar study performed by Alsina et al. [80], fish-oil supplemented high-oleic-sunflower oil group (HOSO-F) supplementation diminished mesenteric, epidydimal, and perirenal fats, which become visceral fat deposits. The group that received HOSO supplemented with fish oil or phytosterols (F) displayed an improvement in lipid serum levels and fat deposits. Moreover, supplementation with F resulted in the inhibition of cholesterol absorption in the gastrointestinal tract. During the digestive process, cholesterol in the diet is solubilized by bile acids, incorporated in mixed micelles, and absorbed in enterocytes through the Niemann-Pick C1 Like-1 transporter [82]. F are metabolized in the same way as cholesterol involved in dynamic competition. Finally, F dislocate cholesterol from micelles and the micelles are eliminated by feces [83].

A study [81] with 96 wistar rats in their experimental study, separated them into four groups according to weight and the concentration of TG in plasma and cholesterol. The standard diet was supplemented with 15% of different sources of fat, with the SFA group with bovine serum, used as control; MUFA, having as source the olive oil; PUFA n-3 using fish oil; and, PUFA n-6 with safflower oil. TG levels showed a significant reduction in the first day of supplementation of MUFA and PUFA-6, which when compared to groups SFA and PUFA, n-3 had higher statistical significance. However, after three weeks of supplementation, the MUFA and n-6 PUFA groups returned to TG levels prior to treatment, increasing. Regarding long-term treatment, there was a reduction in the TG levels only in PUFA-3 supplementation. In this study, plasma cholesterol did not show changes in supplementation at both experimental times, a short- and long-term reduction was observed only in animals supplemented with PUFA-3. This TG reduction was accompanied by a decrease of activities of the lipogenic enzymes acetyl-CoA carboxylase (ACC) and fatty acid synthase (FAS), as well as a decreased activity of the citrate carrier (CIC), a mitochondrial protein linked to lipogenesis [81].

It is believed that inhibition of de novo lipogenesis (DNL) may be a viable approach to treating obesity-related disorders, especially in rodents. The decreased DNL is related to reducing the amount of synthesized fatty acids that enter in the pathway of esterification and, resulting in minor's levels of TG for VLDL assembly [81,84]. The hypotriglyceridemic effect of PUFA is partly caused by the reduced activities of liver lipogenic enzymes and by increased β-oxidation, consistent with increased mitochondrial as compared to peroxisomal oxidation [85].

The therapeutic potential of n-PUFA is important because it mediates the biological processes, such as eicosanoid production [86], which creates signaling molecules including leukotrienes, prostaglandins, thromboxane, and prostacyclins. These molecules are responsible for different cellular functions such as chemotaxis (blood cell migration), platelet aggregation, and cellular growth, demonstrating that the type of fatty acid consumed influences inflammation [87].

4. Inflammatory Process and Intestinal Microbiota

Low-grade chronic inflammation contributes to the inflammatory state in adipose tissue of obese individuals, mediated by innate immunity that leads to the production of proinflammatory cytokines, such as TNF-α, IL-1, IL-6, and IL-1β. The excess of adipose tissue favors the exaggerated release of free fatty acids through the action of catecholamines. This process inhibits the capture of glucose, generating a state of hyperglycemia that may cause hyperinsulinemia. The inflammatory process is characterized by the infiltration of macrophages and lymphocytes into adipose tissue and even into other peripheral organs. It results in an imbalance responsible for increasing the production of inflammatory cytokines that contribute to the onset of other metabolic dysfunctions, such as insulin resistance, since they may inhibit signaling or even insulin receptors [88–90].

Changes in diet quality may then improve inflammatory markers, as observed in 22 obese children and adolescents, with a body mass index (BMI) beyond the 95th percentile for age and sex, before and after the qualitative change in their food consumption [90]. The researchers relied on therapeutic protocols, suggesting a lower consumption of foods high in lipids and sugars and an increase in food sources of fiber, having only quantitative control over the portion sizes consumed, were beneficial. As a result, obese individuals (Table 5), when evaluated prior to intervention, had high values for various inflammatory cytokines, such as IL-1β and IL-18, which are associated with inflammatory and autoimmune disorders. INF-γ, IL-12A, IL-6, and TNF-α also decreased after 18 months of intervention. They also observed a decrease in lipopolyssacharide (LPS) and CD14 even without a significant decrease in BMI [90].

Another study [91] (Table 5) evaluated four types of diets with different FA, and found that postprandial endotoxin is influenced by the FA composition of the diet and not by the fat content itself. The results indicated that subjects consuming n-3 PUFA meals decreased their serum endotoxin levels, unlike those who consumed the n-6 PUFA meals, which increased these levels, but the inflammatory markers themselves did not show any changes. This was justified by the small number of participants, considered healthy, and used only a single meal as a source of evaluation. Nonetheless, lower endotoxin levels agree with Simopoulos [92], who considered n-6 PUFA as being responsible for the increase in cellular triglycerides and for the permeability of membrane, which can lead to the accumulation of adipose tissue fat, which is highly pro-inflammatory, and has pro-thrombotic and pro-adipogenic roles. Therefore, the proportion of consumption in relation to the n-6 PUFA and n-3 PUFA rate should be balanced, with the n-3 PUFA consumption being higher to preserve its protective role for metabolic disorders, especially in relation to the inflammatory state.

In another report [93], the effects of HF diets with different concentrations of palmitic acid and oleic acid on metabolism of obese adults were studied over three weeks of treatment. There was a diet with high content of palmitic acid (HPA) and moderate in oleic acid (OA) (fat, 40.4% kcal; PA, 16.0% kcal; OA, 16.2% kcal), and a diet low in PA and high in OA (HOA) (fat, 40.1% kcal; PA, 2.4% kcal; OA, 28.8% kcal). The HPA diet resulted in a decrease in IL-1B, an inflammatory marker, when compared to the control diet with 15.9% OA. This diet also resulted in a decrease in TNF-α, IL-18, and IL-10 levels. On the other hand, the HOA diet showed an increase in these same inflammatory markers, showing that the uneven proportion between these two fatty acids (FA) in the diet may increase inflammatory cytokines, thus triggering this process.

Table 5. Effects of different types of fatty acids on the inflammatory process and intestinal microbiota in human studies.

Host	Fatty Acid Composition of the Experiment	Microbiota	Inflammatory Process	References
Adults individuals	Control group (28.4% fat, of which 5.3% was palmitic fatty acid and 15.9% was oleic fatty acid); High fat (40.4% fat, of which 16% was palmitic fatty acid and 16.2% was oleic fatty acid); High fat (40.4% fat, of which 2.4% was palmitic fatty acid and 28.8% was oleic fatty acid)	Not observed	↓ IL-1β, IL-10, IL-18, and TNF-α ↑ IL-1β, IL-10, IL-18, and TNF-α	[93]
Obese children and adolescents (BMI >95th percentile for sex and age)	Therapeutic protocol: ↓ Fat ↓ Sugar ↑ Fibers	Not observed	↓ IFN-γ, IL-12A, IL-18, TNF-α, IL-6, IL-1β.	[90]
Adult individuals	Control group (20% fat/olive oil—MUFA) High fat with n-3 PUFA (35% fat with fish oil) High fat with n-6 PUFA (35% fat and grapeseed oil) High Fat with SFA (35% fat and coconut oil)	Not observed	↓ endotoxins postprandial ↑ endotoxins postprandial	[91]
Obese individuals	Mediterranean Diet (35% fat, 22% monounsaturated) Low-fat, high-complex carbohydrate diet diet (28% fat, 12% monounsaturated)	↑ *Roseburia* and *Oscillospita* and ↓ *Prevotella* ↑ *Prevotella*, ↓ *Roseburia* and ↑ *F. prausnitzii*	Not obeserved	[94]
Metabolic syndrome "at-risk" population	HS: High saturated fatty acids diet High monounsaturated fat (MUFA)/high glycemic index (GI) (HM/HGI) High MUFA/low GI (HM/LGI) High carbohydrate (CHO)/high GI (HC/HGI) High CHO/low GI (HC/LGI)	↑ Bifidobacterium and Bacteroidetes		[95]
Hypercholesterolemic individuals	Virgin olive oil (OO) naturally containing 80 mg of PC/kg, (VOO) Phenolic compound (PC) enriched virgin olive oil containing 500 mg PC/kg, from OO (FVOO) PC-enriched virgin olive oil containing a mixture of 500 mg PC/kg from OO and thyme 1:1 (FVOOT)	↑ Bifidobacterium, Parascardovia denticolens and Roseburia		[96]
DM 2 subjects	Control group Sardine group (SG)	↓ Firmicutes/Bacteroidetes ↓ Firmicutes/Bacteroidetes and ↓ bacteroidetes/prevotella	↑ TNF-α ↑ Adiponectin	[97]

Abbreviation: Interferons-γ (IFN-γ); body mass index (BMI).

Haro et al. [94] aimed to study the changes in microbiota after one year's consumption of a Mediterranean diet (MD) or a low-fat, high-complex carbohydrate diet (LFHCC diet) in an obese population, within the Coronary Diet Intervention With Olive Oil and Cardiovascular Prevention (CORDIOPREV) study, an ongoing prospective, randomized, opened, controlled trial in patients with coronary heart disease. The participants were randomized to receive the MD (35% fat, 22% monounsaturated) and the LFHCC diet (28% fat, 12% monounsaturated). The MD diet consumption and LFHCC diet increases the abundance of the Roseburia genus and F. prausnitzii, respectively. Roseburia is related to produce an inhibitory substance against *Bacillus subtilis* (Hatziioanou), suggesting MD induce some changes in the microbiota mediated by the antimicrobial effect of this genera, which modifies the microbial population in the colon. On the other hand, LFHCC consumption increased the abundance of another diabetes-protective bacterial species, F. prausnitzii (found to be low in patients with DM II). These two changes after MD and LFHCC diets could have a protective influence for the prevention of T2D, suggested by the findings of an improvement in insulin sensitivity after the consumption of the both diets.

A randomized, controlled, double-blind, crossover clinical trial study with 33 hypercholesterolemic volunteers, aged 35–80 years was carried out [96]. Participants ingested 25 mL/day for 3 weeks, preceded by 2-weekwashout periods, three raw virgin olive oils differing in the concentration and origin of phenolic compounds (PC): (1) a virgin olive oil (OO) naturally containing 80 mg of PC/kg, (VOO); (2) a PC enriched virgin olive oil containing 500 mg PC/kg, from OO (FVOO); and (3) a PC-enriched virgin olive oil containing a mixture of 500 mg PC/kg from OO and thyme 1:1 (FVOOT). The OO group did not present changes in microbiota, whereas the FVOOT group presented an increase in the group of Bifidobacteria, Parascardovia denticolens and Roseburia.

Another study evaluated the effects of PUFA n-3 from sardine. The patients with DM2 were randomized to follow either a type 2 diabetes standard diet (control group: CG), or a standard diet enriched with 100 g of sardines 5 days a week (sardine group: SG), which represented a dose of EPA + DHA of 3 g per day, for 6 months. There was a decrease in phylum Firmicutes in both groups and in the Firmicutes/Bacteroidetes ratio in the SG group over time, and a decrease in Bacteroidetes/Prevotella ratio in CG group. The SG presented an increase in adiponectin levels, whereas CG group showed an increase of in TNF-α [97].

Some volunteers at increased Metabolic Syndrome (MetS) [95] risk followed five diets: high saturated fat diet (HS; saturated fatty acids, SFA); high monounsaturated fat (MUFA)/high glycemic index (GI) (HM/HGI); high MUFA/low GI (HM/LGI); high carbohydrate (CHO)/high GI (HC/HGI); and, high CHO/low GI (HC/LGI) for 24 weeks. The reduction of dietary fat intake and increasing dietary carbohydrate consumption increased both faecal *Bacteroides* and *Bifidobacterium* spp., which are linked to improve body energy regulation and reduced risk factors of MetS. Besides that, increased Bacteroides numbers after the HC/HGI diet were directly and significantly correlated with a modest decrease in body weight, waist circumference and body mass index (BMI). An increase in Bifidobacterium was also observed on both low-fat high-CHO diets, and also had showed a modest increase in Atopobium numbers, both within the Actinobacteria phylum, which are dominant members of the human gastrointestinal microbiota, and are considered important degraders of carbohydrate. These bacteria's growth may have been stimulated by the increased bioavailability of dietary carbohydrate.

Moya-Pérez et al. [89] (Table 6) showed that high fat (HF) diets are responsible for increasing the infiltration of lymphocytes B in rats, which are the first cells in the immune system to be recruited from adipose tissue after administration of these diets. Lymphocytes B also increase insulin sensitivity by activating T cells and increasing the release of proinflammatory macrophages, thus contributing to the inflammation process with the production of IL-8 and interferon-γ (IFN-γ) cytokines. In another study, Masi et al. [98] evaluated the effect of high sugar (HS), HF, and HS and HF diets on mice over a period of eight weeks. The caloric intake from the HF groups was lower. All three diets increased the size of adipocytes and hepatocytes when compared to the control group, and only the HS and HF diet showed a significant increase in proinflammatory cytokines (IL-6 and IL-1β), showing that the increase in the consumption of sugar increases the lipogenesis, promoting the storage of the triglycerides.

This increasement in adipocyte size was also observed when high fat diets (HF) were administered to rats [5], in which 51% of the energy was derived from fats, and they observed that an increase in adipocyte size occurred, and as a consequence, an increase in inflammatory cytokines (NF-γ, IL-6 e TNF-α) was observed, as shown in Table 6. Caër et al. [88] reported that adipocytes are exposed to the effects of inflammatory factors, hormones, and even pollutants. This alters their metabolic capacity and cellular functions through the action of IL-1β, IL-17, and TNF-α, and can lead to a greater accumulation of fat. TNF-α, for example, acts on the lipolytic pathway of these adipocytes, maintaining the fat mass, restricting excess adipocyte production and accumulating lipids.

The beneficial role of fiber, in a hyperlipidic diet on inflammatory markers, was also verified in Moran-Ramos et al. [99] (Table 6). They evaluated the effects of Nopal fibers, a medicinally used plant in Mexico, and found a decrease in adipocytes size and Il-6 levels, when administered as part of a HF diet over a six-week period. These fibers were able to alter the intestinal microbiota and increase fermentation rates, showing their role in preventing intestinal inflammation in being able to increase the beneficial forms of microbial diversity.

Table 6. Effects of different types of fatty acids on the inflammatory process and intestinal microbiota in in vivo studies.

Host	Fatty Acid Composition of the Experiment	Microbiota	Inflammatory Process	References
Female rats	Control group (10% kcal fat), high Fat (60% kcal fat, of which 34% was SFA)	↑ Firmicutes and ↓ Bacteroidetes	↑ Inflammatory citokines	[100]
Female mice	Control group (12.6% fat) High fat (60.3% fat) High fat with oleic fatty acid High Fat with n-3 PUFA (EPA and DHA)	↑ Firmicutes and Enterobacteria, ↓ Bifidobacteria ↓ Firmicutes and ↑ Bifidobacteria ↑ Firmicutes	Not observed	[101]
Male rats	Control group with palmitic fatty acid Palmitic fatty acid with DHA Palmitic fatty acid with ALA	↑ Lactobacillus ↑ Lactobacillus and Allobaculum, ↓ Proteobacteria	Not observed	[102]
Elderly male rats	Normolipid diet (12% fat) High Fat (43% fat)	↓ Firmicutes ↓ Lactobacillus	Not observed	[103]
Male rats	Placebo (10% skimmed milk) High Fat with placebo Placebo with 1 × 109 CFU. *B. pseudocatenalatum* High Fat diet with 1 × 109 CFU. *B. pseudocatenalatum*	↑ Firmicutes (65%) and Bacteroidetes (31%) ↑ Firmicutes, ↓ Bacteroidetes, ↑ Proteobacteria ↑ Firmicutes (66%) and Bacteroidetes (31%) ↑ Firmicutes, ↓ Bacteroidetes	↑ CD8$^+$/CD4$^+$, ↑ TNF-α, MCP-1, IL-10, IL-17A, IP-10, IL-6, ↑ LPS ↓ CD8$^+$/CD4$^+$, ↓ TNF-α, MCP-1, IP-10, 1L-17A, IL-6, ↓ LPS	[90]
Male rats	Normolipid diet (10% fat) with Nopal (4% fiber) High fat (46% fat) with Nopal (4% fiber)	↑ Firmicutes ↑ Bacteroidetes	↑ IL-6 ↓ IL-6, ↓ in adipocyte size	[99]
Male rats	Control group Control group with high sugar (HS) High fat High fat with HS	Not observed	↑ size of adipocytes and hepatocytes ↑ TNF-α ↑ IL-6, ↑ IL-1 β	[98]

Abbreviations: Saturated fatty acids (SFA); docosahexaenoic (DHA) fatty acids; eicosanoic acid (EPA); colony-forming unit (CFU); CD4 and CD8 T cell surface molecules; tumor necrosis factor alpha (TNF-α); monocyte chemoattractant protein-1 (MCP-1); interleukin(IL); interferon induced protein (IP); lipopolyssacharide (LPS).

The administration of n-3 PUFAs have also shown beneficial anti-inflammatory action. The main metabolites of this essential fatty acid are EPA and DHA, considered polyunsaturated long chain fatty acids, with the first double bond in the third carbon of its chain. It is found in large quantities in fish, such as tuna and salmon [104]. Some studies point to this protective factor following the administration of fish oil, with a decrease in the production of TNF-α, IL-1β, and IL-6 by monocytes that were stimulated by endotoxins or mononuclear cells (Table 6). These fatty acids (FA) are responsible for inducing a change in inflammation activity through their incorporation into the phospholipids of inflammatory cells that cause a greater membrane fluidity, modifying the lipid derivatives that will be formed. Thus, it has effect on various anti-inflammatory responses, such as the production of eicosanoids and cytokines, and also on various types of cells, such as monocytes and macrophages [104].

The isolated use of EPA with 1% supplementation in HF given to C57BL/6J mice for 16 weeks was beneficial in the reduction of total cholesterol, and in the reduction of adipocyte size. In addition, it reduced plasma levels of leptin by approximately 60%, considered a pro-inflammatory cytokine [105]. Besides that, another study showed that EPA ameliorates HF-diet effects in mice and cultured adipocytes, which EPA increased the oxygen consumption and fatty acid oxidation and reducing adipocyte size, adipogenesis, and adipose tissue inflammation, independent of obesity [106].

A hyperlipidic diet, associated with the use of antibiotics, can lead to intestinal dysbiosis. Dysbiosis is an imbalance that causes an increase in bacterial growth, production of toxins, and an increase in intestinal permeability, affecting the transient microbiota, thus causing some disorders [107]. In addition, individuals predisposed to obesity may be present with intestinal microbial communities that promote the storage of energy, different than in lean individuals. Different compositions and even administration of strains, such as bifidiobacteria, may influence the production of proinflammatory cytokines [108]. Moya-Pérez et al. [89] administered strains of *B. pseudocatenalatum* in both a placebo and an obese group, with a HF diet over a six-week period. These strains were able to decrease inflammatory markers such as TNF-α, IL-6 and INF-γ in the HF group, which also resulted in a weight reduction. They suggested that the reduction of INF-γ occurred due to the action of the bacteria regardless of the type of diet offered.

The gastrointestinal bacteria, such as *Bacteroides thetaiotaomicron*, are responsible for the digestion of fibers. They produce short chain fatty acids (SCFA), such as butyrate, propionate, and acetate, which serve as energy substrates for other bacteria [108]. Butyrate affects inflammatory mediators since they are able to inhibit the expression of pro-inflammatory cytokines by inhibiting nuclear factor κB (NF-κB). They may also cause changes in the intestinal epithelium, leading to increased intestinal permeability. Acetate is the main SCFA in the colon and acts as a substrate for cholesterol reduction. Propionate is the neoglycogen substrate for the liver, acting to increase adipogenesis and inhibit lipolysis in adipose tissues, which can neutralize cholesterol synthesis and lipogenesis in the liver. In addition, bacteria hydrolyze the urea that comes from the liver, forming ammonia and from it synthesize amino acids. They still synthesize vitamins, such as complex B and vitamin K [103].

A study evaluated the effects of diets rich in palmitic acid supplemented with DHA or ALA oil on the microbiota of rats [109]. They observed that the diet with an addition of 10% ALA by weight was responsible for an increase in the content of *Lactobacillus* and *Allobaculum*, which are species responsible for improving intestinal health and promoting the production of SCFA. These SCFAs increased their concentrations by 41.9% when compared to the group that received only palmitic acid [109].

Lecomte et al. [103] (Table 6) found that mice fed a HF diet (43% lipids) had a lower amount of Firmicutes and an increase in Bacteroidetes as compared to a group with a normolipid diet (12% lipids). This is correlated to the drastic decrease of *Lactobacillus* in the HF group, and appear to mainly decrease in obese phenotypes, as found in the experimental group of study. On the other hand, in Lam et al. [100] rats received one of two types of a diet, either a control (10% lipid energy) or a HF diet (60% energy derived from lipids where 24% was from SFA). The HF group showed an alteration in intestinal microbiota, with a decrease in Bacteroidetes strains and an increase in Firmicutes, as well as an increase in the inflammatory cytokines parameter. This finding was verified in an earlier study by Filippo et al. [110], in which they evaluated children who consumed two types of diets: one traditionally rural and one urban. In children consuming an urban diet, which included higher values of animal protein, starch, sugars, fats, and was poor in fiber, there was a predominance of Firmicutes and Preoteobacterias.

Another study [101] evaluated the effects HF diets supplemented with n-3 (EPA and DHA) or oleic acid would have on the metabolism of mice. The study consisted of two steps. In the first step, the mice were administered HF diets (60.3% of kcal from lipids) over an eight-week period. The second step consisted of a seven-week administration of these HF diets with the addition of either n-3 or oleic acid. As a result, they observed that the HF diet was responsible for increasing the concentration of Firmicutes and Enterobacteria, and decreasing the concentration of Bifidobacteria, but the second step did not present significant results. However, the n-3 group showed an increase of Firmicutes, while the group that received oleic acid decreased the concentration of Firmicutes as well as increasing the Bifidobacteria.

These microbial signals are responsible for regulating the release of Fasting Adipose Factor (Fiaf), which inhibits the action of lipoprotein lipase (LPL). The LPL hydrolyzes the triglycerides in a molecule of monoacylglycerol and two free fatty acids. When they enter the adipocyte, they are re-esterified and stored as fat, regulating this storage by Fiaf. SCFAs control the inflammatory response from a process in which they bind to the G protein conjugate receptors (GPCRs), thereby regulating the energy from the hormones that are derived from the gut [107].

Diets with n-6 PUFA are responsible for increasing the concentrations of Firmicutes, Actinobacteria, and Proteobacteria species and for decreasing the concentrations of Bifidobacteria [111]. Bifidobacteria are related to the increase in intestinal permeability that causes an increase in the circulation of LPS. LPS is associated with chronic systemic inflammation and metabolic syndrome, which includes the metabolic disorders of glucose and hypertriglyceridemia [111].

5. Fatty Acids and Non-Alcoholic Fatty Liver Disease

Non-alcoholic fatty liver disease (NAFLD) is another important disorder which contributes to obesity [112]. The exact NAFLD pathophysiology is unknown since it is a multi-factorial disease that encompasses one or more conditions which contribute to the metabolic syndrome, including diabetes mellitus, obesity, hypertension, and dyslipidemia [113]. NAFLD is considered a public health issue because it is one of the common chronic liver diseases in developed countries, found in, 20% to 30% of the population worldwide [114,115]. There are two pathological conditions with different prognoses: NAFLD is considered a condition without liver inflammation or hepatocytes damage, which may evolve into steatohepatitis with lobular inflammation and hepatocellular injury, called non-alcoholic steatohepatitis (NASH). One of the biggest problems caused by NASH is that many individuals with NASH may develop liver fibrosis. The latter may result in cirrhosis, hepatocyte death, and occasionally hepatocellular carcinoma, which involves a high likelihood of requiring a liver transplantation in the future [116].

Several therapeutic interventions, such as pharmacological and non-pharmacological, are proposed to treat NAFLD. Among the pharmacological therapies there are insulin sensitizers such as thiazolidinedione, lipid lowering drugs such as statins, antioxidants such as α-tocopherol, and vitamin D_3 treatment. However, pharmacological approaches to treat liver steatosis are not always safe and effective [117,118].

Having an unhealthy lifestyle is an important factor influencing the development of NAFLD, mainly associated with a poor nutritional diet and physical inactivity. Therefore, non-pharmacological interventions have also been proposed as a strategy to reduce NAFLD severity. Among these non-pharmacological approaches are weight reduction, which involves strategies like bariatric surgery, some type of diets, and physical activity [119].

Nutritional approaches have been widely studied to reduce NAFLD severity. Dietary animal models and clinical trials in humans have been proposed to study new alternatives to reduce the risks and prevent NAFLD [120]. Although NAFLD pathophysiology is complex, it is strongly associated to oxidative stress, lipotoxicity, and inflammatory biomarkers in the liver. Plasma lipoproteins and fatty acid sources of liver triacylglycerol are derived from lipolysis in adipose tissue as nonesterified fatty acids. De novo *lipogenesis* (DNL) is a process that contributes to this lipotoxicity. During the fasting state, NAFLD patients display 26% of liver triacylglycerol derived from DNL, which is several times higher than the 5% observed in healthy individuals [121].

The quality of dietary fatty acids may have a role in the development of NAFLD, and conversely, may be an alternative source for decreasing deleterious NAFLD effects. Therefore, the composition of liver fatty acids may be involved in hepatic damage [122,123]. Dietary patterns are a combination of foods that are consumed by individuals and the amount of nutrients may produce synergistic health effects. The reason to study dietary patterns is because habitual food consumption is related to the human world diet [124].

The Mediterranean diet (MD) is a kind of dietary strategy that has been widely studied in metabolic dysfunction. According to Trichoppoulou, the MD has been defined as "primarily a plant-based diet characterized by a high ratio of monounsaturated fatty acids (MUFA) to SFAs with total fat accounting for 30–40% of daily energy consumption" [125]. In other words, MD is characterized by a high consumption of olive oil, as the main source of fat, vegetables, legumes, nuts, fruits, whole grains, fish, and seafood, with a low intake of meat and meat products, and moderate ethanol consumption, especially wine [125].

Recent studies have shown that the MD may have clinical nutritional effectiveness on the reduction of NAFLD [120,126] (Table 7). The ideal diet would result in a reduction of steatosis and an improvement in insulin sensitivity. A defect in insulin sensitivity is an important feature of NAFLD and DM II, which are two conditions that are closely related. In a randomized, cross-over six-week dietary intervention study, twelve non-diabetic subjects (six men and six women) with biopsy-proven NAFLD and at least three clinical features of metabolic syndrome (MetS), with the consumption of no more than seven to 10 standard alcoholic drinks per week, and without type 1 or 2 diabetes, were recruited to evaluate the effects of the MD on NAFLD and insulin resistance [126].

Table 7. The effects of dietary fatty acids in humans with non-alcoholic fatty liver disease (NAFLD).

Host	Fatty Acid Composition	Effects	References
Human Clinical Trial: Adults	- Mediterranean diet: olive oil, vegetables, legumes, nuts, fruits, whole grains, fish and seafood, moderate wine - Low-fat-high carbohydrate diet (LF/HCD) Duration: 6 weeks (6-week wash-out period in-between)	- Weight loss was not observed between the two diets - Reduced hepatic steatosis - Improved insulin sensitivity (HOMA-IR) - No differences in peripheral insulin resistance	[126]
Human Clinical Trial: Adults	- Mediterranean diet and Physical activity Duration: 6 months	- Improved BMI, waist circumference, waist-to-rip ratio, ALT, GGT, serum glucose, total cholesterol/HDL, LDL/HDL, TG/HDL, HOMA, NAFLD score	[120]
Human Clinical Trials: Adults	n-3 PUFAs - (50 mL of PUFA with 1:1-DHA: EPA into daily diet) Duration: 6 months	- Reduced ALT and AST levels - Reduced triacylglycerol (TG), total cholesterol (TC) levels - Reduced systemic inflammatory markers: C-reactive protein (PCR) - Reduced pro-oxidant factors: malondialdehyde (MDA) - Reduced fibrosis parameters: type IV collagen and pro-collagen type III pro-peptide	[127]
Human Clinical Trials: Adults	n-3 PUFAs - 2 capsules fish oil 2 times per day (182 mg EPA and 129 mg DHA) - 2 capsules corn oil 2 times per day (without EPA and DHA) Duration: 3 months	- Reduced TG, TC, apolipoprotein B, glucose, ALT, GGT. - Increased serum adiponectin levels. - Reduced NAFLD biomarkers: fibroblast factor growth 21 (FGF-21) and CK18 fragment M30 (CK18-M30). - Reduced pro-inflammatory cytokines: tumor necrosis factor-α (TNF-α), leukotrienes 4, and prostaglandin E2. - Corn oil increased creatinine serum levels, but without other metabolic effects.	[102]
Human Clinical Trials: Adults	n3-PUFAs 4 g/day EPA and DHA - Placebo Duration: 15–18 months	- Erythrocyte DHA enrichment $\geq$2%: no changes in fat liver content. - Fat liver reduction: decrease in hepatic DNL with concomitant increase hepatic FA oxidation and hepatic insulin sensitivity.	[128]

Abbreviations: alanine aminotransferase (ALT); γ-glutamyl transpeptidase (GGT); triacylglycerol (TG); unlike LDL-C (non-HDL); low density lipoprotein (LDL); total cholesterol (TC); high density lipoprotein (HDL); polyunsaturated fatty acids (PUFA); eicosapentaenoic (EPA); docosahexaenoic (DHA); de novo lipogenesis (DNL);

These patients used the MD and a control diet, which was a low-fat high-carbohydrate diet (LF/HCD), in random order with a six-week wash-out period in between. At the baseline, the subjects were obese with metabolic dysfunction parameters, such as elevated fasting concentrations of glucose, insulin, triglycerides, alanine aminotransferase (ALT), γ-glutamyl transpeptidase (GGT), and impaired insulin sensitivity. Weight loss was not observed between the two diets. Hepatic steatosis level after the MD was reduced in comparison to the LF/HCD and insulin sensitivity improved after the MD with a significant improvement in homeostatic model assessment for insulin resistance (HOMA-IR), but not in peripheral insulin resistance, measured by the glucose infusion rate (GINF) [126].

Gelli et al. demonstrated that the MD is associated with physical activity and may be considered as a safe therapeutic approach for reducing the severity of NAFLD. Forty-six adult patients were recruited, ranging from 26–71 years old with NAFLD within the previous six months of diet intervention. Although the MD approach was associated with physical activity, this correlation improved the steatosis grade in nine patients, and 25 out of 46 patients presented with weight reduction or maintenance. Moreover, several metabolic parameters, such as BMI, waist circumference, waist-to-hip ratio, ALT, GGT, serum glucose, total cholesterol/HDL, LDL/HDL, TG/HDL, HOMA, NAFLD score, and others showed a significant improvement between the baselines and the end of treatment [120].

Functional analyses of transcriptome data identified a group of genes from human NASH called Δ9 (stearoyl-coenzyme A desaturase 1 SCD-1), Δ5 (FADS1), and Δ6 (FADS2). Moreover, this study showed that hepatic fatty acid desaturation and unbalanced ω-6 to ω-3 ratio have an important role in the development of NASH. This study observed impaired desaturation fluxes in the ω-3 and ω-6 pathway, with augmented ω-6 to ω-3 ratio and a decreased ω-3 index, in fatty livers in both humans and mice (C57BL/6; six wild type fed with SCD and high fat diet (HFD)). Transgenic *fat-1* mice, which express a ω-3 desaturase, allowing the endogenous conversion of ω-6 into ω-3 fatty acids, were fed HFD [129].

Therefore, HFD-transgenic *fat-1* mice had a significant reduction in hepatic insulin resistance, were resistant to the adipogenic and steatogenic effects of HFD when compared to HFD-wild type mice, reduced macrophage infiltration, necroinflammation, and lipid peroxidation. They also reduced the expressions of genes involved in inflammation, fatty acid oxidation (fatty acid translocase—CD36/FAT and liver fatty acid binding protein L-FABP4), and lipogenesis (ACC, sterol response element-binding protein-1c-SREBP-1C, and fatty acid synthase—FASN). Afterward, they evaluated endogenous and exogenous ω-3 fatty acid enrichment on HFD-induced NASH, and these animals displayed similar findings as in the HFD-transgenic *fat-1* mice. In hepatocytes, CP24879, a Δ5/Δ6 desaturase inhibitor, significantly decreased intracellular lipid accumulation and inflammatory injury, and presented superior anti-inflammatory and antisteatotic actions in *fat-1* and ω-3-treated hepatocytes [129].

Some studies have evaluated the effects of PUFAs in adult individuals [102,127,128]. These human clinical trials demonstrated that PUFA supplementation, especially fish oil, may be an important alternative dietary therapy on NASH. Seventy-eight patients diagnosed with NASH were enrolled and randomly assigned into either the control group or the PUFA treated group (50 mL of PUFA with 1:1 DHA: EPA added to the daily diet) for six months. The group observed that after six months of treatment, these patients displayed a considerable improvement in several NASH parameters, including ALT and AST levels, triacylglycerol (TG), total cholesterol (TC) levels, systemic inflammatory markers, such as C-reactive protein (PCR) and malondialdehyde (MDA), and fibrosis parameters, like type IV collagen and pro-collagen type III pro-peptide, were also significantly reduced after treatment [127].

Similar results were seen in a randomized clinical trial that aimed to assess the effects of fish oil on NAFLD and hyperlipidemic patients. Eighty individuals with NAFLD and hyperlipidemia were randomly assigned to consume either two capsules of fish oil twice per day, including 182 mg EPA and 129 mg DHA, or two capsules of corn oil twice per day, without EPA and DHA, but containing vitamin E, gelatin, glycerin, and water. In addition to vitamin E, gelatin, glycerin, and water, the total capsule weight was 1000 mg. The capsules were taken for three months in a double-blind, randomized clinical trial. This study found a high plasma concentration of EPA and DHA in the fish oil group after intervention and a significant reduction in TG, TC, apolipoprotein B, glucose, ALT, and GGT, and significantly increased serum adiponectin levels. Some NAFLD biomarkers, such as fibroblast factor growth 21 (FGF-21) and CK18 fragment M30 (CK18-M30), and pro-inflammatory cytokines, tumor necrosis factor-α (TNF-α), leukotrienes 4, and prostaglandin E2, decreased after fish oil intervention in NAFLD/dyslipidemic patients. Corn oil increased creatinine serum levels, but had no other metabolic effects [102].

Hodson et al. performed a randomized sub-study with 16 NAFLD participants that received four g/day EPA with DHA, while another group consumed a placebo for 15–18 months. Individuals with

NAFLD, who had an increase in the erythrocyte DHA enrichment of ≥2% with the treatment of ω-3 FA, showed positive changes in hepatic insulin sensitivity and hepatic lipid metabolism. Erythrocyte DHA enrichment is a kind of surrogate marker of changes in tissue enrichment and may be associated with alterations in hepatic DNL, postprandial FA partitioning, and hepatic and peripheral insulin sensitivity. The results demonstrated that although erythrocyte DHA enrichment ≥2% had no effect in diminishing fat liver content, this fat liver reduction may be due to the decrease in hepatic DNL with concomitant increase in hepatic FA oxidation and hepatic insulin sensitivity. This reduction in fat liver was associated with improved hepatic insulin sensitivity, but was not related to peripheral insulin sensitivity [128].

In animal models, several studies have observed beneficial effects of PUFAs on NAFLD. NAFLD may be induced through a HFD diet intervention in mice and rats (Table 8). Wang et al. showed that C57BL/6 mice fed with a HFD for four days induced lipid accumulation, however, short-term n-3 PUFA-enriched HFD (ω-3HFD) reversed this effect. A metabolomics assay was able to determine the reduced plasma content of hydroyeicosapentaenoic acid (HEPEs) and the epoxyeicosatetraenoic acid (EEQ) in short term-HFD animals and, after ω-3 supplementation, these FAs increased. Furthermore, ω-3HFD was able to reduce the macrophage infiltration in adipose tissue and pro-inflammatory cytokines (IL-6, MCP-1, and TNF-α) in the plasma. Primary hepatocytes and peritoneal macrophages were used to evaluate the mechanisms. Therefore, the activation of pro-inflammatory cytokines, as well as the activation of the JNK pathway by palmitate in macrophages, decreased with a mixture of 17,18-EEQ, 5-HEPE, and 9-HEPE, which are identified as the efficient components of these metabolites, including HEPEs and EEQs. Herein, the results have demonstrated that the mixture (17,18-EEQ, 5-HEPE, and 9-HEPE) may be an alternative therapy to prevent the early stages of NAFLD by inhibiting adipose tissue macrophage infiltration and systemic inflammation via cJun-N-terminal-kinase (JNK) signaling [123].

Table 8. The effects of dietary fatty acids in in vivo and in vitro models with non-alcoholic fatty liver disease NAFLD.

Host	Fatty Acid Composition	Effects	References
Mice and In vitro	n-3 PUFAS - HFD-fed mice - n-3 PUFA-enriched HFD (17,18-EEQ, 5-HEPE, 9-HEPE (efficient components of HEPEs and EEQs metabolites) Duration: 4 days - In vitro: Primary hepatocytes and peritoneal macrophages	Mice: Reduced macrophage infiltration in adipose tissue - Reduced pro-inflammatory cytokines (IL-6, MCP-1 and TNF-α) in plasma content In vitro: activation of pro-inflammatory cytokines as well as activation of JNK pathway by palmitate in macrophages were reduced through the mixture of 17,18-EEQ, 5-HEPE, 9-HEPE	[123]
Mice	Corn oil and n3-PUFAs - Corn-oil based HFD - n3-PUFA DHA/EPA-enriched diet Duration: 12 weeks	- The quality of the diet (n3-PUFA) could modulate liver transcriptoma: - corn oil based HFD: modulate PPAR-related gene expression and have induced PPAR-γ gene signatures - DHA/EPA-enriched diet: induced genes known to be regulated by PPAR-α	[130]
Mice	n3-PUFAs - HFD-fed mice - n3 PUFA-enriched HFD Duration: 8 weeks	- n3-PUFA-enriched HFD: without obesity, liver damage, hypertriglyceridemia, hepatic insulin resistance, steatosis - Improved hepatic glucose output - Reduced expression of genes related to lipogenesis: SREBP-1C and FAS - Improved inflammatory markers: increase adiponectin levels - Increased beta oxidation with increased expression of PPARα and PPAR-α target and CPT-1	[131]

Table 8. *Cont.*

Host	Fatty Acid Composition	Effects	References
Mice	n3-PUFAs - HFD-fed mice - DHA/EPA supplementation in HFD (different ratios 1:2, 1:1 and 2:1) Duration: 11 weeks	- Best suggestion: Ratio 1:2 - Increase HDL/C levels - Reduced ALT, AST, MDA levels and increased glutathione (GSH) levels - Reduced the expression of lipid metabolism genes: SREPB-1C, SCD-1, ACC-1 and PPAR-γ - Lowered expression of proteins expression levels c-Jun and c-Fos - Weakened activation of Ap-1 - Reduced inflammatory cytokines (IL-6 and IL-1β)	[132]
Mice	MUFA and n3-PUFAs - Western diet supplemented with olive oil (OO) (WD + OO), - Westerm diet supplemented with EPA (WD + EPA) - Western diet supplemented with DHA (WD + DHA) - Western diet supplemented with DHA + EPA (WD + DHA/EPA) Duration: 16 weeks	- WD + OO: severe NASH phenotype accompanied with inflammation, oxidative stress and fibrosis - WD + DHA/EPA: attenuated ALT and AST levels - WD + DHA: - Reduced cell surface markers for Kupffer cells and macrophages in liver Clec4f; Clec10a; CD68; and F4/80) - Diminished inflammatory markers like IL-1β, TNF-α, TLR4, TLR-9 and genes involved in TLR pathway Cd-14 and MyD88 - Blocked WD-induced accumulation of nuclear factor κ beta (NFκB) in hepatic nuclei - Reduce oxidative stress (NADPH oxidase subunits Nox2, p22phox, p40phox, p47phox, p67phox) - Diminished Procol1α1 - Reduced cytokine TGF-β1	[133]
Mice and In vitro	MUFA and n3-PUFAs - Western diet supplemented with olive oil (OO) (WD + OO), - Westerm diet supplemented with EPA (WD + EPA) - Western diet supplemented with DHA (WD + DHA) - Western diet supplemented with DHA + EPA (WD + DHA/EPA) Duration: 16 weeks In vitro: Human LX2 stellate cells treated with DHA	WD + DHA: No increase in hepatic nuclear abundance (Smad 3) - WD+OO and WD+EPA: Increased Smad3 expression. In vitro: Human LX2 stellate cells: - Blocked TGF-β mediated induction of Col1A1	[134]
Rats	Canola Oil, Soybean Oil, Safflower Oil, Lard - High oleic canola oil (HOC) - Conventional canola oil (C) - Conventional canola oil/flax oil blend (C/F) (3:1 ratio) - High linoleic safflower oil (SF) - Soybean oil (SB) - Lard and soybean oil (L) - Weight-matched group fed lard and soybean oil (WM) Duration: 12 weeks.	- C/F group: - Attenuated hepatic stetatosis—Lower concentration of fat liver - Altered hepatic phospholipids fatty acid profile by increasing EPA and DHA. - HOC, C and C/F groups: - Gained the least of body weight: lowest weight gain without differences in adiposity	[135]
Rats	n3-PUFAs Perilla oil - High-fat diet/high-cholesterol diet (HFD/HC) - Perilla oil-enriched diet (POH)	- POH group: - Improved HFD-induced hyperlipidemia (TG, CT and LDL) - Reduced hepatic steatosis - Diminished activity of ALT and AST enzymes - Reduced hepatic inflammatory infiltration around portal area - Rescued HFD-induced hepatic fibrosis - Abrogated downregulation of ABCG 5 and ABCG 8 - Increased the expression of CYP2A1 and CYP27A1	[136]
Mice	n3-PUFAs EPA - HFD-fed mice - HFD-enriched 3% EPA + 500 mg milidronate/kg/day - HFD-enriched 3% EPA Duration: 10 days	- HFD-enriched 3%: - Accentuated hepatic triglyceride accumulation. - HFD-enriched 3% EPA + 500 mg milidronate/kg/day: - Exacerbation of milidronate-induced triglyceride accumulation - EPA decreased the milidronate-induced mRNA expression of inflammatory genes: MPEG1, COX 2, CD68, F4/80 - Increased GRP120	[137]

Table 8. *Cont.*

Host	Fatty Acid Composition	Effects	References
Mice	*n3-PUFAs and n-9 MUFAs* - Methionine and choline deficient (MCD) diet - MCD-enriched diet n-3 PUFA + n-9 MUFA (EPA/DHA 25 mg + OO 75 mg) (MCD/n-3) - MCD-enriched diet n-9 MUFA alone (OO 100 mg) (MCD/OO) two times a week by intragastric gavage. Duration: 8 weeks	- MCD/n-3 group: higher levels of ALT, severe scores of inflammation - Increased intrahepatic expression of inflammatory markers: TNF-α and CCL2 - Increased expression of profibrogenic genes: TGF-β1 - Increased tissue inhibitor of metalloproteinase (TIMP-1) - Higher portal pressure	[138]
Mice	*n-9 MUFA* - Standard chow diet (SCD) - HFD based on lard (HFD—49 energy % of fat) Duration: 12 weeks HFD-fed mice were divided in four groups: - Unchanged HFD-L (HFD-L) - HFD based on EVOO (HFD-EVOO) - HFD based on EVOO rich in phenols (HFD-OL with same percentage of fat) - R (reversion, LFD) Duration: 24 weeks	- HFD-EVOO: - Reduced body weight - Improved plasma lipid profile - Reduced pro-inflammatory citokynes in epididimal adipose tissue: IFN-γ, IL-6, leptin and macrophage infiltration - Diminished NAFLD activity (NAS) score - Reduced hepatic adiponutrin (Pnpal3) - Increased Cd36 gene	[139]
Mice and In vitro	*Palmitoleate n-7 MUFA* - LFD - LFD + Palmitoleate LFD + Oleate	- LFD+Palmitoleate: -Improved systemic insulin-sensitivity - Induced hepatic steatosis Improved insulin signaling in liver: insulin-stimulates Akt (Ser 473) phosphorylation - Reduced phosphorylation of NFκB p65 (Ser468) - Reduced expression of IL-6 and TNF-α. In vitro: hepatocytes and RAW macrophaged+palmitoleate: - Increased fat deposition' - Stimulated FAS expression - Activated SREBP-1c - Decreased inflammation: NFκB p65 Ser 68, TNF-α, IL-6 in both hepatocytes and RAW macrophages.	[140]
In vitro	Palmitic acid (PA) SAFs In vitro: Kupffer Cells and stellate cells stimulated with TLR2 and palmitic acid	In vitro (Kupffer cells) were more important than HSC in TLR2-mediated progression of NASH - TLR 2 ligand increased NOD3 (inflammasome) in Kupffer cells. - PA together with TLR2 ligand: Induced caspase-1 activation in Kupffer cells - Released IL-1β and IL-1α in Kupffer cells	[141]
Rats and In vitro	Corn Oil - peroxidized Fat - Corn oil peroxidized oil (PO) - Unperoxidized FA (OIL) - Tap water (WA) gavage Duration: 6 days.	- PO group: - Increased pro-oxidant state NOS-2, NO-formation and pronounced lipid peroxidation in liver - Decrease in α- and γ-tocopherol in liver. - Increased inflammatory markers: TNFα, COX-2, IL-1β and macrophage markers cd68 and cd 163 in the liver In vitro: hepatocytes, endothelial and Kupffer cells and incubated with peroxidized linoleic acid: more pronounced in Kupffer cells: - Augmented the secretion of TNF-α, mRNA expression of TNF-α, NOS-2, COX-2 - Increased p38MAPK phosphorylation	[142]

Abbreviations: alanine aminotransferase (ALT); γ-glutamyl transpeptidase (GGT); triacylglycerol (TG); unlike LDL-C (non-HDL); low density lipoprotein (LDL); total cholesterol (TC); high density lipoprotein (HDL); polyunsaturated fatty acids (PUFA); eicosapentaenoic (EPA); docosahexaenoic (DHA); tumor necrosis factor alpha (TNF-α); monocyte chemoattractant protein-1 (MCP-1); interleukin(IL); hydroyeicosapentaenoic acid (HEPEs); cJun-N-terminal-kinase (JNK); epoxyeicosatetraenoic acid (EEQ); peroxisome proliferator-activated receptor (PPAR); Western Diet (WD); olive oil (OO); monounsaturated fatty acids (MUFA); nuclear factor κ beta (NFκB); G protein–coupled receptor 120 (GRP120); C-C motif chemokine ligand 2 (CCL-2); cicloxigenase-2 (COX-2); NO-synthetase-2 (NOS-2); p38 mitogen-activated protein kinases (p38MAPK); ATP-binding cassette hemitransporters *G5* and *G8* (ABCG 5 and 8); Cytochrome P-450 2E1 (CYP2E1); vitamin D$_3$ 25-hydroxylase (CYP27A1) cDNA.

Positive effects of a DHA/EPA-enriched diet on NAFLD after eight or 12 weeks was observed in another study, as the quality of dietary lipids modulated some gene expressions. A liver transcriptoma is an analysis used to evaluate many hepatic processes like transcription (histone methylation/acetylation, chromatin modification), translation (mRNA, rRNA, and tRNA), protein turnover (polyubiquitination), and protein transport, metabolism of lipids and fatty acids, lipid/sterol metabolism, lipid/fatty acid biosynthesis, lipoprotein transport, and cholesterol/phospholipid efflux. After transcriptoma analysis, we concluded that the quality of dietary fat could modulate PPAR-related gene expression, since corn-oil based HFD induced PPAR-γ gene signatures, while DHA/EPA-enriched diets induced genes known to be regulated by PPAR-α [130].

In addition to these positive effects, Bargut et al. investigated if a diet rich in fish oil (HFO n-3 PUFA) for eight weeks could have hepatic alterations in HFD-induced NAFLD. The group that was fed with HFD displayed obesity, liver damage, hypertriglyceridemia, hepatic insulin resistance, and steatosis accompanied with an increase in hepatic lipogenesis and a decrease in beta oxidation. However, the HFO group did not present with metabolic alterations like the HFD group, with improvement in hepatic glucose output with reduced expression of genes related to lipogenesis via SREBP-1C and FAS improved inflammatory markers, with an increase in adiponectin levels as well as elevated beta oxidation with increased expression of PPARα and the PPAR-α target gene, Carnitine palmitoyltransferase I (CPT-1), which is considered the master regulator of mitochondrial beta oxidation [131].

A current study evaluated the ideal ratio of DHA/EPA supplementation in HFD-liver damaged mice. Shang et al. assessed different ratios (1:2, 1:1, and 2:1) of DHA/EPA supplementation for 11 weeks. DHA/EPA supplemented mice displayed a reduction in several parameters, and the best DHA/EPA ratio was found to be 1:2. The results indicated that the DHA/EPA ratio of 1:2 could increase HDL/C levels when compared to the other ratios, with a greater reduction in ALT, AST, and MDA levels, and increased glutathione (GSH) levels. It also reduced the expression of lipid metabolism genes, such as Sterol regulatory element-binding protein-1-C (SREPB-1C), Stearoyl-CoA desaturase-1 (SCD-1), Acetyl-CoA carboxylase (ACC-1), and PPAR-γ, lowered the expression of proteins c-Jun and c-Fos levels, which are proteins related to inflammatory responses of metaflammation, activating protein-1 (Ap-1), and weakening the activation of Ap-1. Additionally, serum levels of pro-inflammatory cytokines (IL-6 and IL-1β) were reduced with the DHA/EPA ratio of 1:2 [132].

Another animal model that demonstrated steatohepatitis is $Ldlr^{-/-}$ mice, which is a Western diet (WD)-induced hepatic fibrosis animal model. This model provides considerable insight into the similarity of processes that are related to cardiovascular diseases and the development of NASH, but are not identical to the process in humans [133]. Some studies focused on evaluating the effects of WD to induce NASH in $Ldlr^{-/-}$ mice [134,143]. Mice were fed with WD supplemented with olive oil (OO) (WD + OO), EPA (WD + EPA), DHA (WD + DHA), and DHA + EPA (WD + DHA/EPA) for 16 weeks. $Ldlr^{-/-}$ mice that were fed with WD + OO displayed a severe NASH phenotype, accompanied with inflammation, oxidative stress, and fibrosis. The results demonstrated that both DHA and EPA were able to decrease ALT and AST in WD + OO groups. However, considering the other parameters that characterize the severity of NASH, WD + DHA could reduce the expression of most of these parameters, such as cell surface markers for Kupffer cells and macrophages in the liver (C-type lectin domain family 4f—Clec4f; C-type lectin domain family 10a—Clec10a; cell determination-68—CD68; and F4/80) when compared to the other groups [133].

Furthermore, MD+DHA have diminished inflammatory markers, such as IL-1β, TNF-α, toll-like receptor-4 (TLR4), and -9 (TLR-9). MD+DHA also had genes involved in the TLR pathway cluster of differentiation-14 (Cd-14) and myeloid differentiation in the primary response gene-88 (MyD88) and had blocked WD-induced accumulation of nuclear factor κ beta (NFκB) in hepatic nuclei. Dietary DHA was more able to reduce oxidative stress (NADPH oxidase subunits Nox2, p22phox, p40phox, p47phox, and p67phox) as compared to EPA, and had diminished procollagen-1a1 (Procol1α1), a marker of stellate cell marker, and had decreased cytokine TGF-β1, which is a cytokine involved in the activation of hepatic stellate cells and Procol1α1 [133].

The effectiveness of DHA in WD-induced NASH Ladlr$^{-/-}$ mice was compared to EPA by a metabolomics analysis that focused on changes in hepatic lipid, amino acid, and vitamin metabolism. In NASH, hepatic sphyngomielin, SFA, MUFA, and n-6 PUFA accumulate, with a depletion in n-3 PUFA. Hence, dietary n3-PUFAs has the ability to reduce hepatic sphyngomielin, SFA, MUFA, and n-6 PUFA and also decrease the hepatic nuclear abundance of NFκB in NASH-linked inflammation [133].

Hepatic fibrosis involves a significant production of extracellular matrix (ECM), from activated hepatic stellate cells, and myofibroblasts that infiltrate the liver. Several subtypes of collagens underlie the connective tissue in the liver; therefore, fibrosis, which is the result of hepatic damage, is connected to an increase ECM deposition of collagen type 1 (collagen 1 A1-Col1A1) and also is associated with a high level of production of proteins from stellate cells and macrophages that are involved in ECM remodeling. Thus, another explanation as to how DHA and EPA differentially affect WD-induced hepatic fibroses is associated to the TGF-β pathway. WD+DHA did not increase the hepatic nuclear abundance of phospho-mothers against decapentaplegic homolog (Smad3) when compared to WD+OO and WD+EPA, which increased Smad3 expression. Smad3 is a key regulator of Col1A1 expression in stellate cells. Human LX2 stellate cells were treated with DHA and there was a blocked TGF-β mediated induction of Col1A1, concluding that DHA decreased the WD-induced fibrosis through the TGF-β-Smad3-Col1A1 pathway [134].

In rats, current studies have evaluated dietary fatty acids on NAFLD. Sprague-Dawley rats were fed with HFD and supplemented with different oils for 12 weeks, divided in different groups: (i) high oleic canola oil (HOC); (ii) conventional canola oil (C); (iii) conventional canola oil/flax oil blend (C/F) (3:1 ratio); (iv) high linoleic safflower oil (SF); (v) soybean oil (SB); (vi) lard and soybean oil (L); and, (vii) a weight-matched group fed lard and soybean oil (WM). The results demonstrated that the C/F group had decreased hepatic steatosis, presented the lowest concentration of fat liver, as did the WM group, and had an altered hepatic phospholipids fatty acid profile by increasing EPA and DHA. All of the groups that contained canola oil (HOC, C, and C/F) gained the least amount of body weight during the study, and after 12 weeks of diet, these groups displayed the lowest weight gain without differences in adiposity, which was assessed by visceral fat mass. The C/F diet contained MUFA and high amounts of alpha-linolenic acid (ALA), a plant-based n-3 PUFA, which was demonstrated to be beneficial for diminishing hepatic steatosis in HFD-Sprague-Dawley rats [135].

One example of a plant that is rich in ALA is *Perilla frutenses*, which is a medicinal plant that is found in East Asia and India, and the oil from the seeds oil contain 60% ALA. Chen et al. investigated the role of perilla oil in high-fat /high-cholesterol diet (HFD/HC), inducing NASH. Two groups of Sprague-Dawley rats were fed either HFD/HC or fed perilla oil-enrichment HFD (POH) for 16 weeks. The results demonstrated that the POH group showed improvement in HFD-induced hyperlipidemia (TG, CT, and LDL), reduced hepatic steatosis with reduced ALT activity, reduced AST enzymes, reduced hepatic inflammatory infiltration around the portal area, and reduced HFD-induced hepatic fibrosis. On the other hand, perilla oil could not modulate the expression of genes that are involved in cholesterol synthesis, but increased cholesterol removed hepatocytes by conversion to bile acids and increased fecal cholesterol excretion. HFD downregulated ABC proteins, including ATP-binding cassette hemitransporters G5 and G8 (ABCG 5 and ABCG 8), which are involved in cholesterol secretion, so these effects were pronounced in the POH group. Moreover, perilla oil increased the expression of Cytochrome P-450 2E1 (CYP2A1) and CYP27A1, which are two key enzymes in bile acid production, whereas the HFD/HC group had reduced the expression of these enzymes [136].

Despite many studies presenting several beneficial effects of n-3 and perilla oil, which contains a large amount of ALA, on NASH, a few studies have reported no benefits after consuming n3-PUFAs on NASH [137,138]. Du et al. demonstrated that EPA supplementation accentuated hepatic triglyceride accumulation in mice with impaired fatty acid oxidation. C57BL/6 mice were fed with HFD, either supplemented or not with 3% EPA, in the presence or absence of 500 mg mildronate/kg/day for 10 days. Milindronate decreases hepatic carnitine concentration and mitochondrial FA β-oxidation. After dietary EPA supplementation, mildronate-induced triglyceride accumulation was exacerbated, with considerable increase in EPA and a decrease in the total n-3/n-6 ratio. Conversely, EPA supplementation decreased the mildronate-induced mRNA expression of inflammatory genes, such as macrophage-expressed gene 1 (MPEG1), cyclooxygenase 2 (COX 2), CD68, F4/80, and increased G protein–coupled receptor 120 (GRP120), a protein related to mediate the anti-inflammatory effects of n-3 PUFA, in adipose tissue [137].

Provenzano et al. observed that Balb/C mice fed a methionine and choline deficient (MCD) diet, an animal model of steatohepatitis, for four or eight weeks. Along with the diet, the animals were either supplemented n-3 PUFA and n-9 MUFA (EPA/DHA 25 mg with OO 75 mg) (MCD/n-3) or supplemented with n-9 MUFA alone (OO 100 mg) (MCD/OO) two times per week by intragastric gavage. After eight weeks, the MCD/n-3 group displayed higher levels of ALT, severe scores for inflammation, increased intrahepatic expression of inflammatory markers, such as TNF-α and C-C motif chemokine ligand 2 (CCL2), increased expression of profibrogenic genes TGF-β1, and tissue inhibition of metalloproteinase (TIMP-1) with higher portal pressure as compared to MCD/OO. Moreover, after hepatic fatty acid profile analysis, t supplementation was confirmed to result in effective n-3 incorporation. The results showed that the addition of specific nutrients may modulate the course or the progress of steatohepatitis, indicating further attention and monitoring is required when administering n-3 PUFA in patients with hepatic inflammation [138].

A current study showed that extra virgin olive oil (EVOO) displayed a protective effect on the inflammatory response and liver damage in a NAFLD-mouse model. C57BL/6 mice were fed with standard chow diet (SCD) and HFD based on lard, where 49% of the energy was from fat, for 12 weeks to NAFLD development. The mice that were fed with HFD were divided into four groups: (i) unchanged HFD-L (HFD-L); (ii) HFD based on EVOO (HFD-EVOO); (iii) HFD based on EVOO rich in phenols (HFD-OL with the same percentage of fat); and, iv) R (reversion, LFD) over a period of 24 weeks. EVOO diets were able to reduce body weight and improve the plasma lipid profile, the pro-inflammatory cytokines in the epidydimal adipose tissue, such as IFN-γ, IL-6, and leptin, and improve the macrophage infiltration [139].

Moreover, EVOO decreased the NAFLD activity (NAS) score and increased the hepatic adiponutrin (Pnpal3), which is a protein that plays a role in triglyceride metabolism by acting as a hydrolase. Also, Cd36 gene expression, which is a gene responsible for fatty acid uptake, esterification into triglycerides, and contributes to fatty liver in HFD-fed mice, was increased in the EVOO groups. Hepatic fat composition showed an increase in MUFAs, especially oleic acid, and a decreased amount of SFAs. In conclusion, the results suggested that methionine metabolism, which influences DNA methylation status may induce the modifications in the expression of selected genes that are central to lipid metabolism in HFD-EVOO mice and to the cell cycle in HFD-OL mice [139].

Palmitoleate is a MUFA (16:1 n7) and is available as a dietary source and is produced by adipose tissue. It is a bioactive lipid and may coordinate metabolic crosstalk between the liver and adipose tissue [144]. Mice were fed with a low-fat diet (LFD) for 12 weeks. One group was supplemented with palmitoleate and the control group with oleate for a period of four weeks. Palmitoleate was able to improve systemic insulin-sensitivity, induce hepatic steatosis, but improve insulin signaling in the liver with a significant increase in insulin-stimulate Akt (Ser 473) phosphorylation. Furthermore, palmitoleate reduced phosphorylation of NFκB p65 (Ser468), IL-6, and TNF-α. In hepatocytes, palmitoleate increased fat deposition, stimulated FAS expression, activated SREBP-1c, and decreased inflammation (NFκB p65 Ser 68, TNF-α, and IL-6) in both hepatocytes and RAW macrophages. Despite palmitoleate inducing hepatic steatosis, this FA may dissociate the liver inflammatory response from hepatic steatosis, and promote insulin-sensitization and its pro-lipogenic effect, by enhancing hepatic FAS expression due to higher expression of SREBP-1c [140].

Conversely, the excess consumption of saturated fatty acids (SFAs) may be a risk factor for NAFLD pathogenesis [121]. Palmitic acid (PA), which is a kind of SFA, in cooperation with receptor toll-like type 2 (TLR2) have been shown in vitro to activate inflammation in the development of NASH. Kupffer cells and hepatic stellate cells (HSC) were isolated from wild type mice and stimulated with TLR2 and palmitic acid. These cells responded to the TLR2 ligand, but when they were stimulated with PA alone, increased TLR2 signaling-targeting genes were not seen, including cytokines and inflammasome components. Kupffer cells were more important than HSC in the TLR2-mediated progression of NASH, since the TLR2 ligand could increase the Nod-like receptor protein 3 (NOD3), which is an inflammasome component in Kuppfer cells. Moreover, PA together with the TLR2 ligand have induced caspase-1 activation and the release of interleukin-1β (IL-1β) and -1α (IL-1α) in Kuppfer cells [141].

Toll-like receptors are a defense of the organism against invading pathogens by proinflammatory cytokines in immune cells, but when TLR signaling is overactivated, altering the TLR tolerance, these conditions may result in a large number of proinflammatory cytokines that lead to tissue damage [145]. On the other hand, inflammasome activation is a pathway that converts pro-interleukin-1β into secreted IL-1β and may be induced by endogenous and exogenous danger signals. Lipopolyssacharide (LPS), a toll-like receptor 4 (TLR4) ligand, activates inflammasome and plays a role in NASH. Other studies have demonstrated that PA has activated inflammasome and induced sensitization in the LPS-induced-IL-1β release in hepatocytes, releasing danger signals from hepatocytes in a caspase-dependent manner. Thus, hepatocytes may orchestrate tissue responses to danger signals in NASH [146].

Another study evaluated the role of peroxidized oil in steatohepatitis and hepatic inflammation. Corn oil (CO), in which linoleic acid is the main FA, contains peroxidized FAs. Han-Wister rats were treated with CO (PO), unperoxidized FA (OIL), or tap water (WA), and applied by gavage over a period of six days. The PO group displayed a pro-oxidant state with enhanced NO-synthetase-2 (NOS-2), NO-formation, pronounced lipid peroxidation, and a decrease in α- and γ-tocopherol in the liver. Furthermore, the PO group had an increase in inflammatory markers, such as TNFα, COX-2, and IL-1β, and macrophage markers cd68 and cd 163 in the liver. In hepatocytes, endothelial and Kupffer cells were isolated from the untreated liver and incubated with peroxidized linoleic acid; the linoleic acid increased the secretion of TNF-α, mRNA expression of TNF-α, NOS-2, COX-2, and p38MAPK phosphorylation expression, especially in Kupffer cells. When p38MAPK was inhibited, an increase in NOS-2 and COX-2 mRNA in linoleic acid-induced Kupffer cells was seen, indicating that p38MAPK activation may be involved in the pro-inflammatory effects of linoleic acid [142].

6. Conclusions

This review evaluated the consumption of saturated and unsaturated fatty acid sources, including MUFAs or PUFAs (EPA and DHA), during in vivo, in vitro, and in human studies. PUFAs may promote benefits for obesity-related comorbidities, such as a reduction in insulin resistance, dyslipidemias, inflammation, and non-alcoholic fatty liver disease markers. The HF diets, with a predominance of saturated fatty acids, influenced intestinal permeability damages, leading to the greater stimulus of endotoxin production and consequently greater inflammatory process. However, due to the different types of SFA sources, this lipid class deserves further study, especially on the dyslipidemia profile. On the other hand, ingesting higher concentrations (1000 mg/day) of EPA and DHA may be a great supplementation option, together with a dietary fatty acid balance, which may promote the prevention and decrease of the metabolic framework of obesity and its disorders.

Acknowledgments: We thank the post-graduate program in health and development in the Central-West Region of Brazil, Federal University of Mato Grosso do Sul-UFMS, and the post-graduate program in biotechnology, Catholic University Dom Bosco for their support.

Author Contributions: Priscila Silva Figueiredo, Aline Carla Inada, Gabriela Marcelino, Carla Maiara Lopez Cardoso, and Rita de Cássia Avellaneda Guimarães: assistance with structuring of the review, writing, and literature review; Valter Aragão do Nascimento, Alinne Pereira de Castro, Priscila Aiko Hiane and Karine de Cássia Freitas: assistance with structuring of the review.

Conflicts of Interest: The authors report no conflict of interest.

References

1. Lyons, C.; Kennedy, E.; Roche, H. Metabolic inflammation-differential modulation by dietary constituents. *Nutrients* **2016**, *8*, 247. [CrossRef] [PubMed]
2. Cinti, S.; Mitchell, G.; Barbatelli, G.; Murano, I.; Ceresi, E.; Faloia, E.; Wang, S.; Fortier, M.; Greenberg, A.S.; Obin, M.S. Adipocyte death defines macrophage localization and function in adipose tissue of obese mice and humans. *J. Lipid Res.* **2005**, *46*, 2347–2355. [CrossRef] [PubMed]
3. Lau, D.C.W.; Dhillon, B.; Yan, H.; Szmitko, P.E.; Verma, S. Adipokines: Molecular links between obesity and atheroslcerosis. *Am. J. Physiol. Heart Circ. Physiol.* **2005**, *288*, H2031–H2041. [CrossRef] [PubMed]
4. Trayhurn, P.; Bing, C.; Wood, I.S. Adipose tissue and adipokines—Energy regulation from the human perspective. *J. Nutr.* **2006**, *136*, 1935S–1939S. [PubMed]
5. Xiao, L.; Yang, X.; Lin, Y.; Li, S.; Jiang, J.; Qian, S.; Tang, Q.; He, R.; Li, X. Large adipocytes function as antigen-presenting cells to activate cd4+ t cells via upregulating mhcii in obesity. *Int. J. Obes.* **2016**, *40*, 112–120. [CrossRef] [PubMed]
6. Chan, K.L.; Pillon, N.J.; Sivaloganathan, D.M.; Costford, S.R.; Liu, Z.; Théret, M.; Chazaud, B.; Klip, A. Palmitoleate reverses high fat-induced proinflammatory macrophage polarization via amp-activated protein kinase (AMPK). *J. Biol. Chem.* **2015**, *290*, 16979–16988. [CrossRef] [PubMed]
7. Kien, C. Dietary interventions for metabolic syndrome: Role of modifying dietary fats. *Curr. Diabetes Rep.* **2009**, *9*, 43–50. [CrossRef]
8. Giacca, A.; Xiao, C.; Oprescu, A.I.; Carpentier, A.C.; Lewis, G.F. Lipid-induced pancreatic β-cell dysfunction: Focus on in vivo studies. *Am. J. Physiol. Endocrinol. Metab.* **2011**. [CrossRef] [PubMed]
9. Blair, H.A.; Dhillon, S. Omega-3 carboxylic acids (epanova): A review of its use in patients with severe hypertriglyceridemia. *Am. J. Cardiovasc. Drugs* **2014**. [CrossRef] [PubMed]
10. Crandell, J.R.; Tartaglia, C.; Tartaglia, J. Lipid effects of switching from prescription epa+dha (omega-3-acid ethyl esters) to prescription epa-only (icosapent ethyl) in dyslipidemic patients. *Postgrad. Med.* **2016**. [CrossRef] [PubMed]
11. Ooi, E.M.M.; Watts, G.F.; Ng, T.W.K.; Hugh, P.; Barrett, R. Effect of dietary fatty acids on human lipoprotein metabolism: A comprehensive update. *Nutrients* **2015**, *7*, 4416–4425. [CrossRef] [PubMed]
12. Nakamura, M.T.; Nara, T.Y. Structure, function, and dietary regulation of delta6, delta5, and delta9 desaturases. *Annu. Rev. Nutr.* **2004**, *24*, 345–376. [CrossRef] [PubMed]
13. Schmitz, G.; Ecker, J. The opposing effects of n-3 and n-6 fatty acids. *Prog. Lipid Res.* **2008**, *47*, 147–155. [CrossRef] [PubMed]
14. Calder, P.C. Polyunsaturated fatty acids and inflammation. *Prostaglandins Leukot. Essent. Fatty Acids* **2006**, *75*, 197–202. [CrossRef] [PubMed]
15. Wallis, J.G.; Watts, J.L.; Browse, J. Polyunsaturated fatty acid synthesis: What will they think of next? *Trends Biochem. Sci.* **2002**, *27*, 467–473. [CrossRef]
16. Diabetes Prevention Program Research Group. Reduction in the Incidence of Type 2 Diabetes with Lifestyle Intervention or Metformin. *N. Engl. J. Med.* **2002**. [CrossRef]
17. Tuomilehto, J.; Lindström, J.; Eriksson, J.G.; Valle, T.T.; Hämäläinen, H.; Ilanne-Parikka, P.; Keinänen-Kiukaanniemi, S.; Laakso, M.; Louheranta, A.; Rastas, M.; et al. Prevention of type 2 diabetes mellitus by changes in lifestyle among subjects with impaired glucose tolerance. *N. Engl. J. Med.* **2001**, *344*, 1343–1350.
18. Arunima, S.; Rajamohan, T. Influence of virgin coconut oil-enriched diet on the transcriptional regulation of fatty acid synthesis and oxidation in rats—A comparative study. *Br. J. Nutr.* **2014**, *111*, 1782–1790. [CrossRef] [PubMed]
19. Kahn, S.E.; Hull, R.L.; Utzschneider, K.M. Mechanisms linking obesity to insulin resistance and type 2 diabetes. *Nature* **2006**. [CrossRef] [PubMed]
20. Meek, S.E.; Nair, K.S.; Jensen, M.D. Insulin regulation of regional free fatty acid metabolism. *Diabetes* **1999**, *48*, 10–14. [CrossRef] [PubMed]
21. Riserus, U. Fatty acids and insulin sensitivity. *Curr. Opin. Clin. Nutr. Metab. Care* **2008**. [CrossRef] [PubMed]
22. Koska, J.; Ozias, M.K.; Deer, J.; Kurtz, J.; Salbe, A.D.; Harman, S.M.; Reaven, P.D. A human model of dietary saturated fatty acid induced insulin resistance. *Metab. Clin. Exp.* **2016**, *65*, 1621–1628. [CrossRef] [PubMed]
23. Xu, Y.; Qian, S.Y. Anti-cancer activities of ω-6 polyunsaturated fatty acids. *Biomed. J.* **2014**. [CrossRef]

24. Bermudez, B.; Ortega-Gomez, A.; Varela, L.M.; Villar, J.; Abia, R.; Muriana, F.J.G.; Lopez, S.; Gillingham, L.G.; Harris-Janz, S.; Jones, P.J.; et al. Clustering effects on postprandial insulin secretion and sensitivity in response to meals with different fatty acid compositions. *Food Funct.* **2014**, *5*, 1374. [CrossRef] [PubMed]
25. Shadman, Z.; Khoshniat, M.; Poorsoltan, N.; Akhoundan, M.; Omidvar, M.; Larijani, B.; Hoseini, S. Association of high carbohydrate versus high fat diet with glycated hemoglobin in high calorie consuming type 2 diabetics. *J. Diabetes Metab. Disord.* **2013**, *12*, 27. [CrossRef] [PubMed]
26. Crochemore, I.C.C.; Souza, A.F.P.; de Souza, A.C.F.; Rosado, E.L. Ω-3 polyunsaturated fatty acid supplementation does not influence body composition, insulin resistance, and lipemia in women with type 2 diabetes and obesity. *Nutr. Clin. Pract.* **2012**, *27*, 553–560. [CrossRef] [PubMed]
27. Müllner, E.; Plasser, E.; Brath, H.; Waldschütz, W.; Forster, E.; Kundi, M.; Wagner, K.H. Impact of polyunsaturated vegetable oils on adiponectin levels, glycaemia and blood lipids in individuals with type 2 diabetes: A randomised, double-blind intervention study. *J. Hum. Nutr. Diet.* **2014**, *27*, 468–478. [CrossRef] [PubMed]
28. Lee, T.C.; Ivester, P.; Hester, A.G.; Sergeant, S.; Case, L.D.; Morgan, T.; Kouba, E.O.; Chilton, F.H. The impact of polyunsaturated fatty acid-based dietary supplements on disease biomarkers in a metabolic syndrome/diabetes population. *Lipids Health Dis.* **2014**, *13*, 196. [CrossRef] [PubMed]
29. Gomes, P.M.; Hollanda-Miranda, W.R.; Beraldo, R.A.; Castro, A.V.B.; Geloneze, B.; Foss, M.C.; Foss-Freitas, M.C. Supplementation of α-linolenic acid improves serum adiponectin levels and insulin sensitivity in patients with type 2 diabetes. *Nutrition* **2015**, *31*, 853–857. [CrossRef] [PubMed]
30. Bozzeto, L.; Prinster, A.; Costagliola, L.; Mangione, A.; Vitelli, A. Liver fat is reduced by an isoenergetic mufa diet in a controlled randomized study in type 2 diabetic patients. *Diabetes Care* **2012**, *35*, 1429–1435. [CrossRef] [PubMed]
31. Garibay-Nieto, N.; Queipo-Garcia, G.; Alvarez, F.; Bustos, M.; Villanueva, E.; Ramirez, F.; Leon, M.; Laresgoiti-Servitje, E.; Duggirala, R.; Macias, T.; et al. Effects of conjugated linoleic acid and metformin on insulin sensitivity in obese children: Randomized clinical trial. *J. Clin. Endocrinol. Metab.* **2017**. [CrossRef]
32. Zhang, W.Y.; Lee, J.J.; Kim, Y.; Kim, I.S.; Park, J.S.; Myung, C.S. Amelioration of insulin resistance by scopoletin in high-glucose-induced, insulin-resistant hepg2 cells. *Horm. Metab. Res.* **2010**, *42*, 930–935. [CrossRef] [PubMed]
33. Vaag, A.A.; Holst, J.J.; Volund, A.; Becknielsen, H. Gut incretin hormones in identical-twins discordant for non- insulin-dependent diabetes-mellitus (niddm)—Evidence for decreased glucagon-like peptide-1 secretion during oral glucose- ingestion in niddm twins. *Eur. J. Endocrinol.* **1996**, *135*, 425–432. [CrossRef] [PubMed]
34. Benjamin, S.; Spener, F. Conjugated linoleic acids as functional food: An insight into their health benefits. *Nutr. Metab.* **2009**. [CrossRef] [PubMed]
35. Zhou, X.-R.; Sun, C.-H.; Liu, J.-R.; Zhao, D. Dietary conjugated linoleic acid increases ppar gamma gene expression in adipose tissue of obese rat, and improves insulin resistance. *Growth Horm. IGF Res.* **2008**. [CrossRef] [PubMed]
36. Perdomo, L.; Beneit, N.; Otero, Y.F.; Escribano, Ó.; Díaz-Castroverde, S.; Gómez-Hernández, A.; Benito, M. Protective role of oleic acid against cardiovascular insulin resistance and in the early and late cellular atherosclerotic process. *Cardiovasc. Diabetol.* **2015**, *14*, 75. [CrossRef] [PubMed]
37. Gao, D.; Griffiths, H.R.; Bailey, C.J. Oleate protects against palmitate-induced insulin resistance in l6 myotubes. *Br. J. Nutr.* **2009**. [CrossRef] [PubMed]
38. Zhou, Y.-J.; Tang, Y.-S.; Song, Y.-L.; Li, A.; Zhou, H.; Li, Y. Saturated fatty acid induces insulin resistance partially through nucleotide-binding oligomerization domain 1 signaling pathway in adipocytes. *Chin. Med. Sci. J.* **2013**, *28*, 211–217. [CrossRef]
39. Malinska, H.; Huttl, M.; Oliyarnyk, O.; Bratova, M.; Kazdova, L. Conjugated linoleic acid reduces visceral and ectopic lipid accumulation and insulin resistance in chronic severe hypertriacylglycerolemia. *Nutrition* **2015**. [CrossRef] [PubMed]
40. Finucane, O.M.; Lyons, C.L.; Murphy, A.M.; Reynolds, C.M.; Klinger, R.; Healy, N.P.; Cooke, A.A.; Coll, R.C.; McAllan, L.; Nilaweera, K.N.; et al. Monounsaturated fatty acid-enriched high-fat diets impede adipose nlrp3 inflammasome-mediated il-1β secretion and insulin resistance despite obesity. *Diabetes* **2015**. [CrossRef] [PubMed]

41. Rocca, A.S.; Lagreca, J.; Kalitsky, J.; Brubaker, P.L. Monounsaturated fatty acid diets improve glycemic tolerance through increased secretion of glucagon-like peptide-1. *Endocrinology* **2001**. [CrossRef] [PubMed]
42. Rocca, A.S.; Brubaker, P.L. Stereospecific effects of fatty acids on proglucagon-derived peptide secretion in fetal rat intestinal cultures. *Endocrinology* **1995**. [CrossRef] [PubMed]
43. Lucero, D.; Olano, C.; Bursztyn, M.; Morales, C.; Stranges, A.; Friedman, S.; Macri, E.V.; Schreier, L.; Zago, V. Supplementation with n-3, n-6, n-9 fatty acids in an insulin-resistance animal model: Does it improve vldl quality? *Food Funct.* **2017**, *8*, 2053–2061. [CrossRef] [PubMed]
44. Sambra Vásquez, V.; Rojas Moncada, P.; Basfi-Fer, K.; Valencia, A.; Codoceo, J.; Inostroza, J.; Carrasco, F.; Ruz Ortiz, M. Impact of dietary fatty acids on lipid profile, insulin sensitivity and functionality of pancreatic β cells in type 2 diabetic subjects. *Nutr. Hosp.* **2015**, *32*, 1107–1115. [CrossRef] [PubMed]
45. Storlien, L.H.; Kraegen, E.W.; Chisholm, D.J.; Ford, G.L.; Bruce, D.G.; Pascoe, W.S.; Chisholm, D.J.; Ford, G.L.; Bruce, D.G.; Pascoe, W.S. Fish oil prevents insulin resistance induced by high-fat feeding in rats. *Science* **1987**, *237*, 885–888. [CrossRef] [PubMed]
46. Neves Ribeiro, D.; De Cássia, R.; Alfenas, G.; Bressan, J.; Brunoro Costa, N.M. The effect of oilseed consumption on appetite and on the risk of developing type 2 diabetes mellitus. *Nutr. Hosp.* **2013**, *28*, 296–305. [CrossRef] [PubMed]
47. Vessby, B.; Uusitupa, M.; Hermansen, K.; Riccardi, G.; Rivellese, A.A.; Tapsell, L.C.; Nälsén, C.; Berglund, L.; Louheranta, A.; Rasmussen, B.M.; et al. Substituting dietary saturated for monounsaturated fat impairs insulin sensitivity in healthy men and women: The kanwu study. *Diabetologia* **2001**. [CrossRef]
48. Lopez-Ridaura, R.; Willett, W.C.; Rimm, E.B.; Liu, S.; Stampfer, M.J.; Manson, J.E.; Hu, F.B. Magnesium intake and risk of type 2 diabetes in men and women. *Diabetes Care* **2004**, *27*, 134–140. [CrossRef] [PubMed]
49. Rodriguez-Moran, M.; Guerrero-Romero, F. Oral magnesium supplementation improves insulin sensitivity and metabolic control in type 2 diabetic subjects. *Diabetes Care* **2003**, *26*, 1147–1152. [CrossRef] [PubMed]
50. Kaline, K.; Bornstein, S.R.; Bergmann, A.; Hauner, H.; Schwarz, P.E.H. The importance and effect of dietary fiber in diabetes prevention with particular consideration of whole grain products. *Horm. Metab. Res.* **2007**, *39*, 687–693. [CrossRef] [PubMed]
51. Schulze, M.B. Fiber and magnesium intake and incidence of type 2 diabetes. *Arch. Intern. Med.* **2007**. [CrossRef] [PubMed]
52. Thomas, D.; Elliott, E.J.; Baur, L. Low glycaemic index, or low glycaemic load, diets for overweight and obesity. *Cochrane Libr.* **2005**. [CrossRef]
53. Schulze, M.B.; Liu, S.; Rimm, E.B.; Manson, J.E.; Willett, W.C.; Hu, F.B. Glycemic index, glycemic load, and dietary fiber intake and incidence of type 2 diabetes in younger and middle-aged women. *Am. J. Clin. Nutr.* **2004**, *80*, 348–356. [PubMed]
54. Okuyama, H.; Langsjoen, P.H.; Ohara, N.; Hashimoto, Y.; Hamazaki, T.; Yoshida, S.; Kobayashi, T.; Langsjoen, A.M. Medicines and vegetable oils as hidden causes of cardiovascular disease and diabetes. *Pharmacology* **2016**, *98*, 134–170. [CrossRef] [PubMed]
55. Sun, H.; Samarghandi, A.; Zhang, N.; Yao, Z.; Xiong, M.; Teng, B.B. Proprotein convertase subtilisin/kexin type 9 interacts with apolipoprotein b and prevents its intracellular degradation, irrespective of the low-density lipoprotein receptor. *Arterioscler. Thromb. Vasc. Biol.* **2012**, *32*, 1585–1595. [CrossRef] [PubMed]
56. Jorgensen, A.B.; Frikke-Schmidt, R.; Nordestgaard, B.G.; Tybjaerg-Hansen, A. Loss-of-function mutations in apoc3 and risk of ischemic vascular disease. *N. Engl. J. Med.* **2014**, *371*, 32–41. [CrossRef] [PubMed]
57. Musunuru, K.; Kathiresan, S. Surprises from genetic analyses of lipid risk factors for atherosclerosis. *Circ. Res.* **2016**, *118*, 579–585. [CrossRef] [PubMed]
58. Hurtubise, J.; McLellan, K.; Durr, K.; Onasanya, O.; Nwabuko, D.; Ndisang, J.F. The different facets of dyslipidemia and hypertension in atherosclerosis. *Curr. Atheroscler. Rep.* **2016**, *18*, 82. [CrossRef] [PubMed]
59. Stocker, R.; Keaney, J.F. Role of oxidative modifications in atherosclerosis. *Physiol. Rev.* **2004**, *84*, 1381–1478. [CrossRef] [PubMed]
60. Sanin, V.; Pfetsch, V.; Koenig, W. Dyslipidemias and cardiovascular prevention: Tailoring treatment according to lipid phenotype. *Curr. Cardiol. Rep.* **2017**, *19*, 61. [CrossRef] [PubMed]
61. Lopez-Garcia, E.; Schulze, M.B.; Meigs, J.B.; Manson, J.E.; Rifai, N.; Stampfer, M.J.; Willett, W.C.; Hu, F.B. Consumption of trans fatty acids is related to plasma biomarkers of inflammation and endothelial dysfunction. *J. Nutr.* **2005**, *135*, 562–566. [PubMed]

62. Benes, L.B.; Bassi, N.S.; Davidson, M.H. Omega-3 carboxylic acids monotherapy and combination with statins in the management of dyslipidemia. *Vasc. Health Risk Manag.* **2016**. [CrossRef] [PubMed]

63. Singh, S.; Arora, R.R.; Singh, M.; Khosla, S. Eicosapentaenoic acid versus docosahexaenoic acid as options for vascular risk prevention. *Am. J. Therap.* **2016**, *23*, e905–e910. [CrossRef] [PubMed]

64. Shearer, G.C.; Savinova, O.V.; Harris, W.S. Fish oil—How does it reduce plasma triglycerides? *Biochim. Biophys. Acta* **2012**, *1821*, 843–851. [CrossRef] [PubMed]

65. De Mattos, A.M.; da Costa, J.A.C.; Jordão Júnior, A.A.; Chiarello, P.G. Omega-3 fatty acid supplementation is associated with oxidative stress and dyslipidemia, but does not contribute to better lipid and oxidative status on hemodialysis patients. *J. Renal Nutr.* **2017**, *27*, 333–339. [CrossRef] [PubMed]

66. Sawada, T.; Tsubata, H.; Hashimoto, N.; Takabe, M.; Miyata, T.; Aoki, K.; Yamashita, S.; Oishi, S.; Osue, T.; Yokoi, K.; et al. Effects of 6-month eicosapentaenoic acid treatment on postprandial hyperglycemia, hyperlipidemia, insulin secretion ability, and concomitant endothelial dysfunction among newly-diagnosed impaired glucose metabolism patients with coronary artery disease. An open label, single blinded, prospective randomized controlled trial. *Cardiovasc. Diabetol.* **2016**. [CrossRef]

67. Wang, F.; Wang, Y.; Zhu, Y.; Liu, X.; Xia, H.; Yang, X.; Sun, G. Treatment for 6 months with fish oil-derived n-3 polyunsaturated fatty acids has neutral effects on glycemic control but improves dyslipidemia in type 2 diabetic patients with abdominal obesity: A randomized, double-blind, placebo-controlled trial. *Eur. J. Nutr.* **2016**. [CrossRef] [PubMed]

68. Dittrich, M.; Jahreis, G.; Bothor, K.; Drechsel, C.; Kiehntopf, M.; Blüher, M.; Dawczynski, C. Benefits of foods supplemented with vegetable oils rich in α-linolenic, stearidonic or docosahexaenoic acid in hypertriglyceridemic subjects: A double-blind, randomized, controlled trail. *Eur. J. Nutr.* **2015**, *54*, 881–893. [CrossRef] [PubMed]

69. Harris, W.S.; Bulchandani, D. Why do omega-3 fatty acids lower serum triglycerides? *Curr. Opin. Lipidol.* **2006**. [CrossRef] [PubMed]

70. Miller, M.; Motevalli, M.; Westphal, D.; Kwiterovich, P.O. Incorporation of oleic acid and eicosapentaenoic acid into glycerolipids of cultured normal human fibroblasts. *Lipids* **1993**, *28*, 1–5. [CrossRef] [PubMed]

71. Rosenson, R.S.; Brewer, H.B.; Davidson, W.S.; Fayad, Z.A.; Fuster, V.; Goldstein, J.; Hellerstein, M.; Jiang, X.C.; Phillips, M.C.; Rader, D.J.; et al. Cholesterol efflux and atheroprotection: Advancing the concept of reverse cholesterol transport. *Circulation* **2012**. [CrossRef] [PubMed]

72. Hashmi, S.; Wang, Y.; Parhar, R.S.; Collison, K.S.; Conca, W.; Al-Mohanna, F.; Gaugler, R. A c. Elegans model to study human metabolic regulation. *Nutr. Metab. (Lond.)* **2013**, *10*, 31. [CrossRef] [PubMed]

73. Zhukova, N.V.; Novgorodtseva, T.P.; Denisenko, Y.K.; Gonzalez, D.E.; Mustad, V.A.; Kris-Etherton, P.M.; Rise, P.; Eligini, S.; Ghezzi, S.; Colli, S.; et al. Effect of the prolonged high-fat diet on the fatty acid metabolism in rat blood and liver. *Lipids Health Dis.* **2014**. [CrossRef] [PubMed]

74. Barrows, B.R.; Parks, E.J. Contributions of different fatty acid sources to very low-density lipoprotein-triacylglycerol in the fasted and fed states. *J. Clin. Endocrinol. Metab.* **2006**, *91*, 1446–1452. [CrossRef] [PubMed]

75. Parlevliet, E.T.; Wang, Y.; Geerling, J.J.; Schröder-Van der Elst, J.P.; Picha, K.; O'Neil, K.; Stojanovic-Susulic, V.; Ort, T.; Havekes, L.M.; Romijn, J.A.; et al. Glp-1 receptor activation inhibits vldl production and reverses hepatic steatosis by decreasing hepatic lipogenesis in high-fat-fed apoe*3-leiden mice. *PLoS ONE* **2012**. [CrossRef] [PubMed]

76. Figueiredo, P.S.; Candido, C.J.; Jaques, J.A.S.; Nunes, Â.A.; Caires, A.R.L.; Michels, F.S.; Almeida, J.A.; Filiú, W.F.O.; Hiane, P.A.; Nascimento, V.A.; et al. Oxidative stability of sesame and flaxseed oils and their effects on morphometric and biochemical parameters in an animal model. *J. Sci. Food Agric.* **2017**, *97*, 3359–3364. [CrossRef] [PubMed]

77. Yang, L.G.; Song, Z.X.; Yin, H.; Wang, Y.Y.; Shu, G.F.; Lu, H.X.; Wang, S.K.; Sun, G.J. Low n-6/n-3 pufa ratio improves lipid metabolism, inflammation, oxidative stress and endothelial function in rats using plant oils as n-3 fatty acid source. *Lipids* **2016**, *51*, 49–59. [CrossRef] [PubMed]

78. Li, F.; Duan, Y.; Li, Y.; Tang, Y.; Geng, M.; Oladele, O.A.; Kim, S.W.; Yin, Y. Effects of dietary n-6:N-3 pufa ratio on fatty acid composition, free amino acid profile and gene expression of transporters in finishing pigs. *Br. J. Nutr.* **2015**. [CrossRef] [PubMed]

79. Macri, E.V.; Lifshitz, F.; Alsina, E.; Juiz, N.; Zago, V.; Lezón, C.; Rodriguez, P.N.; Schreier, L.; Boyer, P.M.; Friedman, S.M. Monounsaturated fatty acids-rich diets in hypercholesterolemic-growing rats. *Int. J. Food Sci. Nutr.* **2015**. [CrossRef] [PubMed]

80. Alsina, E.; Macri, E.V.; Lifshitz, F.; Bozzini, C.; Rodriguez, P.N.; Boyer, P.M.; Friedman, S.M. Efficacy of phytosterols and fish-oil supplemented high-oleic-sunflower oil rich diets in hypercholesterolemic growing rats. *Int. J. Food Sci. Nutr.* **2016**. [CrossRef] [PubMed]

81. Gnoni, A.; Giudetti, A.M. Dietary long-chain unsaturated fatty acids acutely and differently reduce the activities of lipogenic enzymes and of citrate carrier in rat liver. *J. Physiol. Biochem.* **2016**, *72*, 485–494. [CrossRef] [PubMed]

82. Altmann, S.W.; Davis, H.R.; Zhu, L.-J.; Yao, X.; Hoos, L.M.; Tetzloff, G.; Iyer, S.P.N.; Maguire, M.; Golovko, A.; Zeng, M.; et al. Niemann-pick c1 like 1 protein is critical for intestinal cholesterol absorption. *Science (N. Y.)* **2004**. [CrossRef] [PubMed]

83. Ikeda, I.; Tanaka, K.; Sugano, M.; Vahouny, G.V.; Gallo, L.L. Inhibition of cholesterol absorption in rats by plant sterols. *J. Lipid Res.* **1988**, *29*, 1573–1582. [PubMed]

84. Strable, M.S.; Ntambi, J.M. Genetic control of de novo lipogenesis: Role in diet-induced obesity. *Crit. Rev. Biochem. Mol. Biol.* **2010**, *45*, 199–214. [CrossRef] [PubMed]

85. Eissing, L.; Scherer, T.; Todter, K.; Knippschild, U.; Greve, J.W.; Buurman, W.A.; Pinnschmidt, H.O.; Rensen, S.S.; Wolf, A.M.; Bartelt, A.; et al. De novo lipogenesis in human fat and liver is linked to chrebp-beta and metabolic health. *Nat. Commun.* **2013**, *4*, 1528. [CrossRef] [PubMed]

86. Borkman, M.; Storlien, L.H.; Pan, D.A.; Jenkins, A.B.; Chisholm, D.J.; Campbell, L.V. The relation between insulin sensitivity and the fatty-acid composition of skeletal-muscle phospholipids. *N. Engl. J. Med.* **1993**. [CrossRef] [PubMed]

87. Rustan, A.C. Fatty acids: Structures and properties. *Encycl. Life Sci.* **2009**. [CrossRef]

88. Caër, C.; Rouault, C.; Roy, T.L.; Poitou, C.; Aron, J.; Adriana, T.; Bic, J.-C.; Clément, K. Immune cell-derived cytokines contribute to obesity-related inflammation, fibrogenesis and metabolic deregulation in human adipose tissue. *Sci. Rep.* **2017**. [CrossRef]

89. Moya-Pérez, A.; Neef, A.; Sanz, Y. Bifidobacterium pseudocatenulatum cect 7765 reduces obesity-associated inflammation by restoring the lymphocyte-macrophage balance and gut microbiota structure in high-fat diet-fed mice. *PLoS ONE* **2015**, *10*. [CrossRef] [PubMed]

90. Rainone, V.; Schneider, L.; Saulle, I.; Ricci, C.; Biasin, M.; Al-Daghri, N.M.; Giani, E.; Zuccotti, G.V.; Clerici, M.; Trabattoni, D. Upregulation of inflammasome activity and increased gut permeability are associated with obesity in children and adolescents. *Int. J. Obes.* **2016**, *40*, 1026–1033. [CrossRef] [PubMed]

91. Lyte, J.M.; Gabler, N.K.; Hollis, J.H. Postprandial serum endotoxin in healthy humans is modulated by dietary fat in a randomized, controlled, cross-over study. *Lipids Health Dis.* **2016**, *15*, 186. [CrossRef] [PubMed]

92. Simopoulos, A.P. An increase in the omega-6/omega-3 fatty acid ratio increases the risk for obesity. *Nutrients* **2016**, *8*, 128. [CrossRef] [PubMed]

93. Kien, C.L.; Bunn, J.Y.; Fukagawa, N.K.; Anathy, V.; Matthews, D.E.; Crain, K.I.; Ebenstein, D.B.; Tarleton, E.K.; Pratley, R.E.; Poynter, M.E. Lipidomic evidence that lowering the typical dietary palmitate to oleate ratio in humans decreases the leukocyte production of proinflammatory cytokines and muscle expression of redox-sensitive genes. *J. Nutr. Biochem.* **2015**, *26*, 1599–1606. [CrossRef] [PubMed]

94. Haro, C.; Montes-Borrego, M.; Rangel-Zuniga, O.A.; Alcala-Diaz, J.F.; Gomez-Delgado, F.; Perez-Martinez, P.; Delgado-Lista, J.; Quintana-Navarro, G.M.; Tinahones, F.J.; Landa, B.B.; et al. Two healthy diets modulate gut microbial community improving insulin sensitivity in a human obese population. *J. Clin. Endocrinol. Metab.* **2016**, *101*, 233–242. [CrossRef] [PubMed]

95. Fava, F.; Gitau, R.; Griffin, B.A.; Gibson, G.R.; Tuohy, K.M.; Lovegrove, J.A. The type and quantity of dietary fat and carbohydrate alter faecal microbiome and short-chain fatty acid excretion in a metabolic syndrome 'at-risk' population. *Int. J. Obes.* **2013**, *37*, 216–223. [CrossRef] [PubMed]

96. Martin-Pelaez, S.; Mosele, J.I.; Pizarro, N.; Farras, M.; de la Torre, R.; Subirana, I.; Perez-Cano, F.J.; Castaner, O.; Sola, R.; Fernandez-Castillejo, S.; et al. Effect of virgin olive oil and thyme phenolic compounds on blood lipid profile: Implications of human gut microbiota. *Eur. J. Nutr.* **2017**, *56*, 119–131. [CrossRef] [PubMed]

97. Balfego, M.; Canivell, S.; Hanzu, F.A.; Sala-Vila, A.; Martinez-Medina, M.; Murillo, S.; Mur, T.; Ruano, E.G.; Linares, F.; Porras, N.; et al. Effects of sardine-enriched diet on metabolic control, inflammation and gut microbiota in drug-naive patients with type 2 diabetes: A pilot randomized trial. *Lipids Health Dis.* **2016**, *15*, 78. [CrossRef] [PubMed]

98. Masi, L.N.; Martins, A.R.; Crisma, A.R.; do Amaral, C.T.L.; Davanso, M.R.; Serdan, T.D.A.; da Cunha de S, R.D.C.; Cruz, M.M.; Alonso-Vale, M.I.C.; Torres, R.N.P.; et al. Combination of a high-fat diet with sweetened condensed milk exacerbates inflammation and insulin resistance induced by each separately in mice. *Sci. Rep.* **2017**, *7*, 3937. [CrossRef] [PubMed]

99. Moran-Ramos, S.; He, X.; Chin, E.L.; Tovar, A.R.; Torres, N.; Slupsky, C.M.; Raybould, H.E. Nopal feeding reduces adiposity, intestinal inflammation and shifts the cecal microbiota and metabolism in high-fat fed rats. *PLoS ONE* **2017**, *12*, e0171672. [CrossRef] [PubMed]

100. Lam, Y.Y.; Ha, C.W.; Campbell, C.R.; Mitchell, A.J.; Dinudom, A.; Oscarsson, J.; Cook, D.I.; Hunt, N.H.; Caterson, I.D.; Holmes, A.J.; et al. Increased gut permeability and microbiota change associate with mesenteric fat inflammation and metabolic dysfunction in diet-induced obese mice. *PLoS ONE* **2012**, *7*, e34233. [CrossRef] [PubMed]

101. Mujico, J.R.; Baccan, G.C.; Gheorghe, A.; Diaz, L.E.; Marcos, A. Changes in gut microbiota due to supplemented fatty acids in diet-induced obese mice. *Br. J. Nutr.* **2013**, *110*, 711–720. [CrossRef] [PubMed]

102. Qin, Y.; Zhou, Y.; Chen, S.H.; Zhao, X.L.; Ran, L.; Zeng, X.L.; Wu, Y.; Chen, J.L.; Kang, C.; Shu, F.R.; et al. Fish oil supplements lower serum lipids and glucose in correlation with a reduction in plasma fibroblast growth factor 21 and prostaglandin e2 in nonalcoholic fatty liver disease associated with hyperlipidemia: A randomized clinical trial. *PLoS ONE* **2015**, *10*, e0133496. [CrossRef] [PubMed]

103. Lecomte, V.; Kaakoush, N.O.; Maloney, C.A.; Raipuria, M.; Huinao, K.D.; Mitchell, H.M.; Morris, M.J. Changes in gut microbiota in rats fed a high fat diet correlate with obesity-associated metabolic parameters. *PLoS ONE* **2015**, *10*, e0126931. [CrossRef] [PubMed]

104. Calder, P. Mechanisms of action of (n-3) fatty acids. *J. Nutr.* **2012**, 1–8. [CrossRef] [PubMed]

105. Pinel, A.; Pitois, E.; Rigaudiere, J.P.; Jouve, C.; De Saint-Vincent, S.; Laillet, B.; Montaurier, C.; Huertas, A.; Morio, B.; Capel, F. Epa prevents fat mass expansion and metabolic disturbances in mice fed with a western diet. *J. Lipid Res.* **2016**, *57*, 1382–1397. [CrossRef] [PubMed]

106. LeMieux, M.J.; Kalupahana, N.S.; Scoggin, S.; Moustaid-Moussa, N. Eicosapentaenoic acid reduces adipocyte hypertrophy and inflammation in diet-induced obese mice in an adiposity-independent manner. *J. Nutr.* **2015**, *145*, 411–417. [CrossRef] [PubMed]

107. Carvalho, B.M.; Guadagnini, D.; Tsukumo, D.M.L.; Schenka, A.A.; Latuf-Filho, P.; Vassallo, J.; Dias, J.C.; Kubota, L.T.; Carvalheira, J.B.C.; Saad, M.J.A. Modulation of gut microbiota by antibiotics improves insulin signalling in high-fat fed mice. *Diabetologia* **2012**. [CrossRef] [PubMed]

108. Tremaroli, V.; Bäckhed, F. Functional interactions between the gut microbiota and host metabolism. *Nature* **2012**, *489*, 242–249. [CrossRef] [PubMed]

109. Wan, J.; Hu, S.; Jacoby, J.J.; Liu, J.; Zhang, Y.; Yu, L. The impact of dietary sn-2 palmitic triacylglycerols in combination with docosahexaenoic acid or arachidonic acid on lipid metabolism and host faecal microbiota composition in sprague dawley rats. *Food Funct.* **2017**, *8*, 1793–1802. [CrossRef] [PubMed]

110. De Filippo, C.; Cavalieri, D.; Di Paola, M.; Ramazzotti, M.; Poullet, J.B.; Massart, S.; Collini, S.; Pieraccini, G.; Lionetti, P. Impact of diet in shaping gut microbiota revealed by a comparative study in children from europe and rural africa. *Proc. Natl. Acad. Sci. USA* **2010**, *107*, 14691–14696. [CrossRef] [PubMed]

111. Bibbó, S.; Ianiro, G.; Giorgio, V.; Scaldaferri, F.; Masucci, L.; Gasbarrini, A.; Cammarota, G. The role of diet on gut microbiota composition. *Eur. Rev. Med. Pharmacol. Sci.* **2016**, *20*, 4742–4749. [PubMed]

112. Deol, P.; Evans, J.R.; Dhahbi, J.; Chellappa, K.; Han, D.S.; Spindler, S.; Sladek, F.M. Soybean oil is more obesogenic and diabetogenic than coconut oil and fructose in mouse: Potential role for the liver. *PLoS ONE* **2015**, *10*, e0132672. [CrossRef] [PubMed]

113. Lonardo, A.; Ballestri, S.; Marchesini, G.; Angulo, P.; Loria, P. Nonalcoholic fatty liver disease: A precursor of the metabolic syndrome. *Dig. Liver Dis.* **2015**, *47*, 181–190. [CrossRef] [PubMed]

114. Papamiltiadous, E.S.; Roberts, S.K.; Nicoll, A.J.; Ryan, M.C.; Itsiopoulos, C.; Salim, A.; Tierney, A.C. A randomised controlled trial of a mediterranean dietary intervention for adults with non alcoholic fatty liver disease (medina): Study protocol. *BMC Gastroenterol.* **2016**, *16*, 14. [CrossRef] [PubMed]

115. Wah-Kheong, C.; Khean-Lee, G. Epidemiology of a fast emerging disease in the asia-pacific region: Non-alcoholic fatty liver disease. *Hepatol. Int.* **2013**. [CrossRef] [PubMed]

116. Baidal, J.A.W.; Lavine, J.E. The intersection of nonalcoholic fatty liver disease and obesity. *Sci. Transl. Med.* **2016**, *8*. [CrossRef] [PubMed]

117. Del Ben, M.; Polimeni, L.; Baratta, F.; Pastori, D.; Loffredo, L.; Angelico, F. Modern approach to the clinical management of non-alcoholic fatty liver disease. *World J. Gastroenterol.* **2014**, *20*, 8341–8350. [CrossRef] [PubMed]

118. Musso, G.; Cassader, M.; Rosina, F.; Gambino, R. Impact of current treatments on liver disease, glucose metabolism and cardiovascular risk in non-alcoholic fatty liver disease (nafld): A systematic review and meta-analysis of randomised trials. *Diabetologia* **2012**, *55*, 885–904. [CrossRef] [PubMed]

119. Zelber-Sagi, S.; Salomone, F.; Mlynarsky, L. The mediterranean dietary pattern as the diet of choice for non-alcoholic fatty liver disease: Evidence and plausible mechanisms. *Liver Int.* **2017**, *37*, 936–949. [CrossRef] [PubMed]

120. Gelli, C.; Tarocchi, M.; Abenavoli, L.; Di Renzo, L.; Galli, A.; De Lorenzo, A. Effect of a counseling-supported treatment with the mediterranean diet and physical activity on the severity of the non-alcoholic fatty liver disease. *World J. Gastroenterol.* **2017**, *23*, 3150–3162. [CrossRef] [PubMed]

121. Lottenberg, A.M.; Afonso Mda, S.; Lavrador, M.S.; Machado, R.M.; Nakandakare, E.R. The role of dietary fatty acids in the pathology of metabolic syndrome. *J. Nutr. Biochem.* **2012**, *23*, 1027–1040. [CrossRef] [PubMed]

122. Buettner, R.; Ascher, M.; Gäbele, E.; Hellerbrand, C.; Kob, R.; Bertsch, T.; Bollheimer, L.C. Olive oil attenuates the cholesterol-induced development of nonalcoholic steatohepatitis despite increased insulin resistance in a rodent model. *Horm. Metab. Res.* **2013**, *45*, 795–801. [CrossRef] [PubMed]

123. Wang, C.; Liu, W.; Yao, L.; Zhang, X.; Zhang, X.; Ye, C.; Jiang, H.; He, J.; Zhu, Y.; Ai, D. Hydroxyeicosapentaenoic acids and epoxyeicosatetraenoic acids attenuate early occurrence of nonalcoholic fatty liver disease. *Br. J. Pharmacol.* **2017**, *174*, 2358–2372. [CrossRef] [PubMed]

124. Zelber-Sagi, S.; Ratziu, V.; Oren, R. Nutrition and physical activity in nafld: An overview of the epidemiological evidence. *World J. Gastroenterol.* **2011**, *17*, 3377–3389. [CrossRef] [PubMed]

125. Trichopoulou, A.; Martínez-González, M.A.; Tong, T.Y.; Forouhi, N.G.; Khandelwal, S.; Prabhakaran, D.; Mozaffarian, D.; de Lorgeril, M. Definitions and potential health benefits of the mediterranean diet: Views from experts around the world. *BMC Med.* **2014**. [CrossRef] [PubMed]

126. Ryan, M.C.; Itsiopoulos, C.; Thodis, T.; Ward, G.; Trost, N.; Hofferberth, S.; O'Dea, K.; Desmond, P.V.; Johnson, N.A.; Wilson, A.M. The mediterranean diet improves hepatic steatosis and insulin sensitivity in individuals with non-alcoholic fatty liver disease. *J. Hepatol.* **2013**, *59*, 138–143. [CrossRef] [PubMed]

127. Li, Y.H.; Yang, L.H.; Sha, K.H.; Liu, T.G.; Zhang, L.G.; Liu, X.X. Efficacy of poly-unsaturated fatty acid therapy on patients with nonalcoholic steatohepatitis. *World J. Gastroenterol.* **2015**, *21*, 7008–7013. [CrossRef] [PubMed]

128. Hodson, L.; Bhatia, L.; Scorletti, E.; Smith, D.E.; Jackson, N.C.; Shojaee-Moradie, F.; Umpleby, M.; Calder, P.C.; Byrne, C.D. Docosahexaenoic acid enrichment in nafld is associated with improvements in hepatic metabolism and hepatic insulin sensitivity: A pilot study. *Eur. J. Clin. Nutr.* **2017**, *71*, 973–979. [CrossRef] [PubMed]

129. Lopez-Vicario, C.; Gonzalez-Periz, A.; Rius, B.; Moran-Salvador, E.; Garcia-Alonso, V.; Lozano, J.J.; Bataller, R.; Cofan, M.; Kang, J.X.; Arroyo, V.; et al. Molecular interplay between delta5/delta6 desaturases and long-chain fatty acids in the pathogenesis of non-alcoholic steatohepatitis. *Gut* **2014**, *63*, 344–355. [CrossRef] [PubMed]

130. Soni, N.K.; Nookaew, I.; Sandberg, A.-S.; Gabrielsson, B.G. Eicosapentaenoic and docosahexaenoic acid-enriched high fat diet delays the development of fatty liver in mice. *Lipids Health Dis.* **2015**. [CrossRef] [PubMed]

131. Bargut, T.C.L.; Frantz, E.D.C.; Mandarim-De-Lacerda, C.A.; Aguila, M.B. Effects of a diet rich in n-3 polyunsaturated fatty acids on hepatic lipogenesis and beta-oxidation in mice. *Lipids* **2014**, *49*, 431–444. [CrossRef] [PubMed]

132. Shang, T.; Liu, L.; Zhou, J.; Zhang, M.; Hu, Q.; Fang, M.; Wu, Y.; Yao, P.; Gong, Z. Protective effects of various ratios of dha/epa supplementation on high-fat diet-induced liver damage in mice. *Lipids Health Dis.* **2017**, *16*, 65. [CrossRef] [PubMed]

133. Depner, C.M.; Philbrick, K.A.; Jump, D.B. Docosahexaenoic acid attenuates hepatic inflammation, oxidative stress, and fibrosis without decreasing hepatosteatosis in a ldlr$^{-/-}$ mouse model of western diet-induced nonalcoholic steatohepatitis. *J. Nutr.* **2013**, *143*, 315–323. [CrossRef] [PubMed]

134. Lytle, K.A.; Depner, C.M.; Wong, C.P.; Jump, D.B. Docosahexaenoic acid attenuates western diet-induced hepatic fibrosis in ldlr$^{-/-}$ mice by targeting the tgfbeta-smad3 pathway. *J. Lipid Res.* **2015**, *56*, 1936–1946. [CrossRef] [PubMed]

135. Hanke, D.; Zahradka, P.; Mohankumar, S.K.; Clark, J.L.; Taylor, C.G. A diet high in alpha-linolenic acid and monounsaturated fatty acids attenuates hepatic steatosis and alters hepatic phospholipid fatty acid profile in diet-induced obese rats. *Prostaglandins Leukot. Essent. Fatty Acids* **2013**, *89*, 391–401. [CrossRef] [PubMed]

136. Chen, T.; Yuan, F.; Wang, H.; Tian, Y.; He, L.; Shao, Y.; Li, N.; Liu, Z. Perilla oil supplementation ameliorates high-fat/high-cholesterol diet induced nonalcoholic fatty liver disease in rats via enhanced fecal cholesterol and bile acid excretion. *BioMed Res. Int.* **2016**, *2016*, 2384561. [CrossRef] [PubMed]

137. Du, Z.Y.; Ma, T.; Liaset, B.; Keenan, A.H.; Araujo, P.; Lock, E.J.; Demizieux, L.; Degrace, P.; Frøyland, L.; Kristiansen, K.; et al. Dietary eicosapentaenoic acid supplementation accentuates hepatic triglyceride accumulation in mice with impaired fatty acid oxidation capacity. *Biochim. Biophys. Acta Mol. Cell Biol. Lipids* **2013**, *1831*, 291–299. [CrossRef] [PubMed]

138. Provenzano, A.; Milani, S.; Vizzutti, F.; Delogu, W.; Navari, N.; Novo, E.; Maggiora, M.; Maurino, V.; Laffi, G.; Parola, M.; et al. N-3 polyunsaturated fatty acids worsen inflammation and fibrosis in experimental nonalcoholic steatohepatitis. *Liver Int.* **2014**, *34*, 918–930. [CrossRef] [PubMed]

139. Jurado-Ruiz, E.; Varela, L.M.; Luque, A.; Berna, G.; Cahuana, G.; Martinez-Force, E.; Gallego-Duran, R.; Soria, B.; de Roos, B.; Romero Gomez, M.; et al. An extra virgin olive oil rich diet intervention ameliorates the nonalcoholic steatohepatitis induced by a high-fat "western-type" diet in mice. *Mol. Nutr. Food Res.* **2017**, *61*. [CrossRef]

140. Guo, X.; Li, H.; Xu, H.; Halim, V.; Zhang, W.; Wang, H.; Ong, K.T.; Woo, S.L.; Walzem, R.L.; Mashek, D.G.; et al. Palmitoleate induces hepatic steatosis but suppresses liver inflammatory response in mice. *PLoS ONE* **2012**, *7*, e39286. [CrossRef] [PubMed]

141. Miura, K.; Yang, L.; van Rooijen, N.; Brenner, D.A.; Ohnishi, H.; Seki, E. Toll-like receptor 2 and palmitic acid cooperatively contribute to the development of nonalcoholic steatohepatitis through inflammasome activation in mice. *Hepatology* **2013**, *57*, 577–589. [CrossRef] [PubMed]

142. Böhm, T.; Berger, H.; Nejabat, M.; Riegler, T.; Kellner, F.; Kuttke, M.; Sagmeister, S.; Bazanella, M.; Stolze, K.; Daryabeigi, A.; et al. Food-derived peroxidized fatty acids may trigger hepatic inflammation: A novel hypothesis to explain steatohepatitis. *J. Hepatol.* **2013**, *59*, 563–570. [CrossRef] [PubMed]

143. Depner, C.M.; Traber, M.G.; Bobe, G.; Kensicki, E.; Bohren, K.M.; Milne, G.; Jump, D.B. A metabolomic analysis of omega-3 fatty acid-mediated attenuation of western diet-induced nonalcoholic steatohepatitis in ldlr$^{-/-}$ mice. *PLoS ONE* **2013**, *8*, e83756. [CrossRef] [PubMed]

144. Cao, H.; Gerhold, K.; Mayers, J.R.; Wiest, M.M.; Steve, M.; Hotamisligil, G.S. Identification of a lipokine, a lipid hormone linking adipose tissue to systemic metabolism. *Cell* **2009**, *134*, 933–944. [CrossRef] [PubMed]

145. Seki, E.; Brenner, D.A. Toll-like receptors and adaptor molecules in liver disease: Update. *Hepatology* **2008**, *48*, 322–335. [CrossRef] [PubMed]

146. Csak, T.; Ganz, M.; Pespisa, J.; Kodys, K.; Dolganiuc, A.; Szabo, G. Fatty acid and endotoxin activate inflammasomes in mouse hepatocytes that release danger signals to stimulate immune cells. *Hepatology* **2011**, *54*, 133–144. [CrossRef] [PubMed]

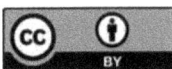

nutrients

MDPI

Commentary

The Role of the Japanese Traditional Diet in Healthy and Sustainable Dietary Patterns around the World

Ana San Gabriel *, Kumiko Ninomiya and Hisayuki Uneyama

Science Group, Global Communications Department, Ajinomoto Co., Inc., 15-1, Kyobashi 1-Chome, Chuo-ku, Tokyo 104-8315, Japan; kumiko_ninomiya@ajinomoto.com (K.N.); hisayuki_uneyama@ajinomoto.com (H.U.)
* Correspondence: ana_sangabriel@ajinomoto.com; Tel.: +81-3-5250-5140

Received: 29 November 2017; Accepted: 31 January 2018; Published: 3 February 2018

Abstract: As incomes steadily increase globally, traditional diets have been displaced by diets that are usually animal-based with a high content of "empty calories" or refined sugars, refined fats, and alcohol. Dietary transition coupled with the expansion of urbanization and lower physical activity have been linked to the global growth in the prevalence of obesity, overweight and life style-related non-communicable diseases. The challenge is in how to reverse the trend of high consumption of less healthy food by more healthful and more environmentally sustainable diets. The increasing recognition that each individual has specific needs depending on age, metabolic condition, and genetic profile adds complexity to general nutritional considerations. If we were to promote the consumption of low-energy and low salt but nutritious diets, taste becomes a relevant food quality. The Japanese traditional diet (Washoku), which is characterized by high consumption of fish and soybean products and low consumption of animal fat and meat, relies on the effective use of umami taste to enhance palatability. There may be a link between Washoku and the longevity of the people in Japan. Thus Washoku and umami may be valuable tools to support healthy eating.

Keywords: healthy dietary patterns; Washoku; umami; glutamate; taste; Japanese cuisine; traditional diets; vegetables; taste receptors; dietary guidelines

---

1. The Traditional Japanese Diet and Its Potential Health Benefits

1.1. The Importance of Umami Taste in Foods and Its Application

Much has been written in the last twenty years about umami as the fifth basic taste, also known in English as the "savory" taste. Umami taste is elicited primarily by the free amino acid glutamate, which is commercially prepared as sodium salt, hence its shortened name, MSG or monosodium glutamate. This savory taste characterizes many traditional Japanese foods. It is now believed that there are several identifiable receptor mechanisms responsible for detecting the taste of glutamate on the tongue and the palate [1–3].

Ikeda [4], who first identified glutamate as the primary umami taste compound, proposed that it served to identify sources of protein and consequently, some have proposed that protein status may be important for the sensitivity to umami. Early studies showed that both, well-nourished and malnourished infants preferred a soup with the seasoning MSG [5]. However, recently, Masic and Yeomans analyzed the liking for umami among high and low protein consumers and they found that the liking for MSG was rated as more pleasant when high protein consumers were in protein deficit [6]. More work is needed to understand the relationship between umami sensation preference and nutritional needs. Interestingly, even though no link has been found between the perception of umami taste with specific health outcomes, Pepino and colleagues [7] reported a lower sensitivity to MSG among obese women who preferred higher levels of MSG compared to normal-weight women.

Thanks to the extensive analysis in food ingredients of the levels of glutamate and two of the most abundant 5′-ribonucleotides, inosine monophosphate (IMP) and guanosine monophosphate (GMP), which synergize with glutamate to increase umami taste in foods, food technologists have identified foods that are naturally rich in umami substances, such as soup stocks, mushrooms, tomatoes, and fermented cheeses [8]. However, the characteristics of umami taste in complex food systems need to be studied in more detail. Thus, the authors here will focus on the evidence that explains the unique role that umami plays in the Japanese traditional diet, known as Washoku. We also discuss its potential application in other diets.

The Japanese soup stock *dashi* contains a significant amount of glutamate and IMP or GMP, depending of the type of *dashi*. It is believed that the particular profile of umami substances in *dashi* enhances the original flavors of foods and increases their palatability [9,10]. The effect of umami substances is described as "meaty and mouthful", "coating sensation" or even tactile. How can umami compounds exert this function in foods? From a food technology and physiological point of view, the exact mechanism by which glutamate and 5′-ribonucleotides function to create this effect cannot be fully explained by the activation of glutamate receptors on the tongue.

Glutamate plays an important role in the palatability of foods, and its palatability is not entirely due to learning. Early behavioral studies based on the analysis of facial expressions in neonates showed that the addition of 0.5% MSG was able to reverse the typical aversive response of spitting and gaping to a clear vegetable soup. In fact, newborn infants displayed a similar response to soup with added MSG as they do to sweet solutions: sucking and positive facial expressions [11]. This reaction of acceptance of MSG in soups by newborns is representative of the effect of glutamate in other foods in adults as well as children. Strangely, in an aqueous solution, MSG is unpalatable to both adults and infants. The reason for this is obscure [12]. In short, the optimal concentration of MSG, which usually ranges from 0.04% to 1.6%, has the ability to increase the acceptability of foods by changing the sensory and consequently, hedonic or pleasant properties of food.

Added glutamate also increases the liking of novel flavors, in much the same way that fat and sugar do [13]. Sugar and fat are thought to influence liking via their caloric content and reward effect. It is not clear in the case of MSG how umami influences liking. The increase in palatability by MSG is so robust that it can maintain the acceptability of food with reduced salt, which also works by improving the perception and flavor intensity in food [14–18]. That is, studies have confirmed that the partial substitution of salt by MSG allows for an overall decrease in sodium without reducing food palatability. Thus, added MSG could be an effective strategy to decrease sodium concentration in foods. Prescott and Young [19] illustrated how MSG increases the acceptability of soups, even among consumers that have a negative outlook towards MSG. Consumers rated the flavor of foods with added MSG as significantly better liked, richer, saltier, and more natural tasting. This higher food acceptability after adding MSG also influences food choices and, consequently, food intake. This property has been used to improve the nutritional status of older individuals [20,21]. Altogether, substantial research indicates that MSG and natural glutamates from *dashi* or other foods rich in umami could play a role in enhancing the palatability and promoting the consumption of nutritious foods with low sodium content. It thus has the potential to be strategically used to decrease the intake of animal-based ingredients and enhance intake of others that promote overall health, such as vegetables, as is done in Washoku. There is a long history for the use of MSG as a flavor enhancer, which the Food and Drug Administration of the United States has categorize as generally recognized as safe (GRAS) [22,23].

1.2. How Does Umami Enhances the Palatability of Foods?

The answer to this question is still unclear but there are several possible explanations. Part of the effect of MSG in foods could be explained by the content of sodium in MSG. However, Okiyama and Beauchamp [24] found that when comparing two soups with the same amount of sodium, subjects still preferred the one with MSG. The interaction of umami with other tastes modalities could be another reason. This interaction can work in two ways, either on taste intensity or on the temporal evolution of a taste sensation, also known as temporal dominance of sensation (TDS) [25,26]. In regard to taste intensity, umami sensation can enhance the perception of saltiness and make sourness more pleasant. There is also some evidence to suggest that glutamate can augment the perception of sweetness and suppress the intensity of some bitter compounds [25]. Recently, umami taste interaction with salty and sour tastes have also have been analyzed from a temporal point of view [26]. One study has shown that when MSG is combined with either NaCl (salty taste) or lactic acid (sour taste) the duration of the umami sensation was altered. IMP and NaCl decrease the duration of umami taste, whereas MSG suppresses the duration of the sourness of lactic acid.

Umami sensation increases salivary secretion, and this increase over 10 min is larger than that elicited by sour stimuli [27,28]. This property may be another way for glutamate to enhance food palatability. Saliva serves as a vehicle to dissolve the taste substances from foods and protect the proper functioning of taste sensation [29]. Hyposalivation can alter taste perception, which may result in poor appetite, weight loss and poor general health. Umami taste stimulation has been employed therapeutically to improve the flow of salivary secretion in elderly patients who have deficient umami taste sensation [30].

Another important physiological function of glutamate worth mentioning is its role as a signaling molecule in the gastrointestinal tract. Glutamate receptors have been found in the stomach and the gut [31,32], and studies suggest that glutamate may enhance food signaling to the brain by stimulating the vagus nerve and the secretion of neuroendocrine hormones and digestive juices that support the digestion of proteins [33,34].

And lastly, recently, it has been found that the umami sensation interacts with odors, as sweet and sour tastes do, by enhancing the intensity of aromas, such as that of chicken soup or celery (phthalide compounds), especially when these foods are swallowed [35]. Altogether, in addition to the modality of 'mouth feel' of umami that influences the body and thickness of a dish, it seems that glutamate enhances appetitive sensorial traits in a complex food context while masking the negative ones. At the same time umami is involved in the regulation of various gastrointestinal functions (review, [36]). This could partially explain why there is no need in Japanese traditional diets to use large amounts of animal fat or meats for optimal palatability—the meat-like sensation of traditional Japanese dishes with umami is sufficient.

1.3. The Traditional Japanese Cuisine, Washoku: Why Is It Thought to Be Healthy?

The traditional dietary cultures of Japan are collectively known as Washoku. In 2013, Washoku was named in the UNESCO list of Intangible Cultural Heritage. According to Professor Kumakura Isao, the President of the National Assembly on the Preservation and Continuation of Washoku culture, the guiding principles of Washoku are a staple food—rice—which is complemented by a variety of side dishes, soup, and pickles. Together these form the basic structure of a meal, customarily eaten using chopsticks, wooden bowls known as "wan", and the like (Figure 1, Table 1). This menu benefits fully from the distinctive flavor (combination of taste, smell, and tactile sensations) of each ingredient.

This style of eating a main staple food with side dishes interchangeably, is unique to Washoku, mixes, and harmonizes all flavors inside the mouth. Small bites, due to the use of chopsticks, together with the combination of foods inside the mouth seem to contribute to satiety. There is evidence showing that multiple alternation of foods decreases food consumption at the end of the meal [37]. The relatively small portion size of the main and side dishes is another trait that helps to avoid overeating, since studies have shown that big portions encourage the consumption of larger meals [38,39]. Frequent intake of soup by Japanese men has been correlated with a lower body mass index (BMI), waist circumference, and waist-to-hip ratio, all physical factors related to obesity [40]. Others have also demonstrated that soups have a satiating effect [41,42]. In fact, the core flavor of Japanese food is umami taste from *dashi* stock, which is the base of many Japanese recipes. To heighten the distinctive flavor of many ingredients, cooks in Japan have mastered the techniques of extracting umami substances from dried kelp and dried bonito flakes in *dashi* stock with traditional flavoring products, such as soy sauce, miso, and vinegar [9].

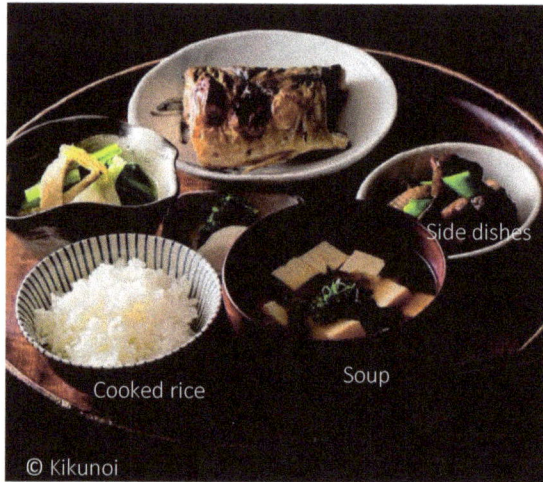

Figure 1. The basic structure of Washoku, comprised of one soup, cooked rice, and three side dishes, deliciously prepared with *dashi* stock as accompaniment for the rice.

Table 1. Characteristic dishes and ingredients of the Japanese traditional diet.

Dishes	Ingredients	Elements
Staple food	Grains, mainly rice (noodles or glutinous rice)	Recipes with cooked rice (sushi or curry rice)
Soup	Miso Soup (seaweed, shellfish, vegetables)	*Dashi* soup stock (fermented soybeans)
Main dish	Fish, seafood, sometimes meats	Great variety of edible fishes
Side dishes	Vegetables, wild plants, mushrooms, seaweed, shellfish	Change with the season and locality

Water is another important ingredient in traditional diets. As rivers in Japan are short, water is soft and quite free of impurities. Thanks to the work of culinary professionals at the Japanese Culinary Academy, it is known that soft water functions not only to reduce or remove bitterness but it also efficiently brings out the umami sensation from dried kelp and dried bonito flakes. This *dashi* stock is used to boil vegetables and serves two functions: It reduces the volume and increases the palatability of vegetables. This facilitates the inclusion of larger quantities of vegetables within the Japanese menu and thereby increases their consumption, which has been shown to lead to a lower the risk of cardiovascular diseases (CVD) and all causes of mortality and morbidity [43]. Moreover, the main cooking methods in Washoku are steaming, boiling, and stewing, thereby enhancing the water content of Japanese dishes. This incorporation of water into food seems to be more efficient that drinking water to decrease the overall intake of energy in a meal [44].

Altogether, the style of eating in Washoku—a large variety of foods, small portions, the inclusion of soups, abundant vegetables, the cooking method, the large content of water, and the effective usage of umami taste—promotes not only the pleasant experience of eating, combined with the large incorporation of bioactive compounds from vegetables, but also ensures an adequate signal for satiety that prevents overeating. Another parameter to take into account as a potential healthful trait of the Japanese diet is the frequent consumption of fish. Side dishes in Washoku include many types of fish that are a rich source of high quality protein as well as eicosapentaenoic acid (EPA) and docosahexaenoic acid (DHA), ω-3 fatty acids that are believed to be beneficial for health [45]. Soy bean-based foods, in the form of fermented miso and tofu, are common in Japanese traditional diets, and are known to reduce blood pressure and blood glucose [46,47]. Additional factors to consider are the energy and sodium content of the Japanese diet. Several studies have found consistent low calorie ingestion among men and women from Japan, compared to those in China, the United States, Italy or the UK [48,49]. This may partly explain the lower BMI among Japanese compared to other populations. In reference to sodium, a high urinary excretion has been reported for Japanese people, accompanied by a high estimated sodium consumption—between 11 mg for men and 9 mg for women daily. Although salt intake in Japan, especially in certain regions, has considerably decreased from the 1950s and 1960s, the current consumption is still higher than the recommended amount to reduce mortality by stroke (<6 mg per day) [50,51]. The most common dietary sources of sodium in the Japanese diet are miso soup and salted vegetables as well as soy sauce and commercially processed fish or seafood. However, in spite of a high sodium intake, Japanese have an overall low incidence of CVD, probably due to a higher potassium intake with vegetables [52]. Finally, families strengthen their bonds by sharing meals together, which is important for usual communication [53]. In summary, the main elements of Washoku that promote positive health outcomes are: (1) the great variety of seasonal foodstuffs, including vegetables and fishes; (2) the way of cooking dishes based on large amounts of high quality water; (3) the well-balanced nutrition; and finally (4) the value of its connection with health and family ties (Tables 2 and 3) [9].

Table 2. Basic elements of the Japanese traditional diet [1].

Elements	Contents	Description
Foodstuffs	Seasonal foods	Rice, vegetables, wild plants, mushrooms, variety of fish
Dishes	Cooking methods with abundant water, *dashi* stock, delicious meals, with vegetables and seafood	Steaming, boiling, and stewing
Nutrition	Relative low-calorie density, low total fat, high quality protein, variety of ingredients, easy to eat different nutrients	Nutritionally well-balanced
Hospitality	Health and family ties	The joy of eating together and caring for one another

[1] The traditional Japanese diet starts with the selection of foodstuffs, and includes the way foods are prepared, how ingredients contribute to balanced nutrition, and finally, the attitude of appreciation.

Table 3. Potential health traits of Washoku.

Element	Effect	Health Consequences
Small portion size	Smaller meal size	Prevents overeating [38,39].
Soup and dishes with high water content	Lower total energy intake	Lower [1] BMI, waist circumference and waist-to-hip ratio [40–42,48,49].
Soy sauce, salted vegetables and fruits, miso soup, and salted fish	High sodium consumption, with a high sodium/potassium ratio	The high vegetable intake seems to protect against CVD [50–52].
High [2] EPA and [3] DHA, low animal fat, low total fat	Modulation of the membranes of cells, lipid signaling and gene expression	Supports optimal health, low risk of [1,4] CVD, cancer and inflammation [45]
Foods based on beans	Decrease blood pressure and blood glucose	Protects against CVD [46,47]
Variety of seasonal vegetables and green tea	Intestinal bulk and protection against inflammation and high blood pressure	Low risk of CVD and all causes of mortality [43].
Umami taste	Enhances flavor, food palatability and salivation	Promotes chewing and swallowing, and maintains adequate taste sensation [27,28,30].

[1] Body Mass Index [BMI]; [2] Eicosapentaenoic acid (EPA); [3] Docosahexaenoic acid (DHA); [4] Cardiovascular diseases (CVD).

2. Food Polyphenols and Their Sensory Properties

The sensorial properties of foods depend basically on two major factors: the amount and type of taste active compounds from foods and the distinct sensitivity and taste experience of each individual. Flavonoid phenols, such as flavonols, which are present in several fruits, nuts, chocolate and beverages like tea, cider, and red wine, provide a characteristic bitterness and the tactile feeling of astringency (puckering, rough or drying mouth-feel). Although astringent molecules may have protective effects in our body, excess astringency can be unpalatable. These sensorial properties are best known to arise from the monomers of flavan-3-ol that are called proanthocyanidins, and also condensed tannins (epigallocatechin, epicatechin gallate, epigallocatechin gallate, catechin and epicatechin) [54]. They can be found in wine and tea and are thought to be responsible for the bitterness and astringency of both drinks. Small changes in the chemical structure of flavonoids can induce significant differences in sensory properties. For example, catechin is less bitter and astringent than its chiral isomer, epicatechin. On the other hand, bitterness declines, whereas astringency intensifies, with increasing polymerization of flavonoids. Moreover, the interactions between flavonoids and other food compounds, such as ethanol, can enhance the intensity of bitterness in wine without affecting its astringency. Oral sensory perception of astringency comes, in part, from the reduction of oral lubrication after the precipitation of certain salivary proline-rich proteins that show a strong binding affinity for polyphenols, like tannins [55]. However, astringency involves an intricate mechanism that gives a complex sensation that is not yet fully understood [56,57].

The sensorial properties of other phenolic compounds have also been studied. Over the past ten years, the peculiar pharyngeal pungency of a phenolic constituent present in newly pressed extra virgin olive oils (EVOOs), known as oleocanthal (OC) [(−)-decarboxymethyl ligstroside aglycone], has been investigated by Beauchamp and colleagues [58]. OC appears to have very similar pharmacological activity to ibuprofen in the inflammatory pathways and also a similar oropharyngeal irritation. This makes OC a natural nonsteroidal anti-inflammatory compound and could partly explain the beneficial effects of the Mediterranean diet, together with protective effects of other antioxidant polyphenols of olive oil [59]. The sensory properties of OC seem to be mediated by a type of transient receptor potential receptor (TRPA1) that has been shown to be involved in the transduction of pain, due to thermal, mechanical, and chemical signals [60,61].

3. Why Taste Matters?

Taste matters for food selection and utilization, for several reasons. Firstly, taste is considered the nutrition gatekeeper, thereby helping individuals determine food acceptability, which is lifesaving for all animals, including humans. Most taste researchers believe that there are five basic or primary taste qualities: sweet, salty, sour, bitter, and umami (savory or meat-like). Sweet and umami taste perception probably functions to sense energetic sources, in particular, to recognize carbohydrates and proteins, respectively. A strong sour taste may serve to identify spoiled foods, while a salty taste acts to recognize the presence of sodium, which is necessary for the homeostasis of body fluids. Finally, strong bitter tastes aid in detecting the presence of toxicity [62–64], while a mild bitterness might potentially indicate the presence of medicinal compounds.

Taste remains important in food selection, even in developed cultures. This is indicated by results of study of food-related values that individuals use to make food choices. According to the Food Choice Process Model, these values include health, cost, time and social relationships. Of these, taste is among the top motives [65]. Thus, it is expected that taste perception and preference significantly influence food intake behaviors [66–68]. Taste perception varies among individuals due to genetic variations of taste receptors that can lead to adverse eating behaviors among some individuals and consequently, to a greater risk of chronic diseases [64,69]. This is discussed in greater detail below. On the other hand, some researchers think that it is necessary to have prolonged oro-sensory exposures to taste for a sufficient cephalic phase and satiety responses [70]. This would be the reason why slow eating elicits a robust satiety signal, whereas energy-containing beverages are only briefly tasted and thus provide a weak satiety signal.

3.1. Genetic Variation of Taste Receptors: Bitter Taste

Bitter taste perception is a consequence of certain molecules interacting with bitter taste receptors, called *TAS2Rs*. These receptors are a group of 25 G protein-coupled receptors that transduce the bitter taste sensation [71] The most commonly researched genetic taste variation is the inherited polymorphism of one these bitter taste receptors, *TAS2R38*. By chance, a chemist at DuPont laboratories (Arthus Fox) found in 1932 that some people could not detect certain bitter compounds, whereas others found them extremely bitter [72]. Later, Linda Bartoshuk studied the genetic differences of bitter taste perception in more detail [73]. She found that 25% of the mainly Caucasian population she examined was particularly sensitive to a group of bitter organosulfur thiourea compounds—phenylthiocarbamide (PTC) and 6-n-propylthiouracil (PROP). They contain a phenyl ring and are considered to be potent disruptors of several enzymes produced by the thyroid gland (goitrogens). Although neither PTC nor PROP is present in foods, cruciferous vegetables such as cabbage, broccoli and brussel sprouts contain chemically related glucosinolates with distinctive thiourea moieties [74]. Those who could not taste PTC or PROP, except at very high concentrations, accounted for approximately 25% to 30% of this population and were termed non-tasters. In marked contrast, approximately 25% of this population was extremely sensitive to these compounds. This extremely sensitive group she called "super-tasters". The remaining 45 to 50% of the population was average in their ability to taste PROP.

The major factor explaining individual variation in bitter taste perception of these compounds is genetic polymorphism at the taste receptor level, or at the messenger RNA expression level of the receptor. There are three major polymorphisms of the *TAS2R38* gene that are responsible for the perception of PROP, PTC, and other thiourea related compounds. These combine to form most of the taster haplotypes. However, changes in the thresholds of perception may also be related to the differences in the expression of *TAS2R38* [75].

Previous surveys have already noted that individuals who have a higher taste sensitivity to PTC or PROP are prone to disliking pungent foods with strong tasting qualities, compared to non-tasters who, having lower taste sensitivity, experience more pleasant taste sensations from foods in general. Some studies have shown that there seems to be a link between the sensitivity to PROP, food perception, food preference, and finally food choice, which could potentially predict the risk of chronic diseases [66,74]. As attractive as this hypothesis linking differences in genetic sensitivity to food choice might be, taste sensitivity, or PROP genotype, are not the only aspects that influence food choice or dietary intake. Other factors, such as culture or experience, education, socioeconomic status, peers, individual characteristics in relation to health, sex, age and body weight, also influence the food we prefer to eat [74].

3.2. Other Taste Receptor Variants and Taste Perception

Single nucleotide polymorphisms (SNPs) have been also found in other taste genes. Among these are potential fatty acid taste receptor cluster determinant 36 (CD36), the umami heterodimer taste receptors, type 1 member 1 (T1R1) and T1R3, the heterodimer sweet taste receptors (T1R2 & T1R3), the salt taste epithelial sodium channel (ENaC), and the transient receptor potential cation channels (TRPV1) (reviews: [1,64]). Although fat taste (oleogustus), the taste of triacylgrycerols, as a basic taste, is still in dispute, energy-dense foods that are high in fat may contribute to a higher palatability and predispose individuals to metabolic diseases [64]. This palatability could be different from the sensation of non-esterified, long chain fatty acids (NEFA), which are part of fatty foods in small amounts. Evidence points to the possibility that humans taste NEFA as a unique sensation [76]. A substantial individual variability has been reported for the sensitivity of NEFA in humans [77,78]. Some studies have found that a lower sensitivity to NEFA perception is linked to a higher energy and fat consumption, and consequently, a higher BMI [79–81]. Differences in sensitivity could be in part due to SNPs or the expression level of CD36 that is involved not only in taste but also in lipid metabolism and the risk of CVD [80,82]. Low sensitivity for the taste associated with CD36 seems to promote fat intake, which would explain, in part, why obese individuals eat fatty foods more often [68]. However, more studies are necessary for a better understanding of differences in taste sensitivity between lean and obese individuals [83].

For the sweet taste receptor, *TAS1R2* seems to be the human gene with one of the highest polymorphic rates [84]. Most of the SNPs seem to be located at the sequence where ligands bind to the receptor. Some studies have associated T1R2 and T1R3 receptor variations with taste sensitivity to sweet and sugar intake, obesity and dental caries [85–87].

Umami taste is represented most prominently by the taste of monosodium glutamate (MSG) and by its synergistic interaction with the 5'ribonucleotides: inosine monophosphate (IMP), guanosine monophosphate (GMP), and adenosine monophosphate (AMP). For MSG, there are also studies that show individual differences in sensitivity [88]. Some of these differences may come partly from SNPs in T1R1 and T1R3 receptors [89].

In contrast to the lack of studies showing a link between umami taste and diseases, excess sodium intake presents a major public health concern because of its relationship with the development of high blood pressure. As indicated before, supertasters report a stronger perception of the saltiness of concentrated salt solutions than do non-tasters [67]. However, sensory habituation to high dietary sodium appears to play a greater role in defining inter-individual differences for salt preference [90]. Unfortunately, salt taste receptors are not sufficiently characterized to draw conclusive implications on their role in behavioral preference to sodium and health effects. Currently, it is accepted that there are two responses to sodium. The appealing taste sensation of low-to-moderate sodium concentration seems to be mediated by the protein ENaC, whereas the TRPV1 system may be more related to aversive reactions to the taste of very high concentrations of sodium [91]. Polymorphisms related to the perception of salty taste intensity have been reported for both ENaC and TRVP1 [92]. Further research is needed to understand the extent to which the SNPs of salt taste receptors are involved in the preference for salty foods.

Lastly, coding SNPs have been also described in the genes of the presumed sour taste receptors, PKD2L1 and PKD1L3. They belong to a subfamily of transient receptor potential ion channels—polycystic kidney diseases-like (PKDL). However, the effect of these SNPs in the perception of sour taste is not yet well known (for review [64]). Altogether, current research shows that particular genetic variations of the fat, salty, sweet, and bitter taste receptors may predispose individuals to eat less vegetables (healthy foods) and overconsume fat, salt, and sugar (unhealthy foods), Table 4.

Table 4. Taste receptor genes with single nucleotide polymorphisms (SNPs) and their corresponding taste qualities.

Taste Quality	Taste Receptors with SNPs	Citation
Bitter	*TAS2R38*	[71]
Fatty Acids	*CD36*	[77,82]
Sweet	*TAS1R2/TAS1R3*	[84]
Umami	*TAS1R1/TAS1R3*	[89]
Salty	*ENaC*	[91,92]
Sour	*PKD2L1/PKD1L3*	[64]

4. Is the Current Diet of the Japanese People Healthy?

Japan is among the nations with the highest average life span for both, men and women, a fact consistent with the potential benefits of the traditional Japanese diet [93–95]. The culture of the traditional diet has been broadly maintained with a high intake of fish and soybean products and low intake of fat. At the same time, it has been also characterized by a high salt consumption [96]. However, in spite of a higher sodium intake and prevalence of high blood pressure, Japan still has lower mortality rates caused by CVD than Western nations [97]. For cultural and religious reasons, the Japanese have traditionally avoided the use of animal meats. During the Japanese economic development and the dramatic surge in the variety of available ingredients, the nutritional balance improved considerably in the 1980s, which, for most Japanese, reached an almost ideal balance of protein, fat, and carbohydrates.

In 2005, the Japanese Ministry of Health, Labour and Welfare developed, jointly with the Ministry of Agriculture, Forestry and Fisheries, the Japanese Food Guide Spinning Top, based on the dietary guidelines for Japanese that were formulated in 2000 [98]. However, more recently, the incidence rates of obesity and the metabolic syndrome have increased among middle-aged men. Coincidentally, the rate of underweight young women who want be thin has also increased, while child obesity in both boys and girls is starting to be of concern [99]. In the last forty years, there has been a partial loss in traditional food culture among the Japanese population. They have taken up less healthy dietary habits, such as skipping breakfast, insufficient vegetable intake and excess fat intake, combined with an increase in consumption of meat, eggs, milk, and dairy products.

Following the recent inclusion of "Washoku, traditional dietary cultures of the Japanese" in the list of Intangible Cultural Heritage of UNESCO, the interest in the traditional Japanese diet has increased, with a renewed appreciation for its potential health benefits. This seems to be a positive result, since recent Japanese cohort studies have shown that individuals with greater adherence to the Spinning Top of the Japanese Food Guide have a lower total mortality rate of 15% in both men and women, mainly due to a reduction in cerebrovascular diseases [93]. Others have now created a modified score to measure diet quality for Japanese that is also based on the Japanese food guide Spinning Top, but includes intake of sodium from seasonings, which was not part of previous scores [100].

At the first World Food Summit, held in Rome in 1996, under the auspices of the Food and Agriculture Organization of the United Nations [101], it was acknowledged that the eating habits of Japanese people are unique, compared to those of other nations or regions. Moreover, "Eating deliciously" is a priority of Japanese citizens, according to a 2006 survey by the NHK Broadcasting Research Center [102]. This is facilitated by the wide use of umami rich *dashi* in traditional cuisine. Now, more studies on dietary health scores for Japanese are necessary, to develop specific strategies for improving the dietary habits of younger generations. However, they are also necessary because some of the concepts within the Japanese diet can be useful in increasing healthy dietary habits in other countries.

5. Sustainability of Healthy Diets

The Food and Agriculture Organization of the United Nations (FAO) has defined sustainable diets as those having "low environmental impacts that contribute to food and nutrition security." Sustainable diets are also considered not only culturally acceptable, accessible and affordable, but also able to optimize natural and human resources [103]. The question is whether diets assessed as healthy can be also sustainable, because healthier diets are not necessarily more beneficial for the environment. Many recent studies looking at nutrition indicators, such as energy adequacy, food quality and composition, also address the environmental impact of a diet. [104]. Most of these studies refer to the Mediterranean diet. In general terms, plant-based foods produce fewer emissions of greenhouse gasses than animal-based foods. Sustainable vegetarian diets consist of grains, vegetables and fruits, with few servings of meat or seafood [105]. These are common ingredients in most traditional diets, including the Japanese traditional diet, and it will be necessary in the future to evaluate the impact that any diet may have on the environment in the region where it is implemented.

6. Summary and Conclusions

In this article, we put forward an argument that Japanese traditional diet practices (Washoku), which prominently include the flavoring of foods with umami taste, can be characterized as a healthy diet in the same way that the DASH diet or the Mediterranean diet is so classified (summary in Figure 2). We then discussed the importance of taste in guiding food choice and the important role that genetically-based individual differences in taste perception can have on a person's food selection

Nutrients **2018**, *10*, 173

behavior. We hope that several of the principles of Washoku will be studied and adopted by physicians, nutritionists, dieticians and others engaged in encouraging healthful eating.

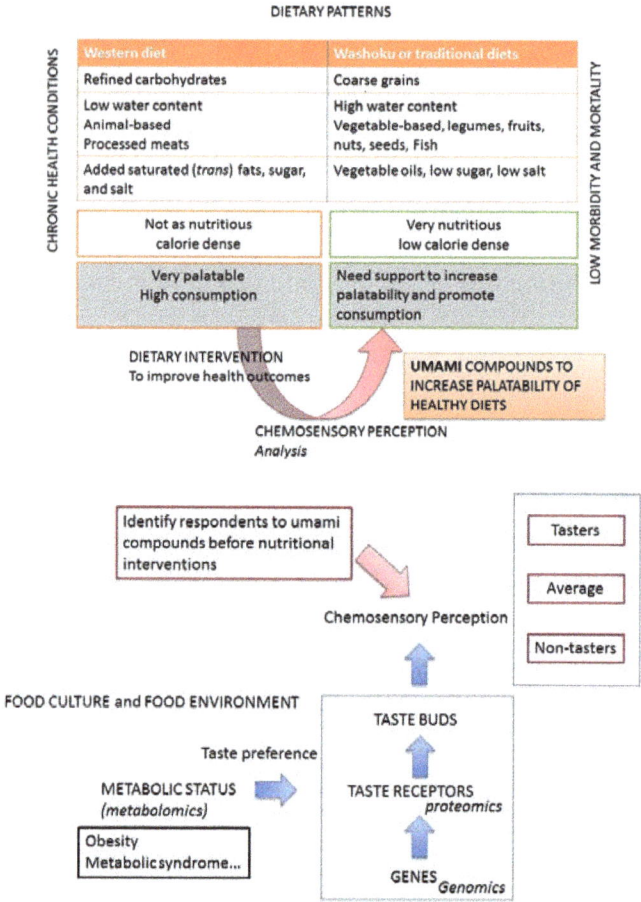

Figure 2. Traditional diets are usually associated with longevity and lower morbidity and mortality, but they are not as palatable as "Western diets". Taking into account data on taste sensitivity in personalized nutrition, together with the better understanding of food consumption behavior, can ensure a better adherence to nutritional interventions.

Acknowledgments: Thanks to Greg de St. Maurice for his contribution on the Japanese Food and Washoku, and to Gary Beauchamp for his support, especially on umami taste, and his critical review of the manuscript. Ajinomoto Co., Inc. will cover all article processing charges.

Author Contributions: Ana San Gabriel selected the focus, performed the literature revision, and wrote the review. Kumiko Ninomiya has overseen the contents of umami taste and Hisayuki Uneyama the contents of health and Japanese diet.

Conflicts of Interest: The authors are employees of Ajinomoto Co., Inc., which is a major producer of umami seasonings.

References

1. Bachmanov, A.A.; Beauchamp, G.K. Taste receptor genes. *Annu. Rev. Nutr.* **2007**, *27*, 389–414. [CrossRef] [PubMed]

2. San Gabriel, A.; Uneyama, H.; Yoshie, S.; Torii, K. Clonning and characterization of a novel mGluR1 variant from vallate papillae that functions as a receptor for L-glutamate stimuli. *Chem. Senses* **2005**, *30* (Suppl. 1), i25–i26. [CrossRef] [PubMed]

3. Yasuo, T.; Kusuhara, Y.; Yasumatsu, K.; Ninomiya, Y. Multiple receptor systems for glutamate detection in the taste organ. *Biol. Pharm. Bull.* **2008**, *31*, 1833–1837. [CrossRef] [PubMed]

4. Lindemann, B.; Ogiwara, Y.; Ninomiya, Y. The Discovery of umami. *Chem. Senses* **2002**, *27*, 843–844. [CrossRef] [PubMed]

5. Vazquez, M.; Pearson, P.B.; Beauchamp, G.K. Flavor preferences in malnourished Mexican infants. *Physiol. Behav.* **1982**, *28*, 513–519. [CrossRef]

6. Masic, U.; Yeomans, M.R. Does acute or habitual protein deprivation influence liking for monosodium glutamate. *Physiol. Behav.* **2017**, *15*, 79–86. [CrossRef] [PubMed]

7. Pepino, M.Y.; Finkbeiner, S.; Beauchamp, G.K.; Mennella, J.A. Obese women have lower monosodium glutamate taste sensitivity and prefer higher concentrations than do normal-weight women. *Obesity* **2010**, *18*, 959–965. [CrossRef] [PubMed]

8. Yamaguchi, S.; Ninomiya, K. Umami and food palatability. *J. Nutr.* **2000**, *130* (4S Suppl.), 921S–926S. [CrossRef] [PubMed]

9. Kumakura, I.; Japanese Culinary Academy. What is Japanese Cuisine. In *Introduction to Japanese Cuisine, Nature, History and Culture*; Kiyota Junji, Shuhari Initiative: Tokyo, Japan, 2015.

10. Ninomiya, K. Science of umami taste: Adaptation to gastronomic culture. *Flavour* **2015**, *4*, 1–5. [CrossRef]

11. Steiner, J. *Umami: A Basic Taste*; Kawamura, Y., Kare, M.R., Eds.; Marcel Dekker: New York, NY, USA, 1987; pp. 97–123.

12. Beauchamp, G.K.; Pearson, P. Human development and umami taste. *Physiol. Behav.* **1991**, *49*, 1009–1012. [CrossRef]

13. Prescott, J. Effects of added glutamate on liking for novel food flavors. *Appetite* **2004**, *42*, 143–150. [CrossRef] [PubMed]

14. Yamaguchi, S.; Takahashi, C. Interactions of monosodium glutamate and sodium chloride on saltiness and palatability. *J. Food Sci.* **1984**, *49*, 82–85. [CrossRef]

15. Roininen, K.; Lahteenmaki, L.; Tuorila, H. Effect of umami taste on pleasantness of low-salt soups during repeated testing. *Physiol. Behav.* **1996**, *60*, 953–958. [CrossRef]

16. Ball, P.; Woodward, D.; Beard, T.; Shoobridge, A.; Ferrier, M. Calcium diglutamate improves taste characteristics of lower-salt soup. *Eur. J. Clin. Nutr.* **2002**, *56*, 519–523. [CrossRef] [PubMed]

17. Carter, B.E.; Monsivais, P.; Drewnowski, A. The sensory optimum of chicken broths supplemented with calcium di-glutamate: A possibility for reducing sodium while maintaining taste. *Food Qual. Prefer.* **2011**, *22*, 699–703. [CrossRef]

18. Leong, J.; Kasamatsu, C.; Ong, E.; Hoi, J.T.; Loong, M.N. A study on sensory properties of sodium reduction and replacement in Asian food using difference-from-control test. *Food Sic. Nutr.* **2015**, *4*, 469–478. [CrossRef] [PubMed]

19. Prescott, J.; Young, A. Does information about MSG (monosodium glutamate) content influence consumer ratings of soups with and without added MSG? *Appetite* **2002**, *39*, 25–33. [CrossRef] [PubMed]

20. Bellisle, F.; Monneuse, M.O.; Chabert, M.; Laure-Achagiotis, C.; Lanteaume, M.T.; Louis-Sylvestre, J. Monosodium glutamate as a palatability enhancer in the European diet. *Physiol. Behav.* **1991**, *49*, 869–873. [CrossRef]

21. Yamamoto, S.; Tomoe, M.; Toyama, K.; Kawai, M.; Uneyama, H. Can dietary supplementation of monosodium glutamate improve the health of the elderly? *Am. J. Clin. Nutr.* **2009**, *90*, 844S–849S. [CrossRef] [PubMed]

22. Beyreuther, K.; Biesalski, H.K.; Fernstrom, J.D.; Grimm, P.; Hammes, W.P.; Heinemann, U.; Kempski, O.; Stehle, P.; Steinhart, H.; Walker, R. Consensus meeting: Monosodium glutamate—And update. *Eur. J. Clin. Nutr.* **2007**, *61*, 304–313. [CrossRef] [PubMed]

23. Henry-Unaeze, H.N. Update on food safety of monosodium L-glutamate (MSG). *Pathophysiology* **2017**, *24*, 243–249. [CrossRef] [PubMed]

24. Okiyama, A.; Beuchamp, G.K. Taste dimensions of monosodium glutamate (MSG) in a food system: Role of glutamate in young American subjects. *Physiol. Behav.* **1998**, *65*, 177–181. [CrossRef]

25. Wilkie, L.M.; Capaldi Phillips, E.D. Heterogeneous binary interactions of taste primaries: Perceptual outcomes, physiology, and future directions. *Neurosci. Biobehav. Rev.* **2014**, *47*, 70–86. [CrossRef] [PubMed]

26. Kawasaki, H.; Sekizaki, Y.; Hirota, M.; Sekine-Hayakawa, Y.; Nonaka, M. Analysis of binary taste-taste interaction of MSG, lactic acid, and NaCl by temporal dominance of sensations. *Food Qual. Pref.* **2016**, *52*, 1–10. [CrossRef]

27. Hodson, N.A.; Linden, R.W. The effect of monosodium glutamate on parotid salivary flow in comparison to response to representatives of the other four basic tastes. *Physiol. Behav.* **2006**, *89*, 711–717. [CrossRef] [PubMed]

28. Sasano, T.; Satoh-Kuriwada, S.; Shoji, N.; Sekine-Hayakawa, Y.; Kawaki, M.; Uneyama, H. Application of umami taste stimulation to remedy hypogeusia based on reflex salivation. *Biol. Pharm. Bull.* **2010**, *33*, 1791–1795. [CrossRef] [PubMed]

29. Mese, H.; Matsuo, R. Salivary secretion, taste and hyposalivation. *J. Oral Rehabil.* **2007**, *34*, 711–723. [CrossRef] [PubMed]

30. Sasano, T.; Satoh-Kuriwada, S.; Shoji, N.; Iikubo, M.; Kawai, M.; Uneyama, H.; Sakamoto, M. Important role of umami taste sensitivity in oral and overall health. *Curr. Pharm. Des.* **2014**, *20*, 2750–2754. [CrossRef] [PubMed]

31. San Gabriel, A.M.; Maekawa, T.; Uneyama, H.; Yoshie, S.; Torii, K. mGluR1 in the fundic glands of rat stomach. *FEBS Lett.* **2007**, *582*, 1119–1123. [CrossRef] [PubMed]

32. Young, R.L.; Sutherland, K.; Pezos, N.; Brierley, S.M.; Horowitz, M.; Rayner, C.K.; Blackshaw, L.A. Expression of taste molecules in the upper gastrointestinal tract in humans with and without type 2 diabetes. *Gut* **2009**, *58*, 337–346. [CrossRef] [PubMed]

33. Uneyama, H.; Niijima, A.; San Gabriel, A.; Torii, K. Luminal amino acid sensing in the rat gastric mucosa. *Am. J. Physiol. Gastrointest. Liver Physiol.* **2006**, *291*, G1163–G1170. [CrossRef] [PubMed]

34. San Gabriel, A.; Uneyama, H. Amino acid sensing in the gastrointestinal tract. *Amino Acids* **2013**, *45*, 451–461. [CrossRef] [PubMed]

35. Nishimura, T.; Goto, S.; Miura, K.; Takakura, Y.; Egusa, A.S.; Wakabayashi, H. Umami compounds enhance the intensity of retronasal sensation of aroma from model chicken soups. *Food Chem.* **2016**, *196*, 577–583. [CrossRef] [PubMed]

36. Prescott, J. Taste hedonics and the role of umami. *Food Aust.* **2001**, *53*, 550–554.

37. Brondel, L.; Lauraine, G.; Van Wymerbeke, V.; Romer, M.; Schaal, B. Alternation between foods within a meal. Influence on satiation and consumption in humans. *Appetite* **2009**, *53*, 203–209. [CrossRef] [PubMed]

38. Ello-Martin, J.A.; Ledikwe, J.H.; Rolls, B.J. The influence of food portion size and energy density on energy intake: Implications for weight management. *Am. J. Clin. Nutr.* **2005**, *82* (1 Suppl.), 236S–241S. [PubMed]

39. Brunstrom, J.M.; Jarvstad, A.; Griggs, R.L.; Potter, C.; Evans, N.R.; Martin, A.A.; Brooks, J.C.; Rogers, P.J. Large portions encourage the selection of palatable rather than filling foods. *J. Nutr.* **2016**, *146*, 2117–2123. [CrossRef] [PubMed]

40. Kuroda, M.; Ohta, M.; Okufuji, T.; Takigami, C.; Eguchi, M.; Hayabuchi, H.; Ikeda, M. Frequency of soup intake is inversely associated with body mass index, waist circumference, and waist-to-hip ratio, but not with other metabolic risk factors in Japanese men. *J. Am. Diet. Assoc.* **2011**, *111*, 137–142. [CrossRef] [PubMed]

41. Rolls, B.J.; Fedoroff, I.C.; Guthrie, J.F.; Laster, L.J. Foods with different satiating effects in humans. *Appetite* **1990**, *15*, 115–126. [CrossRef]

42. Clegg, M.E.; Ranawana, V.; Shafat, A.; Henry, C.J. Soups increase satiety through delayed gastric emptying yet increased glycaemic response. *Eur. J. Clin. Nutr.* **2013**, *67*, 8–11. [CrossRef] [PubMed]

43. Bazzano, L.A.; He, J.; Ogden, L.G.; Loria, C.M.; Vupputuri, S.; Myers, L.; Whelton, P.K. Fruit and vegetable intake and risk of cardiovascular diseases in US adults: The first national health and nutrition examination survey epidemiologic follow-up study. *Am. J. Clin. Nutr.* **2002**, *76*, 93–99. [CrossRef] [PubMed]

44. Rolls, B.J.; Bell, E.A.; Thorwart, M.L. Water incorporated into a food but not served with a food decreases energy intake in lean women. *Am. J. Clin. Nutr.* **1999**, *70*, 448–455. [PubMed]

45. Calder, P.C. Very long-chain n-3 fatty acids and human health: Fact, fiction and the future. *Proc. Nutr. Soc.* **2017**, *17*, 1–21. [CrossRef] [PubMed]

46. Rivas, M.; Garay, R.P.; Escanero, J.F.; Cia, P., Jr.; Cia, P.; Alda, J.O. Soy milk lowers blood pressure in men and women with mild to moderate essential hypertension. *J. Nutr.* **2002**, *132*, 1900–1902. [CrossRef] [PubMed]

47. Jayagopal, V.; Albertazzi, P.; Kilpatrick, E.S.; Howarth, E.M.; Jennings, P.E.; Hepburn, D.A.; Atkin, S.L. Beneficial effects of soy phytoestrogen intake in postmenopausal women with type 2 diabetes. *Diabetes Care* **2002**, *25*, 1709–1714. [CrossRef] [PubMed]

48. Zhou, B.F.; Stamler, J.; Dennis, B.; Moag-Stahlberg, A.; Okuda, N.; Robertson, C.; Zhao, L.; Chan, Q.; Elliott, P.; INTERMAP Research Group. Nutrient intakes of middle-age men and women in China, Japan, United Kingdom, and United States in the late 1990s: The INTERMAP study. *J. Hum. Hypertens.* **2003**, *17*, 623–630. [CrossRef] [PubMed]

49. Zhang, R.; Wang, Z.; Fei, Y.; Zhou, B.; Zheng, S.; Wang, L.; Huang, L.; Jiang, S.; Liu, Z.; Jiang, J.; et al. The difference in nutrient intakes between Chinese and Mediterranean, Japanese and American diets. *Nutrients* **2015**, *7*, 4661–4688. [CrossRef] [PubMed]

50. Ando, K.; Kawarazaki, H.; Miura, K.; Matsuura, H.; Watanabe, Y.; Yoshita, K.; Kawamura, M.; Kusaka, M.; Kai, H.; Tsuchihashi, T.; et al. [Scientific statement] Report of the Salt Reduction Committee of the Japanese Society of Hypertension (1) Role of salt in hypertension and cardiovascular diseases. *Hypertens. Res.* **2013**, *36*, 1009–1019. [CrossRef] [PubMed]

51. Wakasugi, M.; Kazama, J.; Narita, I. Associations between the intake of miso soup and Japanese pickles and the estimated 24-hour unrinary sodium excretion: A population-based cross-sectional study. *Intern. Med.* **2015**, *54*, 903–910. [CrossRef] [PubMed]

52. Anderson, C.A.; Appel, L.J.; Okuda, N.; Brown, I.J.; Chang, Q.; Zhao, L.; Ueshima, H.; Kesteloot, H.; Miura, K.; Curb, J.D.; et al. Dietary sources of sodium in Chaina, Japan, the United Kingdom, and the United States, women and men aged 40 to 59 years: The INTERMAP study. *J. Am. Diet. Assoc.* **2010**, *110*, 736–745. [CrossRef] [PubMed]

53. Ministry of Agriculture, Forestry and Fisheries. Traditional Dietary Cultures of the Japanese. Available online: http://www.maff.go.jp/e/japan_food/washoku/pdf/wasyoku_english.pdf (accessed on 31 December 2013).

54. Lesschaeve, I.; Noble, A.C. Polyphenols: Factors influencing their sensory properties and their effects on food and beverage preferences. *Am. J. Clin. Nutr.* **2005**, *81* (1 Suppl.), 330S–335S. [PubMed]

55. Lee, C.A.; Ismail, B.; Vickers, Z.M. The role of salivary proteins in the mechanism of astringency. *J. Food Sci.* **2012**, *77*, C381–C387. [CrossRef] [PubMed]

56. Breslin, P.A.S.; Gilmore, M.M.; Beauchamp, G.K.; Green, B.G. Psychophysical evidence that oral astringency is a tactile sensation. *Chem. Senses* **1993**, *18*, 405–417. [CrossRef]

57. Gibbins, H.L.; Carpenter, G.H. Alternative mechanisms of astringency—What is the role of saliva? *J. Texture Stud.* **2013**, *44*, 364–375. [CrossRef]

58. Cicerale, S.; Breslin, P.A.; Beauchamp, G.K.; Keast, R.S. Sensory characterization of the irritant properties of oleocanthal, a natural anti-inflammatory agent in extra virgin olive oils. *Chem. Senses* **2009**, *34*, 333–339. [CrossRef] [PubMed]

59. Carluccio, M.A.; Siculella, L.; Ancora, M.A.; Massaro, M.; Scoditti, E.; Storelli, C.; Visioli, F.; Distante, A.; De Caterina, R. Olive oil and red wine antioxidant polyphenols inhibit endothelial activation: Antiatherogenic properties of Mediterranean diet phytochemicals. *Arterioscler. Thromb. Vasc. Biol.* **2003**, *23*, 622–629. [CrossRef] [PubMed]

60. Levine, J.D.; Alessandri-Haber, N. TRP channels: Targets for the relief of pain. *Biochim. Biophys. Acta* **2007**, *1772*, 989–1003. [CrossRef] [PubMed]

61. Peyrot des Gachons, C.; Uchida, K.; Bryant, B.; Shima, A.; Sperry, J.B.; Dankulich-Nagrudny, L.; Tominaga, M.; Smith, A.B., 3rd; Beauchamp, G.K.; Breslin, P.A. Unusual pungency from extra-virgin olive oil is attributable to restricted spatial expression of the receptor of oleocanthal. *J. Neurosci.* **2011**, *31*, 999–1009. [CrossRef] [PubMed]

62. Kim, U.K.; Breslin, P.A.; Reed, D.; Drayna, D. Genetics of human taste perception. *J. Dent. Res.* **2004**, *83*, 448–453. [CrossRef] [PubMed]

63. Tepper, B.J. Nutritional implications of genetic variation: The role of PROP sensitivity and other taste phenotypes. *Ann. Rev. Nutr.* **2008**, *28*, 367–388. [CrossRef] [PubMed]

64. Chamoun, E.; Mutch, D.M.; Allen-Vercoe, E.; Buchholz, A.C.; Duncan, A.M.; Spriet, L.L.; Haines, J.; Ma, D.W.L.; Guelph Family Health Study. A review of the associations between single nucleotide polymorphisms in taste receptors, eating behaviors, and health. *Crit. Rev. Food Sci. Nutr.* **2016**, *31*, 1–14. [CrossRef] [PubMed]

65. Connors, M.; Bisogni, C.A.; Sobal, J.; Devine, C.M. Managing values in personal food systems. *Appetite* **2001**, *36*, 189–200. [CrossRef] [PubMed]

66. Tepper, B.J.; White, E.A.; Koelliker, Y.; Lanzara, C.; d'Adamo, P.; Gasparini, P. Genetic variation in taste sensitivity to 6-n-propylthiouracil and its relationship to taste perception and food selection. *Ann. N. Y. Acad. Sci.* **2009**, *1170*, 126–139. [CrossRef] [PubMed]

67. Hayes, J.E.; Sullivan, B.S.; Duffy, V.B. Explaining variability in sodium intake through oral sensory phenotype, salt and liking. *Physiol. Behav.* **2010**, *100*, 369–380. [CrossRef] [PubMed]

68. Liang, L.C.; Sakimura, J.; May, D.; Breen, C.; Driggin, E.; Tepper, B.J.; Chung, W.K.; Keller, K.L. Fat discrimination: A phenotype with potential implications for studying fat intake behaviors and obesity. *Physiol. Behav.* **2012**, *105*, 470–475. [CrossRef] [PubMed]

69. Feeney, E.; O'Brien, S.; Scannell, A.; Markey, A.; Gibney, E.R. Genetic variation in taste perception: Does it have a role in healthy eating? *Proc. Nutr. Soc.* **2011**, *70*, 135–143. [CrossRef] [PubMed]

70. Graaf, C. Texture and satiation: The role of oro-sensory exposure time. *Physiol. Behav.* **2012**, *107*, 496–501. [CrossRef] [PubMed]

71. Behrens, M.; Reichling, C.; Batram, C.; Brockhoff, A.; Meyerhof, W. Bitter taste receptors and their cells. *Ann. N. Y. Acad. Sci.* **2009**, *1170*, 111–115. [CrossRef] [PubMed]

72. Blakeslee, A.; Fox, A. Our different taste worlds. *J. Hered.* **1932**, *23*, 97–107. [CrossRef]

73. Bartoshuk, L.M. Bitter taste of saccharin related to the genetic ability to taste the bitter substance 6-n-propylthiouracil. *Science* **1979**, *205*, 934–935. [CrossRef] [PubMed]

74. Keller, K.L.; Adise, S. Variation in the ability to taste bitter thiourea compounds: Implications for food acceptance, dietary intake, and obesity risk in children. *Annu. Rev. Nutr.* **2016**, *36*, 157–182. [CrossRef] [PubMed]

75. Lipchock, S.; Mennella, J.; Spielman, A.; Reed, D. Human bitter perception correlates with bitter receptor messenger RNA expression in taste cells. *Am. J. Clin. Nutr.* **2013**, *98*, 1136–1143. [CrossRef] [PubMed]

76. Running, C.A.; Carig, B.A.; Mattes, R.D. Oleogustus: The unique taste of fat. *Chem. Senses* **2015**, *40*, 507–516. [CrossRef] [PubMed]

77. Stewart, J.E.; Feinle-Bisset, C.; Golding, M.; Delahunty, C.; Clifton, P.M.; Keast, R.S. Oral sensitivity to fatty acids, food consumption and BMI in human subjects. *Br. J. Nutr.* **2010**, *104*, 145–152. [CrossRef] [PubMed]

78. Tucker, R.M.; Matter, R.D. Influences of repeated testing on nonesterified fatty acid taste. *Chem. Senses* **2013**, *38*, 325–332. [CrossRef] [PubMed]

79. Martinez-Ruiz, N.R.; Lopez-Diaz, J.A.; Wall-Medrano, A.; Jimenez-Castro, J.A.; Angulo, O. Oral fat perception is related with body mass index, preference and consumption of high-fat foods. *Physiol. Behav.* **2014**, *129*, 36–42. [CrossRef] [PubMed]

80. Pepino, M.Y.; Love-Gregory, L.; Klein, S.; Abumrad, N.A. The fatty acid translocase gene CD36 and lingual lipase influence oral sensitivity to fat in obese subjects. *J. Lipid Res.* **2012**, *53*, 561–566. [CrossRef] [PubMed]

81. Stewart, J.E.; Seimon, R.V.; Otto, B.; Keast, R.S.; Clifton, P.M.; Feinle-Bisset, C. Marked differences in gustatory and gastrointestinal sensitivity to oleic acid between lean and obese men. *Am. J. Clin. Nutr.* **2011**, *93*, 703–711. [CrossRef] [PubMed]

82. Keller, K.L.; Liang, L.C.; Sakimura, J.; May, D.; van Belle, C.; Breen, C.; Driggin, E.; Tepper, B.J.; Deng, L.; Chung, W.K. Common variants in the CD36 gene are associated with oral fat perception, fat preferences, and obesity in African Americans. *Obesity* **2012**, *20*, 1066–1073. [CrossRef] [PubMed]

83. Tucker, R.M.; Kaiser, K.A.; Parman, M.A.; George, B.J.; Allison, D.B.; Mattes, R.D. Comparison of fatty acid taste detection thresholds in people who are lean vs. overweight or obese: A systematic review and meta-analysis. *PLoS ONE* **2017**, *12*, e0169583. [CrossRef] [PubMed]

84. Kim, U.K.; Wooding, S.; Riaz, N.; Jorde, L.B.; Drayna, D. Variation in the human TAS1R taste receptor genes. *Chem. Senses* **2006**, *31*, 599–611. [CrossRef] [PubMed]

85. Reed, D.R.; Bachmanov, A.A.; Beauchamp, G.K.; Tordoff, M.G.; Price, R.A. Heritable variation in food preferences and their contribution to obesity. *Behav. Genet.* **1997**, *27*, 373–387. [CrossRef] [PubMed]

86. Fushan, A.A.; Simons, C.T.; Slack, J.P.; Manichaikul, A.; Drayna, D. Allelic polymorphism within the TAS1R3 promoter is associated with human taste sensitivity to sucrose. *Curr. Biol.* **2009**, *19*, 1288–1293. [CrossRef] [PubMed]

87. Kulkarni, G.V.; Chng, T.; Eny, K.M.; Nielsen, D.; Wessman, C.; El-Sohemy, A. Association of GLUT2 and TAS1R2 genotypes with risk for dental caries. *Caries Res.* **2013**, *47*, 219–225. [CrossRef] [PubMed]

88. Lugaz, O.; Pillias, A.M.; Faurion, A. A new specific ageusia: Some humans cannot taste L-glutamate. *Chem. Senses* **2002**, *27*, 105–115. [CrossRef]

89. Shigemura, N.; Shirosaki, S.; Sanematsu, K.; Yoshida, R.; Ninomiya, Y. Genetic and molecular basis of individual differences in human umami taste. *PLoS ONE* **2009**, *4*, e6717. [CrossRef] [PubMed]

90. Institute of Medicine (IOM). *Sodium Intake in Populations: Assessment of Evidence*; The National Academies Press: Washington, DC, USA, 2013.

91. Yoshida, R.; Horio, N.; Murata, Y.; Yasumatsu, K.; Shigemura, N.; Ninomiya, Y. NaCl responsive taste cells in the mouse fungiform taste buds. *Nueroscience* **2009**, *159*, 795–803. [CrossRef] [PubMed]

92. Dias, A.G.; Rousseau, D.; Duizer, L.; Cockburn, M.; Chiu, W.; Nielsen, D.; El-Sohemy, A. Genetic variation in putative salt taste receptors and salt taste perception in humans. *Chem. Senses* **2013**, *38*, 137–145. [CrossRef] [PubMed]

93. Kurotani, K.; Akter, S.; Kashino, I.; Goto, A.; Mizoue, T.; Noda, M.; Sasazuki, S.; Sawada, N.; Tsugane, S.; Japan Public Health Center based Prospective Study Group. Quality of diet and mortality among Japanese men and women: Japan Public health center prospective study. *BMJ* **2016**, *352*, i1209. [CrossRef] [PubMed]

94. Ikeda, N.; Saito, E.; Kondo, N.; Inoue, M.; Ikeda, S.; Satoh, T.; Wada, K.; Stickley, A.; Katanoda, K.; Mizoue, T.; et al. What has made the population of Japan healthy? *Lancet* **2011**, *378*, 1094–1105. [CrossRef]

95. Nakaji, S.; MacAuley, D.; O'Neill, S.; McNally, O.; Baxter, D.; Sugawara, K. Life expectancies in the United Kingdom and Japan. *J. Public Health Med.* **2003**, *25*, 120–124. [CrossRef] [PubMed]

96. Shimazu, T.; Kuriyama, S.; Hozawa, A.; Ohmori, K.; Sato, Y.; Nakaya, N.; Nishino, Y.; Tsubono, Y.; Tsuji, I. Dietary patterns and cardiovascular disease mortality in Japan: A prospective cohort study. *Int. J. Epidemiol.* **2007**, *63*, 600–609. [CrossRef] [PubMed]

97. Lands, W.E.; Hamazaki, T.; Yamazaki, K.; Okuyama, H.; Sakai, K.; Goto, Y.; Hubbard, V.S. Changing dietary patterns. *Am. J. Clin. Nutr.* **1990**, *51*, 991–993. [CrossRef] [PubMed]

98. Yoshiike, N.; Hayashi, F.; Takemi, Y.; Mizoguchi, K.; Seino, F. A new food guide in Japan: The Japanese food guide Spinning Top. *Nutr. Rev.* **2007**, *65*, 149–154. [CrossRef] [PubMed]

99. Miyoshi, M.; Tsuboyama-Kasaoka, N.; Nishi, N. School-based "Shokuiku" program in Japan: Application to nutrition education in Asian countries. *Asia Pac. J. Clin. Nutr.* **2012**, *21*, 159–162. [PubMed]

100. Kuriyama, N.; Murakami, K.; Livingstone, M.B.E.; Okubo, H.; Kobayashi, S.; Suga, H.; Sasaki, S.; Three-Generation Study of Women on Diets and Health Study Group. Development of a food-based diet quality score for Japanese: Associations of the score with nutrient intakes in young, middle-age and older Japanese women. *J. Nutr. Sci.* **2016**, *5*, e41. [CrossRef] [PubMed]

101. Food and Agriculture Organization of the United Nations. Statistics Yearbook (Food Balance Sheet for the Data of Japan). Available online: http://faostat.fao.org/static/syb/syb_110.pdf (accessed on 31 December 2017).

102. Ministry of Agriculture, Forestry and Fisheries (MAFF) of Japan. Relationship between Diet, Health, and Life Expectancy. Available online: http://www.maff.go.jp/j/keikaku/syokubunka/culture/eiyo.html (accessed on 31 December 2008). (In Japanese)

103. Food and Agriculture Organization of the United Nations. International Scientific Symposium. Biodiversity and Sustainable Diets—United against Hunger. Available online: http://www.fao.org/docrep/016/i3004e/i3004e.pdf (accessed on 31 December 2012).

104. Donini, L.M.; Dernini, S.; Lairon, D.; Serra-Majem, L.; Amiot, M.J.; Del Balzo, V.; Giusti, A.M.; Burlingame, B.; Belahsen, R.; Maiani, G.; et al. A consensus proposal for nutritional indicators to assess the sustainability of a healthy diet: The Mediterranean diet as a case study. *Food Nutr.* **2016**, *3*, 37. [CrossRef] [PubMed]

105. Tilman, D.; Clark, M. Global diets link environmental sustainability and human health. *Nature* **2014**, *515*, 518–522. [CrossRef] [PubMed]

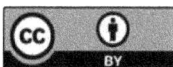

MDPI

St. Alban-Anlage 66

4052 Basel, Switzerland

Tel. +41 61 683 77 34

Fax +41 61 302 89 18

http://www.mdpi.com

Nutrients Editorial Office

E-mail: nutrients@mdpi.com

http://www.mdpi.com/journal/nutrients